hCGChica's

HCG DIET REFILL WORKBOOK

PHASE 2
DAILY TRACKER

RAYZEL LAM

ISBN-13: 978-1517291815

ISBN-10: 151729181X

Disclaimer: This book is not intended to treat or diagnose any medical conditions. The author is not a medical professional, is not qualified to give medical advice, and is just sharing what worked from personal experience. Anyone considering this protocol should consult directly with their doctor or medical healthcare provider. The author assumes no responsbility for the use or misuse of the information in this book. Anyone doing the hCG diet does so at their own risk.

FDA required statement: The FDA has not approved the use of HCG for weight loss and reports no evidence that HCG is effective for the treatment of obesity.

Lots of free guidance and tips
for the hCG diet at:
hcgchica.com
or scan this QR code:

Table of CONTENTS

A Quick HELLO HOW YA DOIN'

WELCOME BACK!

So you're back for more eh? This is the follow-up refill Phase 2 workbook that contains only what you need to track your round, now that you are familiar with the hCG protocol itself and just need a place to keep track of your stats and notes.

As you continue on your journey - **I'd love to hear what you find works for you as you go through this process**- little tips, tricks or organizational things that make this possible.

Why share what helps you? Because **there are others out there, like you, struggling to find a way to make this happen amidst a crazy life - whether it's while raising 4 kids or working 16 hours shifts at a hospital.**

Each of you are finding ways to make this work, and the more tips I can continue to share on hcgchica.com, the more people will be able to have the tools to get through the rough patches.

So please, would love to hear your tips!

Email me here:
hcgchica@hcgchica.com

- Rayzel

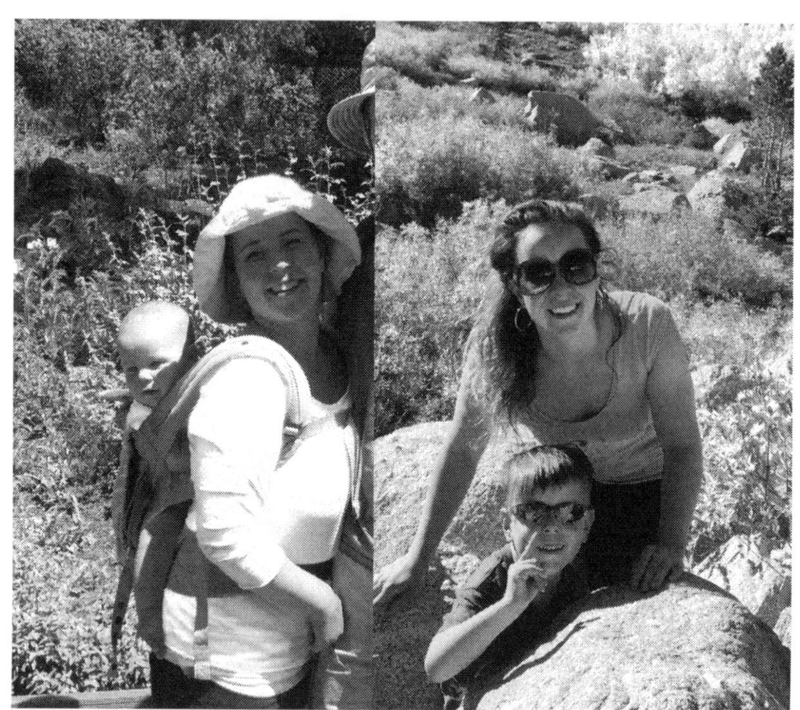

If you'd like to learn more about my personal weight loss story (and what I'm up to now!) go to

HCGCHICA.COM/MYSTORY

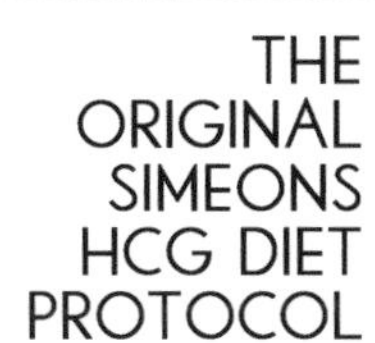
THE ORIGINAL SIMEONS HCG DIET PROTOCOL

PHASE 2 FOODS the 500 Calorie Diet

Non-protocol foods that some now use are shown in grey boxes.

Approved FOOD LIST

Remove all visible fat
Do not cook with skin

PROTEINS:

Meat serving size:
100 grams/3.5 ounces

- Lean Beef
- Chicken breast
- Veal
- Fresh white fish

Types of White Fish:
- Catfish
- Cod
- Flounder
- Halibut
- Sole
- Red Snapper
- Sea Bass
- Tilapia
- Trout

- Lobster
- Crab
- Shrimp

Occasional Meat Replacement:

- 1 egg + 3 egg whites
- 100 grams fat free Cottage Cheese

Off-Protocol PROTEINS

- 99% Fat Free Ham
- Turkey Breast
- Tuna (Water Packed)
- Protein Shake (low carb)

VEGETABLES:

There is no serving size for veggies listed in the original protocol.

- Asparagus
- Beet Greens
- Cabbage
- Celery
- Chard
- Chicory
- Cucumber
- Fennel
- Lettuce
- Onions
- Radishes
- Spinach
- Tomatoes

Off-Protocol VEGGIES

- Bell Pepper
- Broccoli
- Mushrooms
- Yellow Squash
- Zucchini

FRUITS:

- 1 Apple
- ½ Grapefruit
- 1 Orange
- Strawberries *(handful)*

Off-Protocol FRUITS

- Blackberries *(handful)*
- Blueberries *(handful)*
- Raspberries *(handful)*

CARB:

- 1 Grissini Stick
  (Not allowed if these contain olive oil- check ingredients.)
- 1 Melba Toast

SMALL STUFF:

- Juice of 1 lemon/day
- 1 tablespoon milk/day
- Stevia* or saccharin
- Salt, spices, herbs, vinegar etc. ok as long as they don't contain sugar, starch, or oil.

Off-Protocol OTHER

- Miracle Noodles
- Fat Free Greek Yogurt
  (in place of fruits)

*Stevia was not included in the original protocol, since it was written in the 50's before Stevia was even around in most countries. It is a standardly accepted sweetener on this protocol however, and in this day and age, considered to be a healthier option than saccharin.

Please note: I don't necessarily endorse all modifications to the diet. It's your personal choice whether you include them in your Phase 2. To see what modifications I personally used, and under what circumstances I used them, go to: hcgchica.com/modifications

My NOTES

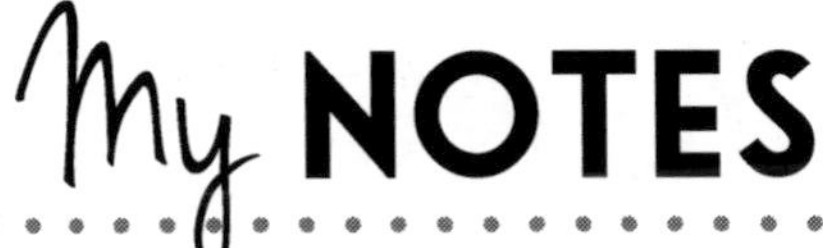
My NOTES

My NOTES

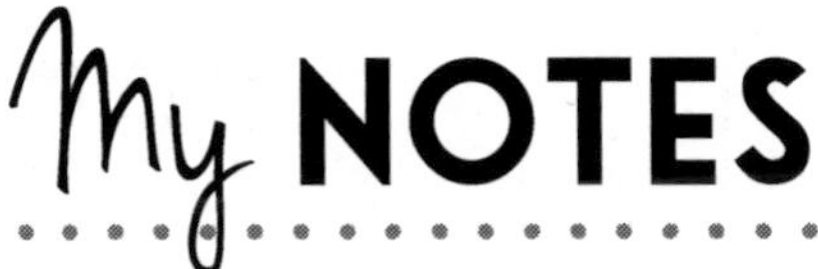

My NOTES

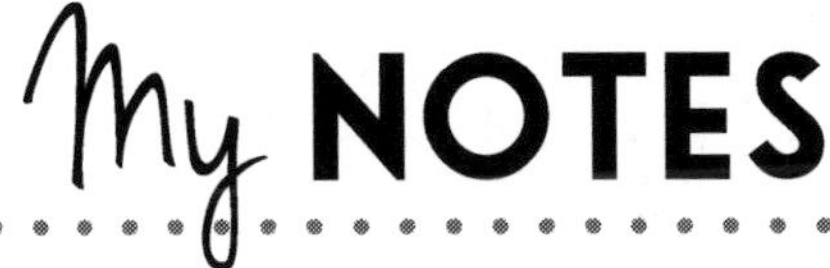

Section 1

QUICK GLANCE PROGRESS

My INCH LOSS RESULTS

"It had long since come to my attention that people of accomplishment rarely sat back and let things happen to them. They went out and happened to things."

–LEONARDO DA VINCI

ROUND# ☐ 1 ☐ 2 ☐ 3 ☐ 4 ☐ 5 ☐ 6 ☐ 7 **OTHER:** ____

Starting **MEASUREMENTS**				
VLCD 0	**DATE**	**A.M. WEIGHT**		
NECK		HIPS		
BICEP		UPPER THIGH	L	R
WRIST		MID THIGH	L	R
BUST		KNEE	L	R
UNDER BUST		CALF	L	R
Smallest part of WAIST		ANKLE	L	R
BELLY BUTTON		OTHER		
BELLY		OTHER		

End **OF ROUND** Last Dose Weight Measurements				
VLCD DAY: ____	**DATE**	**A.M. WEIGHT**		
NECK		HIPS		
BICEP		UPPER THIGH	L	R
WRIST		MID THIGH	L	R
BUST		KNEE	L	R
UNDER BUST		CALF	L	R
Smallest part of WAIST		ANKLE	L	R
BELLY BUTTON		OTHER		
BELLY		OTHER		

My INCH LOSS

Location	DATE VLCD# WEIGHT		DATE VLCD# WEIGHT		DATE VLCD# WEIGHT		DATE VLCD# WEIGHT		DATE VLCD# WEIGHT		DATE VLCD# WEIGHT		DATE VLCD# WEIGHT		DATE VLCD# WEIGHT		INCH LOSS TOTALS
NECK																	
BICEP																	
WRIST																	
BUST																	
Under BUST																	
WAIST																	
Belly BUTTON																	
BELLY																	
HIPS																	
Mid THIGH	L	R	L	R	L	R	L	R	L	R	L	R	L	R	L	R	
Upper THIGH	L	R	L	R	L	R	L	R	L	R	L	R	L	R	L	R	
KNEE	L	R	L	R	L	R	L	R	L	R	L	R	L	R	L	R	
CALF	L	R	L	R	L	R	L	R	L	R	L	R	L	R	L	R	
ANKLE	L	R	L	R	L	R	L	R	L	R	L	R	L	R	L	R	
OTHER:																	
OTHER:																	

Tracking INCHES AFTER HCG

Location	DATE WEIGHT		DATE WEIGHT		DATE WEIGHT		DATE WEIGHT		DATE WEIGHT		DATE WEIGHT		DATE WEIGHT		DATE WEIGHT	
NECK																
BICEP																
WRIST																
BUST																
Under BUST																
WAIST																
Belly BUTTON																
BELLY																
HIPS																
Mid THIGH	L	R	L	R	L	R	L	R	L	R	L	R	L	R	L	R
Upper THIGH	L	R	L	R	L	R	L	R	L	R	L	R	L	R	L	R
KNEE	L	R	L	R	L	R	L	R	L	R	L	R	L	R	L	R
CALF	L	R	L	R	L	R	L	R	L	R	L	R	L	R	L	R
ANKLE	L	R	L	R	L	R	L	R	L	R	L	R	L	R	L	R
OTHER:																
OTHER:																

Quick Glance WEIGHT TRACKING CHART: **PRE–HCG DIET**

The 7-10 day Pre-hCG Diet, as discussed at **hcgchica.com/prehcgdiet**, is an ***optional*** method I found useful for addressing sugar addiction in the quickest, most effective, and least painful manner possible. If sugar/carb addiction is not something you struggle with, this may not be an important thing for you to do.

If you ***do*** choose to implement this tactic, you ***may*** lose a little weight, but you may not. Either result is perfectly normal. The point of this really is helping to alleviate cravings for sugar and carbs prior to the start of the low calorie portion of the diet.

DATE	TIME	DAY	WEIGHT	+ OR –	TOTAL LOSS	NOTES
7–10 DAY PRE–HCG DIET						
		DAY 1				
		DAY 2				
		DAY 3				
		DAY 4				
		DAY 5				
		DAY 6				
		DAY 7				
		DAY 8				
		DAY 9				
		DAY 10				

Quick Glance WEIGHT TRACKING CHART- PHASE 2

My hCG RESULTS:

FINAL RESULTS			
TOTAL LOADING GAIN:			
STARTING WEIGHT:		LDW (last dose weight):	
WEIGHT LOSS - GROSS:			
WEIGHT LOSS - NET:			

Let's get this show on the road!

Please note! I chose to label the first day of the low calorie diet as day 0 for the following reason: Weight loss doesn't start adding up until *after* the first vlcd day. The morning of the eighth day on the diet, your written entry will show how much you've lost after seven full days, one full week, on the 500 calorie diet.

DATE	TIME	DAY	WEIGHT	+ OR -	TOTAL LOSS	NOTES	INJECTION #
		LOAD DAY 1		- WEEK 1 -			
		LOAD DAY 2					
		LOAD DAY 3 (if applicable)					
		VLCD 0					
		VLCD 1					
		VLCD 2					
		VLCD 3					
		VLCD 4					
		VLCD 5					
		VLCD 6					
		VLCD 7				Take Measurements Day	
WEEK 1 WEIGHT LOSS TOTAL:							

Remember! There is often a good portion of weight loss at the start of any diet that is water weight loss - this will often lead to an epic looking first week. The weight loss will naturally decrease in general once the excess water weight is gone. This is normal and expected. The ensuing weeks will be accomplishing a lot of fat loss for you which will greatly change your body, even if the "pounds" lost seem like less than the first week.

Quick Glance WEIGHT TRACKING CHART- PHASE 2

DATE	TIME	DAY	WEIGHT	+ OR –	TOTAL LOSS	NOTES	INJECTION #
WEEK 1 ENDING WEIGHT:				– WEEK 2 –			
		VLCD 8					
		VLCD 9					
		VLCD 10					
		VLCD 11					
		VLCD 12					
		VLCD 13					
		VLCD 14				Take Measurements Day	
WEEK 2 WEIGHT LOSS TOTAL:							

DATE	TIME	DAY	WEIGHT	+ OR –	TOTAL LOSS	NOTES	INJECTION #
WEEK 2 ENDING WEIGHT:				– WEEK 3 –			
		VLCD 15					
		VLCD 16					
		VLCD 17					
		VLCD 18					
		VLCD 19					
		VLCD 20					
		VLCD 21				Take Measurements Day	
WEEK 3 WEIGHT LOSS TOTAL:							

Quick Glance WEIGHT TRACKING CHART- PHASE 2

DATE	TIME	DAY	WEIGHT	+ OR –	TOTAL LOSS	NOTES	INJECTION #
WEEK 3 ENDING WEIGHT:				– WEEK 4 –			
		VLCD 22					
		VLCD 23					
		VLCD 24					
		VLCD 25					
		VLCD 26					
		VLCD 27					
		VLCD 28				Take Measurements Day	
WEEK 4 WEIGHT LOSS TOTAL:							

DATE	TIME	DAY	WEIGHT	+ OR –	TOTAL LOSS	NOTES	INJECTION #
WEEK 4 ENDING WEIGHT:				– WEEK 5 –			
		VLCD 29					
		VLCD 30					
		VLCD 31					
		VLCD 32					
		VLCD 33					
		VLCD 34					
		VLCD 35				Take Measurements Day	
WEEK 5 WEIGHT LOSS TOTAL:							

Quick Glance WEIGHT TRACKING CHART- **PHASE 2**

DATE	TIME	DAY	WEIGHT	+ OR –	TOTAL LOSS	NOTES	INJECTION #
		WEEK 5 ENDING WEIGHT:		– WEEK 6 –			
		VLCD 36					
		VLCD 37					
		VLCD 38					
		VLCD 39					
		VLCD 40					
		VLCD 41					
		VLCD 42				Take Measurements Day	
WEEK 6 WEIGHT LOSS TOTAL:							

Quick Glance WEIGHT TRACKING CHART- PHASE 3

DATE	TIME	DAY	WEIGHT	+ OR –	NOTES
		P3 DAY 1			
		P3 DAY 2			
		P3 DAY 3			
		P3 DAY 4			
		P3 DAY 5			
		P3 DAY 6			
		P3 DAY 7			
		P3 DAY 8			
		P3 DAY 9			
		P3 DAY 10			
		P3 DAY 11			
		P3 DAY 12			
		P3 DAY 13			
		P3 DAY 14			
		P3 DAY 15			
		P3 DAY 16			
		P3 DAY 17			
		P3 DAY 18			
		P3 DAY 19			
		P3 DAY 20			
		P3 DAY 21			

TROUBLESHOOTING *log*

Even though the majority of your experience on the hCG protocol is just the natural way that things go, and I definitely don't encourage over-analyzing, there are times when there may be a legitimate ***thang*** going on that may be inhibiting you in some way. This is a place to consider possible reasons for trouble you may be having. It could be dealing with constipation, trouble sleeping, weight loss issues, possible food intolerances, not drinking enough water, etc. Most importantly, this will help you give thought to what adjustments you can try out to remedy the problem.

DATE: _______
VLCD #: ______

Possible **PROBLEM:**	

Possible Causes	Adjustments to Try	Results

DATE: _______
VLCD #: ______

Possible **PROBLEM:**	

Possible Causes	Adjustments to Try	Results

DATE: ________
VLCD #: ______

Possible PROBLEM:	

Possible Causes	Adjustments to Try	Results

DATE: ________
VLCD #: ______

Possible PROBLEM:	

Possible Causes	Adjustments to Try	Results

DATE: ________
VLCD #: ______

Possible PROBLEM:	

Possible Causes	Adjustments to Try	Results

DATE: ______
VLCD #: ______

Possible PROBLEM:	

Possible Causes	Adjustments to Try	Results

DATE: ______
VLCD #: ______

Possible PROBLEM:	

Possible Causes	Adjustments to Try	Results

DATE: ______
VLCD #: ______

Possible PROBLEM:	

Possible Causes	Adjustments to Try	Results

DATE: ________
VLCD #: ______

Possible PROBLEM:	

Possible Causes	Adjustments to Try	Results

• • • • • • • • • • • • • • •

DATE: ________
VLCD #: ______

Possible PROBLEM:	

Possible Causes	Adjustments to Try	Results

• • • • • • • • • • • • • • •

DATE: ________
VLCD #: ______

Possible PROBLEM:	

Possible Causes	Adjustments to Try	Results

• • • • • • • • • • • • • • •

Section

2

DAILY TRACKING AREA

SOME DAYS WILL CERTAINLY FEEL *hard*.

BUT TRY TO REMEMBER THAT MOST OF THE TIME THOSE FEELINGS **WILL** *pass* AND THE ENSUING DAYS WILL BE MORE DOABLE.

Week 1

"DREAMS ARE RENEWABLE. No matter what age or condition, there are still untapped possibilities within us and new beauty waiting to be born."

- Dr. Dale Turner

Phase 1 - Load **TRACKING**

Please note! Most only do the loading phase for two days. The third day is optional/not usually necessary.

LIFE BEGINS
AT THE END
OF YOUR
COMFORT ZONE.

A flower
does not
think of competing
with the flower
next to it -
IT JUST BLOOMS.

LOAD DAY 1 (Date): ______________

WEIGHT: ______________

HCG DOSAGE: ______________

TOTAL CALORIES: ______________

SUPPLEMENTS: ______________________

☐ Multivitamin ☐ B12 Shot ☐ Lipo Shot

LOADING FOODS/MEALS EATEN

Letting go becomes easier, **WHEN YOU SEE** not what you lose, but all that you gain, in *creating space* for **SOMETHING NEW.**

- Renate Vullings

LOAD DAY **2** (Date): ______________

WEIGHT: ______________

HCG DOSAGE: ______________

TOTAL CALORIES: ______________

SUPPLEMENTS: ______________________

☐ Multivitamin ☐ B12 Shot ☐ Lipo Shot

LOADING FOODS/MEALS EATEN

Don't compare your **BEGINNING** to someone else's MIDDLE.

- Jon Acuff

LOAD DAY **3** (Date): ______________

WEIGHT: ______________

HCG DOSAGE: ______________

TOTAL CALORIES: ______________

SUPPLEMENTS: ______________________

☐ Multivitamin ☐ B12 Shot ☐ Lipo Shot

LOADING FOODS/MEALS EATEN

HCGCHICA TIP:

Don't underestimate the power of sleep in both the quantity and quality (fat vs. muscle) of your weight loss.

VLCD 0 (Date): ______

WEIGHT: ______

HCG DOSAGE: ______

HUNGER LEVEL: ______

BEDTIME/WAKE TIME: ______

HOURS SLEEP: ______

TOTAL CALORIES: ______

SUPPLEMENTS: ______

☐ Multivitamin ☐ B12 Shot ☐ Lipo Shot

INJECTION LOCATION

TIME: ______

☐ Belly ☐ Deltoid ☐ Thigh ☐ Other: ______

DROPS / PELLETS DOSE TIMING

1st Dose: ______ 2nd Dose: ______
3rd Dose: ______ 4th Dose: ______

LIQUIDS:

4 LITERS
3.5 LITERS
3 LITERS
2.5 LITERS
2 LITERS
1.5 LITERS
1 LITER
.5 LITERS

128 oz = 1 GALLON
120 oz
112 oz
104 oz
96 oz = 3 QUARTS
88 oz
80 oz
72 oz
64 oz = 2 QUARTS
56 oz
48 oz
40 oz
32 oz = 1 QUART
24 oz
16 oz
8 oz = 1 CUP

PERSONAL NOTES

BREAKFAST

Time:

☐ None ☐ Fruit: ______ ☐ Protein: ______ Calories: ______

Serving Size: ______ Serving Size: ______

LUNCH Time:

WAS AN ITEM EATEN AS A SNACK? WHICH? Time:

Protein:

- [ ] Chicken breast
- [ ] Beef
- [ ] Veal
- [ ] Shrimp
- [ ] Lobster
- [ ] White fish: ___________
- [ ] Protein Shake
- [ ] Other: ___________

Serving Size:

- [ ] 100 grams/3.5 oz
- [ ] Other: ___________

Calories: ___________

Vegetable:

- [ ] Asparagus
- [ ] Beet Greens
- [ ] Cabbage
- [ ] Celery
- [ ] Chard
- [ ] Cucumber
- [ ] Fennel
- [ ] Lettuce
- [ ] Onions
- [ ] Radishes
- [ ] Spinach
- [ ] Tomatoes
- [ ] Other: ___________
- [ ] Other: ___________
- [ ] Other: ___________

Calories: ___________

Fruit:

- [ ] Strawberries
- [ ] ½ Grapefruit
- [ ] Apple
- [ ] Orange
- [ ] Other: ___________

Starch:

- [ ] Grissini
- [ ] Melba
- [ ] Other: ___________

Calories: ___________

Other:

- [ ] TBS. Milk
- [ ] Juice of 1 Lemon
- [ ] Stevia
- [ ] Shirataki/Miracle Noodles
- [ ] Other: ___________
- [ ] Other: ___________
- [ ] Other: ___________

Calories: ___________

DINNER Time:

WAS AN ITEM EATEN AS A SNACK? WHICH? Time:

Protein:

- [ ] Chicken
- [ ] Beef
- [ ] Veal
- [ ] Shrimp
- [ ] Lobster
- [ ] White fish: ___________
- [ ] Protein Shake
- [ ] Other: ___________

Serving Size:

- [ ] 100 grams
- [ ] Other: ___________

Calories: ___________

Vegetable:

- [ ] Asparagus
- [ ] Beet Greens
- [ ] Cabbage
- [ ] Celery
- [ ] Chard
- [ ] Cucumber
- [ ] Fennel
- [ ] Lettuce
- [ ] Onions
- [ ] Radishes
- [ ] Spinach
- [ ] Tomatoes
- [ ] Other: ___________
- [ ] Other: ___________
- [ ] Other: ___________

Calories: ___________

Fruit:

- [ ] Strawberries
- [ ] ½ Grapefruit
- [ ] Apple
- [ ] Orange
- [ ] Other: ___________

Starch:

- [ ] Grissini
- [ ] Melba
- [ ] Other: ___________

Calories: ___________

Other:

- [ ] TBS. Milk
- [ ] Juice of 1 Lemon
- [ ] Stevia
- [ ] Shirataki/Miracle Noodles
- [ ] Other: ___________
- [ ] Other: ___________
- [ ] Other: ___________

Calories: ___________

FELLOW HCGER TIP:
Sprinkling cinnamon & stevia on your P2 apple slices is the bomb.

VLCD 1 (Date): ____________

WEIGHT: ____________

HCG DOSAGE: ____________

HUNGER LEVEL: ____________

BEDTIME/WAKE TIME: ____________

HOURS SLEEP: ____________

TOTAL CALORIES: ____________

SUPPLEMENTS: ____________

☐ Multivitamin ☐ B12 Shot ☐ Lipo Shot

INJECTION LOCATION

TIME: ________

☐ Belly ☐ Deltoid ☐ Thigh ☐ Other: ____________

DROPS / PELLETS DOSE TIMING

1st Dose: ____________ 2nd Dose: ____________

3rd Dose: ____________ 4th Dose: ____________

LIQUIDS:

☐	4 LITERS
☐	3.5 LITERS
☐	3 LITERS
☐	2.5 LITERS
☐	2 LITERS
☐	1.5 LITERS
☐	1 LITER
☐	.5 LITERS

☐	128 oz = 1 GALLON
☐	120 oz
☐	112 oz
☐	104 oz
☐	96 oz = 3 QUARTS
☐	88 oz
☐	80 oz
☐	72 oz
☐	64 oz = 2 QUARTS
☐	56 oz
☐	48 oz
☐	40 oz
☐	32 oz = 1 QUART
☐	24 oz
☐	16 oz
☐	8 oz = 1 CUP

PERSONAL NOTES

BREAKFAST

Time:

☐ None ☐ Fruit: ____________ ☐ Protein: ____________ Calories: ________

Serving Size: ____________ Serving Size: ____________

LUNCH Time:

WAS AN ITEM EATEN AS A SNACK? WHICH? Time:

Protein:

- ☐ Chicken breast
- ☐ Beef
- ☐ Veal
- ☐ Shrimp
- ☐ Lobster
- ☐ White fish: ____________
- ☐ Protein Shake
- ☐ Other: ____________

Serving Size:

- ☐ 100 grams/3.5 oz
- ☐ Other: ____________

Calories: ____________

Vegetable:

- ☐ Asparagus
- ☐ Beet Greens
- ☐ Cabbage
- ☐ Celery
- ☐ Chard
- ☐ Cucumber
- ☐ Fennel
- ☐ Lettuce
- ☐ Onions
- ☐ Radishes
- ☐ Spinach
- ☐ Tomatoes
- ☐ Other: ____________
- ☐ Other: ____________
- ☐ Other: ____________

Calories: ____________

Fruit:

- ☐ Strawberries
- ☐ ½ Grapefruit
- ☐ Apple
- ☐ Orange
- ☐ Other: ____________

Starch:

- ☐ Grissini
- ☐ Melba
- ☐ Other: ____________

Calories: ____________

Other:

- ☐ TBS. Milk
- ☐ Juice of 1 Lemon
- ☐ Stevia
- ☐ Shirataki/Miracle Noodles
- ☐ Other: ____________
- ☐ Other: ____________
- ☐ Other: ____________

Calories: ____________

DINNER Time:

WAS AN ITEM EATEN AS A SNACK? WHICH? Time:

Protein:

- ☐ Chicken
- ☐ Beef
- ☐ Veal
- ☐ Shrimp
- ☐ Lobster
- ☐ White fish: ____________
- ☐ Protein Shake
- ☐ Other: ____________

Serving Size:

- ☐ 100 grams
- ☐ Other: ____________

Calories: ____________

Vegetable:

- ☐ Asparagus
- ☐ Beet Greens
- ☐ Cabbage
- ☐ Celery
- ☐ Chard
- ☐ Cucumber
- ☐ Fennel
- ☐ Lettuce
- ☐ Onions
- ☐ Radishes
- ☐ Spinach
- ☐ Tomatoes
- ☐ Other: ____________
- ☐ Other: ____________
- ☐ Other: ____________

Calories: ____________

Fruit:

- ☐ Strawberries
- ☐ ½ Grapefruit
- ☐ Apple
- ☐ Orange
- ☐ Other: ____________

Starch:

- ☐ Grissini
- ☐ Melba
- ☐ Other: ____________

Calories: ____________

Other:

- ☐ TBS. Milk
- ☐ Juice of 1 Lemon
- ☐ Stevia
- ☐ Shirataki/Miracle Noodles
- ☐ Other: ____________
- ☐ Other: ____________
- ☐ Other: ____________

Calories: ____________

> Success means doing the best we can with what we have. Success is THE DOING, not the getting; in THE TRYING, not the triumph. Success is a personal standard, reaching for the highest that is in us, becoming all that we can be.
>
> \- Zig Ziglar

VLCD 2 (Date): ____________

WEIGHT: ____________

HCG DOSAGE: ____________

HUNGER LEVEL: ____________

BEDTIME/WAKE TIME: ____________

HOURS SLEEP: ____________

TOTAL CALORIES: ____________

SUPPLEMENTS: ____________

☐ Multivitamin ☐ B12 Shot ☐ Lipo Shot

INJECTION LOCATION

TIME: ________

☐ Belly ☐ Deltoid ☐ Thigh ☐ Other: ____________

DROPS / PELLETS DOSE TIMING

1st Dose: ____________ 2nd Dose: ____________

3rd Dose: ____________ 4th Dose: ____________

LIQUIDS:

☐	4 LITERS
☐	3.5 LITERS
☐	3 LITERS
☐	2.5 LITERS
☐	2 LITERS
☐	1.5 LITERS
☐	1 LITER
☐	.5 LITERS

☐	128 oz = 1 GALLON
☐	120 oz
☐	112 oz
☐	104 oz
☐	96 oz = 3 QUARTS
☐	88 oz
☐	80 oz
☐	72 oz
☐	64 oz = 2 QUARTS
☐	56 oz
☐	48 oz
☐	40 oz
☐	32 oz = 1 QUART
☐	24 oz
☐	16 oz
☐	8 oz = 1 CUP

PERSONAL NOTES

BREAKFAST

Time:

☐ None ☐ Fruit: ____________ ☐ Protein: ____________ Calories: ____________

Serving Size: ____________ Serving Size: ____________

LUNCH Time:

WAS AN ITEM EATEN AS A SNACK? WHICH? Time:

Protein:

- ☐ Chicken breast
- ☐ Beef
- ☐ Veal
- ☐ Shrimp
- ☐ Lobster
- ☐ White fish: ____________
- ☐ Protein Shake
- ☐ Other: ____________

Serving Size:

- ☐ 100 grams/3.5 oz
- ☐ Other: ____________

Calories: ____________

Vegetable:

- ☐ Asparagus
- ☐ Beet Greens
- ☐ Cabbage
- ☐ Celery
- ☐ Chard
- ☐ Cucumber
- ☐ Fennel
- ☐ Lettuce
- ☐ Onions
- ☐ Radishes
- ☐ Spinach
- ☐ Tomatoes
- ☐ Other: ____________
- ☐ Other: ____________
- ☐ Other: ____________

Calories: ____________

Fruit:

- ☐ Strawberries
- ☐ ½ Grapefruit
- ☐ Apple
- ☐ Orange
- ☐ Other: ____________

Starch:

- ☐ Grissini
- ☐ Melba
- ☐ Other: ____________

Calories: ____________

Other:

- ☐ TBS. Milk
- ☐ Juice of 1 Lemon
- ☐ Stevia
- ☐ Shirataki/Miracle Noodles
- ☐ Other: ____________
- ☐ Other: ____________
- ☐ Other: ____________

Calories: ____________

DINNER Time:

WAS AN ITEM EATEN AS A SNACK? WHICH? Time:

Protein:

- ☐ Chicken
- ☐ Beef
- ☐ Veal
- ☐ Shrimp
- ☐ Lobster
- ☐ White fish: ____________
- ☐ Protein Shake
- ☐ Other: ____________

Serving Size:

- ☐ 100 grams
- ☐ Other: ____________

Calories: ____________

Vegetable:

- ☐ Asparagus
- ☐ Beet Greens
- ☐ Cabbage
- ☐ Celery
- ☐ Chard
- ☐ Cucumber
- ☐ Fennel
- ☐ Lettuce
- ☐ Onions
- ☐ Radishes
- ☐ Spinach
- ☐ Tomatoes
- ☐ Other: ____________
- ☐ Other: ____________
- ☐ Other: ____________

Calories: ____________

Fruit:

- ☐ Strawberries
- ☐ ½ Grapefruit
- ☐ Apple
- ☐ Orange
- ☐ Other: ____________

Starch:

- ☐ Grissini
- ☐ Melba
- ☐ Other: ____________

Calories: ____________

Other:

- ☐ TBS. Milk
- ☐ Juice of 1 Lemon
- ☐ Stevia
- ☐ Shirataki/Miracle Noodles
- ☐ Other: ____________
- ☐ Other: ____________
- ☐ Other: ____________

Calories: ____________

FELLOW HCGER TIP:

Delicious Gingery Soup

Shave slices of fresh ginger, cherry tomatoes, and chicken or shrimp into homemade chicken de-fatted broth.

VLCD 3 (Date): ____________

WEIGHT: ____________

HCG DOSAGE: ____________

HUNGER LEVEL: ____________

BEDTIME/WAKE TIME: ____________

HOURS SLEEP: ____________

TOTAL CALORIES: ____________

SUPPLEMENTS: ____________

☐ Multivitamin ☐ B12 Shot ☐ Lipo Shot

INJECTION LOCATION

TIME: ________

☐ Belly ☐ Deltoid ☐ Thigh ☐ Other: ____________

DROPS / PELLETS DOSE TIMING

1st Dose: ____________ 2nd Dose: ____________

3rd Dose: ____________ 4th Dose: ____________

LIQUIDS:

4 LITERS
3.5 LITERS
3 LITERS
2.5 LITERS
2 LITERS
1.5 LITERS
1 LITER
.5 LITERS

128 oz = 1 GALLON
120 oz
112 oz
104 oz
96 oz = 3 QUARTS
88 oz
80 oz
72 oz
64 oz = 2 QUARTS
56 oz
48 oz
40 oz
32 oz = 1 QUART
24 oz
16 oz
8 oz = 1 CUP

PERSONAL NOTES

BREAKFAST

Time:

☐ None ☐ Fruit: ____________ ☐ Protein: ____________ Calories: ____________

Serving Size: ____________ Serving Size: ____________

LUNCH Time :

WAS AN ITEM EATEN AS A SNACK? WHICH? Time:

Protein:

- [ ] Chicken breast
- [ ] Beef
- [ ] Veal
- [ ] Shrimp
- [ ] Lobster
- [ ] White fish: ___________
- [ ] Protein Shake
- [ ] Other: ___________

Serving Size:

- [ ] 100 grams/3.5 oz
- [ ] Other: ___________

Calories: ___________

Vegetable:

- [ ] Asparagus
- [ ] Beet Greens
- [ ] Cabbage
- [ ] Celery
- [ ] Chard
- [ ] Cucumber
- [ ] Fennel
- [ ] Lettuce
- [ ] Onions
- [ ] Radishes
- [ ] Spinach
- [ ] Tomatoes
- [ ] Other: ___________
- [ ] Other: ___________
- [ ] Other: ___________

Calories: ___________

Fruit:

- [ ] Strawberries
- [ ] ½ Grapefruit
- [ ] Apple
- [ ] Orange
- [ ] Other: ___________

Starch:

- [ ] Grissini
- [ ] Melba
- [ ] Other: ___________

Calories: ___________

Other:

- [ ] TBS. Milk
- [ ] Juice of 1 Lemon
- [ ] Stevia
- [ ] Shirataki/Miracle Noodles
- [ ] Other: ___________
- [ ] Other: ___________
- [ ] Other: ___________

Calories: ___________

DINNER Time :

WAS AN ITEM EATEN AS A SNACK? WHICH? Time:

Protein:

- [ ] Chicken
- [ ] Beef
- [ ] Veal
- [ ] Shrimp
- [ ] Lobster
- [ ] White fish: ___________
- [ ] Protein Shake
- [ ] Other: ___________

Serving Size:

- [ ] 100 grams
- [ ] Other: ___________

Calories: ___________

Vegetable:

- [ ] Asparagus
- [ ] Beet Greens
- [ ] Cabbage
- [ ] Celery
- [ ] Chard
- [ ] Cucumber
- [ ] Fennel
- [ ] Lettuce
- [ ] Onions
- [ ] Radishes
- [ ] Spinach
- [ ] Tomatoes
- [ ] Other: ___________
- [ ] Other: ___________
- [ ] Other: ___________

Calories: ___________

Fruit:

- [ ] Strawberries
- [ ] ½ Grapefruit
- [ ] Apple
- [ ] Orange
- [ ] Other: ___________

Starch:

- [ ] Grissini
- [ ] Melba
- [ ] Other: ___________

Calories: ___________

Other:

- [ ] TBS. Milk
- [ ] Juice of 1 Lemon
- [ ] Stevia
- [ ] Shirataki/Miracle Noodles
- [ ] Other: ___________
- [ ] Other: ___________
- [ ] Other: ___________

Calories: ___________

> Plan your hours to be productive, plan your weeks to be educational, plan your years to be purposeful, plan your life to be an experience of growth. *Plan to change.* PLAN TO GROW.
>
> \- *Iyanla Vanzant*

VLCD 4 (Date): ____________

WEIGHT: ____________

HCG DOSAGE: ____________

HUNGER LEVEL: ____________

BEDTIME/WAKE TIME: ____________

HOURS SLEEP: ____________

TOTAL CALORIES: ____________

SUPPLEMENTS: ____________

☐ Multivitamin ☐ B12 Shot ☐ Lipo Shot

INJECTION LOCATION

TIME: ________

☐ Belly ☐ Deltoid ☐ Thigh ☐ Other: ____________

DROPS / PELLETS DOSE TIMING

1st Dose: ____________ 2nd Dose: ____________

3rd Dose: ____________ 4th Dose: ____________

LIQUIDS:

☐	4 LITERS
☐	3.5 LITERS
☐	3 LITERS
☐	2.5 LITERS
☐	2 LITERS
☐	1.5 LITERS
☐	1 LITER
☐	.5 LITERS

☐	128 OZ = 1 GALLON
☐	120 OZ
☐	112 OZ
☐	104 OZ
☐	96 OZ = 3 QUARTS
☐	88 OZ
☐	80 OZ
☐	72 OZ
☐	64 OZ = 2 QUARTS
☐	56 OZ
☐	48 OZ
☐	40 OZ
☐	32 OZ = 1 QUART
☐	24 OZ
☐	16 OZ
☐	8 OZ = 1 CUP

PERSONAL NOTES

....

....

....

....

....

....

....

....

BREAKFAST

Time:

☐ None ☐ Fruit: ____________ ☐ Protein: ____________ *Calories:* ____________

Serving Size: ____________ *Serving Size:* ____________

LUNCH Time:

WAS AN ITEM EATEN AS A SNACK? WHICH? Time:

Protein:

- ☐ Chicken breast
- ☐ Beef
- ☐ Veal
- ☐ Shrimp
- ☐ Lobster
- ☐ White fish: ________
- ☐ Protein Shake
- ☐ Other: ________

Serving Size:

- ☐ 100 grams/3.5 oz
- ☐ Other: ________

Calories: ________

Vegetable:

- ☐ Asparagus
- ☐ Beet Greens
- ☐ Cabbage
- ☐ Celery
- ☐ Chard
- ☐ Cucumber
- ☐ Fennel
- ☐ Lettuce
- ☐ Onions
- ☐ Radishes
- ☐ Spinach
- ☐ Tomatoes
- ☐ Other: ________
- ☐ Other: ________
- ☐ Other: ________

Calories: ________

Fruit:

- ☐ Strawberries
- ☐ ½ Grapefruit
- ☐ Apple
- ☐ Orange
- ☐ Other: ________

Starch:

- ☐ Grissini
- ☐ Melba
- ☐ Other: ________

Calories: ________

Other:

- ☐ TBS. Milk
- ☐ Juice of 1 Lemon
- ☐ Stevia
- ☐ Shirataki/Miracle Noodles
- ☐ Other: ________
- ☐ Other: ________
- ☐ Other: ________

Calories: ________

DINNER Time:

WAS AN ITEM EATEN AS A SNACK? WHICH? Time:

Protein:

- ☐ Chicken
- ☐ Beef
- ☐ Veal
- ☐ Shrimp
- ☐ Lobster
- ☐ White fish: ________
- ☐ Protein Shake
- ☐ Other: ________

Serving Size:

- ☐ 100 grams
- ☐ Other: ________

Calories: ________

Vegetable:

- ☐ Asparagus
- ☐ Beet Greens
- ☐ Cabbage
- ☐ Celery
- ☐ Chard
- ☐ Cucumber
- ☐ Fennel
- ☐ Lettuce
- ☐ Onions
- ☐ Radishes
- ☐ Spinach
- ☐ Tomatoes
- ☐ Other: ________
- ☐ Other: ________
- ☐ Other: ________

Calories: ________

Fruit:

- ☐ Strawberries
- ☐ ½ Grapefruit
- ☐ Apple
- ☐ Orange
- ☐ Other: ________

Starch:

- ☐ Grissini
- ☐ Melba
- ☐ Other: ________

Calories: ________

Other:

- ☐ TBS. Milk
- ☐ Juice of 1 Lemon
- ☐ Stevia
- ☐ Shirataki/Miracle Noodles
- ☐ Other: ________
- ☐ Other: ________
- ☐ Other: ________

Calories: ________

FELLOW HCGER TIP:

Flavored teas...

with stevia, can save you. No joke. When choosing one, just double check ingredients as some acually contain juice - not a good idea.

VLCD 5 (Date): ____________

WEIGHT: ____________

HCG DOSAGE: ____________

HUNGER LEVEL: ____________

BEDTIME/WAKE TIME: ____________

HOURS SLEEP: ____________

TOTAL CALORIES: ____________

SUPPLEMENTS: ____________

☐ Multivitamin ☐ B12 Shot ☐ Lipo Shot

INJECTION LOCATION

TIME: ________

☐ Belly ☐ Deltoid ☐ Thigh ☐ Other: ____________

DROPS / PELLETS DOSE TIMING

1st Dose: ____________ 2nd Dose: ____________

3rd Dose: ____________ 4th Dose: ____________

LIQUIDS:

☐	4 LITERS
☐	3.5 LITERS
☐	3 LITERS
☐	2.5 LITERS
☐	2 LITERS
☐	1.5 LITERS
☐	1 LITER
☐	.5 LITERS

☐	128 OZ = 1 GALLON
☐	120 OZ
☐	112 OZ
☐	104 OZ
☐	96 OZ = 3 QUARTS
☐	88 OZ
☐	80 OZ
☐	72 OZ
☐	64 OZ = 2 QUARTS
☐	56 OZ
☐	48 OZ
☐	40 OZ
☐	32 OZ = 1 QUART
☐	24 OZ
☐	16 OZ
☐	8 OZ = 1 CUP

PERSONAL NOTES

BREAKFAST

Time:

☐ None ☐ Fruit: ____________ ☐ Protein: ____________ Calories: ____________

Serving Size: ____________ Serving Size: ____________

LUNCH Time:

WAS AN ITEM EATEN AS A SNACK? WHICH? Time:

Protein:

- ☐ Chicken breast
- ☐ Beef
- ☐ Veal
- ☐ Shrimp
- ☐ Lobster
- ☐ White fish: ___________
- ☐ Protein Shake
- ☐ Other: ___________

Serving Size:

- ☐ 100 grams/3.5 oz
- ☐ Other: ___________

Calories: ___________

Vegetable:

- ☐ Asparagus
- ☐ Beet Greens
- ☐ Cabbage
- ☐ Celery
- ☐ Chard
- ☐ Cucumber
- ☐ Fennel
- ☐ Lettuce
- ☐ Onions
- ☐ Radishes
- ☐ Spinach
- ☐ Tomatoes
- ☐ Other: ___________
- ☐ Other: ___________
- ☐ Other: ___________

Calories: ___________

Fruit:

- ☐ Strawberries
- ☐ ½ Grapefruit
- ☐ Apple
- ☐ Orange
- ☐ Other: ___________

Starch:

- ☐ Grissini
- ☐ Melba
- ☐ Other: ___________

Calories: ___________

Other:

- ☐ TBS. Milk
- ☐ Juice of 1 Lemon
- ☐ Stevia
- ☐ Shirataki/Miracle Noodles
- ☐ Other: ___________
- ☐ Other: ___________
- ☐ Other: ___________

Calories: ___________

DINNER Time:

WAS AN ITEM EATEN AS A SNACK? WHICH? Time:

Protein:

- ☐ Chicken
- ☐ Beef
- ☐ Veal
- ☐ Shrimp
- ☐ Lobster
- ☐ White fish: ___________
- ☐ Protein Shake
- ☐ Other: ___________

Serving Size:

- ☐ 100 grams
- ☐ Other: ___________

Calories: ___________

Vegetable:

- ☐ Asparagus
- ☐ Beet Greens
- ☐ Cabbage
- ☐ Celery
- ☐ Chard
- ☐ Cucumber
- ☐ Fennel
- ☐ Lettuce
- ☐ Onions
- ☐ Radishes
- ☐ Spinach
- ☐ Tomatoes
- ☐ Other: ___________
- ☐ Other: ___________
- ☐ Other: ___________

Calories: ___________

Fruit:

- ☐ Strawberries
- ☐ ½ Grapefruit
- ☐ Apple
- ☐ Orange
- ☐ Other: ___________

Starch:

- ☐ Grissini
- ☐ Melba
- ☐ Other: ___________

Calories: ___________

Other:

- ☐ TBS. Milk
- ☐ Juice of 1 Lemon
- ☐ Stevia
- ☐ Shirataki/Miracle Noodles
- ☐ Other: ___________
- ☐ Other: ___________
- ☐ Other: ___________

Calories: ___________

When you're trying to motivate yourself, *appreciate* the fact that you're even **THINKING** about making a change. And as you move forward, **ALLOW** yourself to be good enough.

- *Alice Domar*

VLCD 6 (Date): ______________

WEIGHT: ______________

HCG DOSAGE: ______________

HUNGER LEVEL: ______________

BEDTIME/WAKE TIME: ______________

HOURS SLEEP: ______________

TOTAL CALORIES: ______________

SUPPLEMENTS: ______________

☐ Multivitamin ☐ B12 Shot ☐ Lipo Shot

INJECTION LOCATION

TIME: ________

☐ Belly ☐ Deltoid ☐ Thigh ☐ Other: ____________

DROPS / PELLETS DOSE TIMING

1st Dose: ____________ 2nd Dose: ____________

3rd Dose: ____________ 4th Dose: ____________

LIQUIDS:

☐	4 LITERS
☐	3.5 LITERS
☐	3 LITERS
☐	2.5 LITERS
☐	2 LITERS
☐	1.5 LITERS
☐	1 LITER
☐	.5 LITERS

☐	128 oz = 1 GALLON
☐	120 oz
☐	112 oz
☐	104 oz
☐	96 oz = 3 QUARTS
☐	88 oz
☐	80 oz
☐	72 oz
☐	64 oz = 2 QUARTS
☐	56 oz
☐	48 oz
☐	40 oz
☐	32 oz = 1 QUART
☐	24 oz
☐	16 oz
☐	8 oz = 1 CUP

PERSONAL NOTES

BREAKFAST

Time:

☐ None ☐ Fruit: ____________ ☐ Protein: ____________ Calories: ____________

Serving Size: ____________ Serving Size: ____________

LUNCH Time:

WAS AN ITEM EATEN AS A SNACK? WHICH? Time:

Protein:

- [ ] Chicken breast
- [ ] Beef
- [ ] Veal
- [ ] Shrimp
- [ ] Lobster
- [ ] White fish: ________
- [ ] Protein Shake
- [ ] Other: ________

Serving Size:

- [ ] 100 grams/3.5 oz
- [ ] Other: ________

Calories: ________

Vegetable:

- [ ] Asparagus
- [ ] Beet Greens
- [ ] Cabbage
- [ ] Celery
- [ ] Chard
- [ ] Cucumber
- [ ] Fennel
- [ ] Lettuce
- [ ] Onions
- [ ] Radishes
- [ ] Spinach
- [ ] Tomatoes
- [ ] Other: ________
- [ ] Other: ________
- [ ] Other: ________

Calories: ________

Fruit:

- [ ] Strawberries
- [ ] ½ Grapefruit
- [ ] Apple
- [ ] Orange
- [ ] Other: ________

Starch:

- [ ] Grissini
- [ ] Melba
- [ ] Other: ________

Calories: ________

Other:

- [ ] TBS. Milk
- [ ] Juice of 1 Lemon
- [ ] Stevia
- [ ] Shirataki/Miracle Noodles
- [ ] Other: ________
- [ ] Other: ________
- [ ] Other: ________

Calories: ________

DINNER Time:

WAS AN ITEM EATEN AS A SNACK? WHICH? Time:

Protein:

- [ ] Chicken
- [ ] Beef
- [ ] Veal
- [ ] Shrimp
- [ ] Lobster
- [ ] White fish: ________
- [ ] Protein Shake
- [ ] Other: ________

Serving Size:

- [ ] 100 grams
- [ ] Other: ________

Calories: ________

Vegetable:

- [ ] Asparagus
- [ ] Beet Greens
- [ ] Cabbage
- [ ] Celery
- [ ] Chard
- [ ] Cucumber
- [ ] Fennel
- [ ] Lettuce
- [ ] Onions
- [ ] Radishes
- [ ] Spinach
- [ ] Tomatoes
- [ ] Other: ________
- [ ] Other: ________
- [ ] Other: ________

Calories: ________

Fruit:

- [ ] Strawberries
- [ ] ½ Grapefruit
- [ ] Apple
- [ ] Orange
- [ ] Other: ________

Starch:

- [ ] Grissini
- [ ] Melba
- [ ] Other: ________

Calories: ________

Other:

- [ ] TBS. Milk
- [ ] Juice of 1 Lemon
- [ ] Stevia
- [ ] Shirataki/Miracle Noodles
- [ ] Other: ________
- [ ] Other: ________
- [ ] Other: ________

Calories: ________

FELLOW HCGER TIP:

Go-to Breakfast Smoothie

Strawberries, whizzed with ice, water, stevia and 1 tbs. milk. Put in a takeout bottle to go.

VLCD 7 (Date): ____________

WEIGHT: ____________

HCG DOSAGE: ____________

HUNGER LEVEL: ____________

BEDTIME/WAKE TIME: ____________

HOURS SLEEP: ____________

TOTAL CALORIES: ____________

SUPPLEMENTS: ____________

☐ Multivitamin ☐ B12 Shot ☐ Lipo Shot

INJECTION LOCATION

TIME: ________

☐ Belly ☐ Deltoid ☐ Thigh ☐ Other: ____________

DROPS / PELLETS DOSE TIMING

1st Dose: ____________ 2nd Dose: ____________

3rd Dose: ____________ 4th Dose: ____________

LIQUIDS:

4 LITERS
3.5 LITERS
3 LITERS
2.5 LITERS
2 LITERS
1.5 LITERS
1 LITER
.5 LITERS

128 oz = 1 GALLON
120 oz
112 oz
104 oz
96 oz = 3 QUARTS
88 oz
80 oz
72 oz
64 oz = 2 QUARTS
56 oz
48 oz
40 oz
32 oz = 1 QUART
24 oz
16 oz
8 oz = 1 CUP

PERSONAL NOTES

BREAKFAST

Time:

☐ None ☐ Fruit: ____________ ☐ Protein: ____________ Calories: ____________

Serving Size: ____________ Serving Size: ____________

LUNCH Time:

WAS AN ITEM EATEN AS A SNACK? WHICH? Time:

Protein:

- ☐ Chicken breast
- ☐ Beef
- ☐ Veal
- ☐ Shrimp
- ☐ Lobster
- ☐ White fish: ___________
- ☐ Protein Shake
- ☐ Other: ___________

Serving Size:

- ☐ 100 grams/3.5 oz
- ☐ Other: ___________

Calories: ___________

Vegetable:

- ☐ Asparagus
- ☐ Beet Greens
- ☐ Cabbage
- ☐ Celery
- ☐ Chard
- ☐ Cucumber
- ☐ Fennel
- ☐ Lettuce
- ☐ Onions
- ☐ Radishes
- ☐ Spinach
- ☐ Tomatoes
- ☐ Other: ___________
- ☐ Other: ___________
- ☐ Other: ___________

Calories: ___________

Fruit:

- ☐ Strawberries
- ☐ ½ Grapefruit
- ☐ Apple
- ☐ Orange
- ☐ Other: ___________

Starch:

- ☐ Grissini
- ☐ Melba
- ☐ Other: ___________

Calories: ___________

Other:

- ☐ TBS. Milk
- ☐ Juice of 1 Lemon
- ☐ Stevia
- ☐ Shirataki/Miracle Noodles
- ☐ Other: ___________
- ☐ Other: ___________
- ☐ Other: ___________

Calories: ___________

DINNER Time:

WAS AN ITEM EATEN AS A SNACK? WHICH? Time:

Protein:

- ☐ Chicken
- ☐ Beef
- ☐ Veal
- ☐ Shrimp
- ☐ Lobster
- ☐ White fish: ___________
- ☐ Protein Shake
- ☐ Other: ___________

Serving Size:

- ☐ 100 grams
- ☐ Other: ___________

Calories: ___________

Vegetable:

- ☐ Asparagus
- ☐ Beet Greens
- ☐ Cabbage
- ☐ Celery
- ☐ Chard
- ☐ Cucumber
- ☐ Fennel
- ☐ Lettuce
- ☐ Onions
- ☐ Radishes
- ☐ Spinach
- ☐ Tomatoes
- ☐ Other: ___________
- ☐ Other: ___________
- ☐ Other: ___________

Calories: ___________

Fruit:

- ☐ Strawberries
- ☐ ½ Grapefruit
- ☐ Apple
- ☐ Orange
- ☐ Other: ___________

Starch:

- ☐ Grissini
- ☐ Melba
- ☐ Other: ___________

Calories: ___________

Other:

- ☐ TBS. Milk
- ☐ Juice of 1 Lemon
- ☐ Stevia
- ☐ Shirataki/Miracle Noodles
- ☐ Other: ___________
- ☐ Other: ___________
- ☐ Other: ___________

Calories: ___________

Reflections ON WEEK 1

REMEMBER, THIS IS NOT JUST ABOUT LOSING WEIGHT. IT'S ABOUT CHANGING YOUR WHOLE MINDSET ABOUT FOOD AND YOUR BODY.

YOU ARE BREAKING OLD PATTERNS RIGHT NOW. YOU ARE CREATING NEW PATTERNS. TRY NOT TO FOCUS YOUR PROGESS SOLELY ON WEIGHT LOSS.

SO WITH THAT IN MIND, HOW DID THIS WEEK GO?

What are you proud of? Why are you proud of it? What did you struggle with? What would you like to work on changing? What specific logical ways can you think of to make those adjustments? Or maybe you're just burned out at the moment - it's okay to just make it a rant.

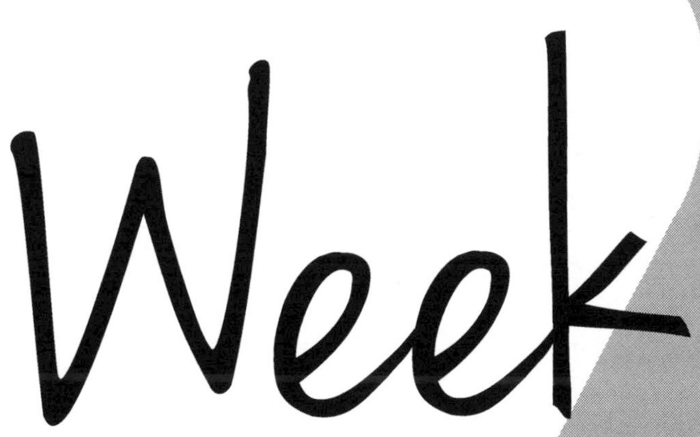

Week 2

"IN MY EXPERIENCE, nothing worthwhile has ever been all that easy. But it certainly has been worthwhile, regardless how difficult it seemed."

- Robert Fanney

When I remove the layers that say I can't, I discover A BURNING EMBER that says I SHOULD, I CAN, AND I WILL.

- Charles F. Glassman

VLCD 8 (Date): ____________

WEIGHT: ____________

HCG DOSAGE: ____________

HUNGER LEVEL: ____________

BEDTIME/WAKE TIME: ____________

HOURS SLEEP: ____________

TOTAL CALORIES: ____________

SUPPLEMENTS: ____________

☐ Multivitamin ☐ B12 Shot ☐ Lipo Shot

INJECTION LOCATION

TIME: ________

☐ Belly ☐ Deltoid ☐ Thigh ☐ Other: ____________

DROPS / PELLETS DOSE TIMING

1st Dose: ____________ 2nd Dose: ____________

3rd Dose: ____________ 4th Dose: ____________

LIQUIDS:

☐	4 LITERS
☐	3.5 LITERS
☐	3 LITERS
☐	2.5 LITERS
☐	2 LITERS
☐	1.5 LITERS
☐	1 LITER
☐	.5 LITERS

☐	128 oz = 1 GALLON
☐	120 oz
☐	112 oz
☐	104 oz
☐	96 oz = 3 QUARTS
☐	88 oz
☐	80 oz
☐	72 oz
☐	64 oz = 2 QUARTS
☐	56 oz
☐	48 oz
☐	40 oz
☐	32 oz = 1 QUART
☐	24 oz
☐	16 oz
☐	8 oz = 1 CUP

PERSONAL NOTES

BREAKFAST

Time:

☐ None ☐ Fruit: ____________ ☐ Protein: ____________ Calories: ____________

Serving Size: ____________ Serving Size: ____________

LUNCH Time :

WAS AN ITEM EATEN AS A SNACK? WHICH? Time:

Protein:

- ☐ Chicken breast
- ☐ Beef
- ☐ Veal
- ☐ Shrimp
- ☐ Lobster
- ☐ White fish: ___________
- ☐ Protein Shake
- ☐ Other: ___________

Serving Size:

- ☐ 100 grams/3.5 oz
- ☐ Other: ___________

Calories: ___________

Vegetable:

- ☐ Asparagus
- ☐ Beet Greens
- ☐ Cabbage
- ☐ Celery
- ☐ Chard
- ☐ Cucumber
- ☐ Fennel
- ☐ Lettuce
- ☐ Onions
- ☐ Radishes
- ☐ Spinach
- ☐ Tomatoes
- ☐ Other: ___________
- ☐ Other: ___________
- ☐ Other: ___________

Calories: ___________

Fruit:

- ☐ Strawberries
- ☐ ½ Grapefruit
- ☐ Apple
- ☐ Orange
- ☐ Other: ___________

Starch:

- ☐ Grissini
- ☐ Melba
- ☐ Other: ___________

Calories: ___________

Other:

- ☐ TBS. Milk
- ☐ Juice of 1 Lemon
- ☐ Stevia
- ☐ Shirataki/Miracle Noodles
- ☐ Other: ___________
- ☐ Other: ___________
- ☐ Other: ___________

Calories: ___________

DINNER Time :

WAS AN ITEM EATEN AS A SNACK? WHICH? Time:

Protein:

- ☐ Chicken
- ☐ Beef
- ☐ Veal
- ☐ Shrimp
- ☐ Lobster
- ☐ White fish: ___________
- ☐ Protein Shake
- ☐ Other: ___________

Serving Size:

- ☐ 100 grams
- ☐ Other: ___________

Calories: ___________

Vegetable:

- ☐ Asparagus
- ☐ Beet Greens
- ☐ Cabbage
- ☐ Celery
- ☐ Chard
- ☐ Cucumber
- ☐ Fennel
- ☐ Lettuce
- ☐ Onions
- ☐ Radishes
- ☐ Spinach
- ☐ Tomatoes
- ☐ Other: ___________
- ☐ Other: ___________
- ☐ Other: ___________

Calories: ___________

Fruit:

- ☐ Strawberries
- ☐ ½ Grapefruit
- ☐ Apple
- ☐ Orange
- ☐ Other: ___________

Starch:

- ☐ Grissini
- ☐ Melba
- ☐ Other: ___________

Calories: ___________

Other:

- ☐ TBS. Milk
- ☐ Juice of 1 Lemon
- ☐ Stevia
- ☐ Shirataki/Miracle Noodles
- ☐ Other: ___________
- ☐ Other: ___________
- ☐ Other: ___________

Calories: ___________

FELLOW HCGER TIP:

Social Settings

"If I'm ever going to be around other people eating during Phase 2, I make *sure* to BRING SOMETHING TO EAT *and* SOMETHING TO DRINK."

VLCD 9 (Date): ____________

WEIGHT: ____________

HCG DOSAGE: ____________

HUNGER LEVEL: ____________

BEDTIME/WAKE TIME: ____________

HOURS SLEEP: ____________

TOTAL CALORIES: ____________

SUPPLEMENTS: ____________

☐ Multivitamin ☐ B12 Shot ☐ Lipo Shot

INJECTION LOCATION

TIME: ________

☐ Belly ☐ Deltoid ☐ Thigh ☐ Other: ____________

DROPS / PELLETS DOSE TIMING

1st Dose: ____________ 2nd Dose: ____________

3rd Dose: ____________ 4th Dose: ____________

LIQUIDS:

4 LITERS
3.5 LITERS
3 LITERS
2.5 LITERS
2 LITERS
1.5 LITERS
1 LITER
.5 LITERS

128 oz = 1 GALLON
120 oz
112 oz
104 oz
96 oz = 3 QUARTS
88 oz
80 oz
72 oz
64 oz = 2 QUARTS
56 oz
48 oz
40 oz
32 oz = 1 QUART
24 oz
16 oz
8 oz = 1 CUP

PERSONAL NOTES

BREAKFAST

Time :

☐ None ☐ Fruit: ____________ ☐ Protein: ____________ Calories: ____________

Serving Size: ____________ Serving Size: ____________

LUNCH Time:

WAS AN ITEM EATEN AS A SNACK? WHICH? Time:

Protein:

- ☐ Chicken breast
- ☐ Beef
- ☐ Veal
- ☐ Shrimp
- ☐ Lobster
- ☐ White fish: ____________
- ☐ Protein Shake
- ☐ Other: ____________

Serving Size:

- ☐ 100 grams/3.5 oz
- ☐ Other: ____________

Calories: ____________

Vegetable:

- ☐ Asparagus
- ☐ Beet Greens
- ☐ Cabbage
- ☐ Celery
- ☐ Chard
- ☐ Cucumber
- ☐ Fennel
- ☐ Lettuce
- ☐ Onions
- ☐ Radishes
- ☐ Spinach
- ☐ Tomatoes
- ☐ Other: ____________
- ☐ Other: ____________
- ☐ Other: ____________

Calories: ____________

Fruit:

- ☐ Strawberries
- ☐ ½ Grapefruit
- ☐ Apple
- ☐ Orange
- ☐ Other: ____________

Starch:

- ☐ Grissini
- ☐ Melba
- ☐ Other: ____________

Calories: ____________

Other:

- ☐ TBS. Milk
- ☐ Juice of 1 Lemon
- ☐ Stevia
- ☐ Shirataki/Miracle Noodles
- ☐ Other: ____________
- ☐ Other: ____________
- ☐ Other: ____________

Calories: ____________

DINNER Time:

WAS AN ITEM EATEN AS A SNACK? WHICH? Time:

Protein:

- ☐ Chicken
- ☐ Beef
- ☐ Veal
- ☐ Shrimp
- ☐ Lobster
- ☐ White fish: ____________
- ☐ Protein Shake
- ☐ Other: ____________

Serving Size:

- ☐ 100 grams
- ☐ Other: ____________

Calories: ____________

Vegetable:

- ☐ Asparagus
- ☐ Beet Greens
- ☐ Cabbage
- ☐ Celery
- ☐ Chard
- ☐ Cucumber
- ☐ Fennel
- ☐ Lettuce
- ☐ Onions
- ☐ Radishes
- ☐ Spinach
- ☐ Tomatoes
- ☐ Other: ____________
- ☐ Other: ____________
- ☐ Other: ____________

Calories: ____________

Fruit:

- ☐ Strawberries
- ☐ ½ Grapefruit
- ☐ Apple
- ☐ Orange
- ☐ Other: ____________

Starch:

- ☐ Grissini
- ☐ Melba
- ☐ Other: ____________

Calories: ____________

Other:

- ☐ TBS. Milk
- ☐ Juice of 1 Lemon
- ☐ Stevia
- ☐ Shirataki/Miracle Noodles
- ☐ Other: ____________
- ☐ Other: ____________
- ☐ Other: ____________

Calories: ____________

Don't let what you cannot do interfere WITH WHAT YOU CAN DO

- John Wooden

VLCD 10 (Date): ______

WEIGHT: ______

HCG DOSAGE: ______

HUNGER LEVEL: ______

BEDTIME/WAKE TIME: ______

HOURS SLEEP: ______

TOTAL CALORIES: ______

SUPPLEMENTS: ______

☐ Multivitamin ☐ B12 Shot ☐ Lipo Shot

INJECTION LOCATION

TIME: ______

☐ Belly ☐ Deltoid ☐ Thigh ☐ Other: ______

DROPS / PELLETS DOSE TIMING

1st Dose: ______ 2nd Dose: ______

3rd Dose: ______ 4th Dose: ______

LIQUIDS:

4 LITERS
3.5 LITERS
3 LITERS
2.5 LITERS
2 LITERS
1.5 LITERS
1 LITER
.5 LITERS

128 oz = 1 GALLON
120 oz
112 oz
104 oz
96 oz = 3 QUARTS
88 oz
80 oz
72 oz
64 oz = 2 QUARTS
56 oz
48 oz
40 oz
32 oz = 1 QUART
24 oz
16 oz
8 oz = 1 CUP

PERSONAL NOTES

BREAKFAST

Time:

☐ None ☐ Fruit: ______ ☐ Protein: ______ Calories: ______

Serving Size: ______ Serving Size: ______

LUNCH Time:

WAS AN ITEM EATEN AS A SNACK? WHICH? Time:

Protein:

- [ ] Chicken breast
- [ ] Beef
- [ ] Veal
- [ ] Shrimp
- [ ] Lobster
- [ ] White fish: ____________
- [ ] Protein Shake
- [ ] Other: ____________

Serving Size:

- [ ] 100 grams/3.5 oz
- [ ] Other: ____________

Calories: ____________

Vegetable:

- [ ] Asparagus
- [ ] Beet Greens
- [ ] Cabbage
- [ ] Celery
- [ ] Chard
- [ ] Cucumber
- [ ] Fennel
- [ ] Lettuce
- [ ] Onions
- [ ] Radishes
- [ ] Spinach
- [ ] Tomatoes
- [ ] Other: ____________
- [ ] Other: ____________
- [ ] Other: ____________

Calories: ____________

Fruit:

- [ ] Strawberries
- [ ] ½ Grapefruit
- [ ] Apple
- [ ] Orange
- [ ] Other: ____________

Starch:

- [ ] Grissini
- [ ] Melba
- [ ] Other: ____________

Calories: ____________

Other:

- [ ] TBS. Milk
- [ ] Juice of 1 Lemon
- [ ] Stevia
- [ ] Shirataki/Miracle Noodles
- [ ] Other: ____________
- [ ] Other: ____________
- [ ] Other: ____________

Calories: ____________

DINNER Time:

WAS AN ITEM EATEN AS A SNACK? WHICH? Time:

Protein:

- [ ] Chicken
- [ ] Beef
- [ ] Veal
- [ ] Shrimp
- [ ] Lobster
- [ ] White fish: ____________
- [ ] Protein Shake
- [ ] Other: ____________

Serving Size:

- [ ] 100 grams
- [ ] Other: ____________

Calories: ____________

Vegetable:

- [ ] Asparagus
- [ ] Beet Greens
- [ ] Cabbage
- [ ] Celery
- [ ] Chard
- [ ] Cucumber
- [ ] Fennel
- [ ] Lettuce
- [ ] Onions
- [ ] Radishes
- [ ] Spinach
- [ ] Tomatoes
- [ ] Other: ____________
- [ ] Other: ____________
- [ ] Other: ____________

Calories: ____________

Fruit:

- [ ] Strawberries
- [ ] ½ Grapefruit
- [ ] Apple
- [ ] Orange
- [ ] Other: ____________

Starch:

- [ ] Grissini
- [ ] Melba
- [ ] Other: ____________

Calories: ____________

Other:

- [ ] TBS. Milk
- [ ] Juice of 1 Lemon
- [ ] Stevia
- [ ] Shirataki/Miracle Noodles
- [ ] Other: ____________
- [ ] Other: ____________
- [ ] Other: ____________

Calories: ____________

VLCD 11 (Date): ______________

HCGCHICA TIP:

Accept Detox

Food addiction is real in my opinion. Understanding that your body may go through detox helps. This passes. On a hard day remember very soon it will feel easier.

WEIGHT: ______________

HCG DOSAGE: ______________

HUNGER LEVEL: ______________

BEDTIME/WAKE TIME: ______________

HOURS SLEEP: ______________

TOTAL CALORIES: ______________

SUPPLEMENTS: ______________

☐ Multivitamin ☐ B12 Shot ☐ Lipo Shot

INJECTION LOCATION

TIME: ________

☐ Belly ☐ Deltoid ☐ Thigh ☐ Other: ____________

DROPS / PELLETS DOSE TIMING

1st Dose: ____________ 2nd Dose: ____________

3rd Dose: ____________ 4th Dose: ____________

LIQUIDS:

4 LITERS
3.5 LITERS
3 LITERS
2.5 LITERS
2 LITERS
1.5 LITERS
1 LITER
.5 LITERS

128 oz = 1 GALLON
120 oz
112 oz
104 oz
96 oz = 3 QUARTS
88 oz
80 oz
72 oz
64 oz = 2 QUARTS
56 oz
48 oz
40 oz
32 oz = 1 QUART
24 oz
16 oz
8 oz = 1 CUP

PERSONAL NOTES

BREAKFAST

Time :

☐ None ☐ Fruit: ____________ ☐ Protein: ____________ Calories: ________

Serving Size: ____________ Serving Size: ____________

AN ITEM EATEN AS A SNACK? WHICH? Time:

Fruit:

- ☐ Strawberries
- ☐ ½ Grapefruit
- ☐ Apple
- ☐ Orange
- ☐ Other: ____________

Starch:

- ☐ Grissini
- ☐ Melba
- ☐ Other: ____________

Other:

- ☐ TBS. Milk
- ☐ Juice of 1 Lemon
- ☐ Stevia
- ☐ Shirataki/Miracle Noodles
- ☐ Other: ____________
- ☐ Other: ____________
- ☐ Other: ____________

- ☐ Other: ____________
- ☐ Other: ____________
- ☐ Other: ____________

Calories: ____________ Calories: ____________ Calories: ____________ Calories: ____________

DINNER Time:

WAS AN ITEM EATEN AS A SNACK? WHICH? Time:

Protein:

- ☐ Chicken
- ☐ Beef
- ☐ Veal
- ☐ Shrimp
- ☐ Lobster
- ☐ White fish: ____________
- ☐ Protein Shake
- ☐ Other: ____________

Serving Size:

- ☐ 100 grams
- ☐ Other: ____________

Vegetable:

- ☐ Asparagus
- ☐ Beet Greens
- ☐ Cabbage
- ☐ Celery
- ☐ Chard
- ☐ Cucumber
- ☐ Fennel
- ☐ Lettuce
- ☐ Onions
- ☐ Radishes
- ☐ Spinach
- ☐ Tomatoes
- ☐ Other: ____________
- ☐ Other: ____________
- ☐ Other: ____________

Fruit:

- ☐ Strawberries
- ☐ ½ Grapefruit
- ☐ Apple
- ☐ Orange
- ☐ Other: ____________

Starch:

- ☐ Grissini
- ☐ Melba
- ☐ Other: ____________

Other:

- ☐ TBS. Milk
- ☐ Juice of 1 Lemon
- ☐ Stevia
- ☐ Shirataki/Miracle Noodles
- ☐ Other: ____________
- ☐ Other: ____________
- ☐ Other: ____________

Calories: ____________ Calories: ____________ Calories: ____________ Calories: ____________

FELLOW HCGER TIP:

THE MAGIC OF Bib Lettuce

Butter/bib lettuce is great for making lettuce wraps filled with a P2 protein and thinly sliced P2 veggies.

VLCD 12 (Date): ____________

WEIGHT: ____________

HCG DOSAGE: ____________

HUNGER LEVEL: ____________

BEDTIME/WAKE TIME: ____________

HOURS SLEEP: ____________

TOTAL CALORIES: ____________

SUPPLEMENTS: ____________

☐ Multivitamin ☐ B12 Shot ☐ Lipo Shot

INJECTION LOCATION

TIME: ________

☐ Belly ☐ Deltoid ☐ Thigh ☐ Other: ____________

DROPS / PELLETS DOSE TIMING

1st Dose: ____________ 2nd Dose: ____________

3rd Dose: ____________ 4th Dose: ____________

LIQUIDS:

	Liters
☐	4 LITERS
☐	3.5 LITERS
☐	3 LITERS
☐	2.5 LITERS
☐	2 LITERS
☐	1.5 LITERS
☐	1 LITER
☐	.5 LITERS

	Ounces
☐	128 oz = 1 GALLON
☐	120 oz
☐	112 oz
☐	104 oz
☐	96 oz = 3 QUARTS
☐	88 oz
☐	80 oz
☐	72 oz
☐	64 oz = 2 QUARTS
☐	56 oz
☐	48 oz
☐	40 oz
☐	32 oz = 1 QUART
☐	24 oz
☐	16 oz
☐	8 oz = 1 CUP

PERSONAL NOTES

BREAKFAST

Time:

☐ None ☐ Fruit: ____________ ☐ Protein: ____________ Calories: ____________

Serving Size: ____________ Serving Size: ____________

LUNCH Time :

WAS AN ITEM EATEN AS A SNACK? WHICH?

Time:

Protein:

- [ ] Chicken breast
- [ ] Beef
- [ ] Veal
- [ ] Shrimp
- [ ] Lobster
- [ ] White fish: ___________
- [ ] Protein Shake
- [ ] Other: ___________

Serving Size:

- [ ] 100 grams/3.5 oz
- [ ] Other: ___________

Calories: ___________

Vegetable:

- [ ] Asparagus
- [ ] Beet Greens
- [ ] Cabbage
- [ ] Celery
- [ ] Chard
- [ ] Cucumber
- [ ] Fennel
- [ ] Lettuce
- [ ] Onions
- [ ] Radishes
- [ ] Spinach
- [ ] Tomatoes
- [ ] Other: ___________
- [ ] Other: ___________
- [ ] Other: ___________

Calories: ___________

Fruit:

- [ ] Strawberries
- [ ] ½ Grapefruit
- [ ] Apple
- [ ] Orange
- [ ] Other: ___________

Starch:

- [ ] Grissini
- [ ] Melba
- [ ] Other: ___________

Calories: ___________

Other:

- [ ] TBS. Milk
- [ ] Juice of 1 Lemon
- [ ] Stevia
- [ ] Shirataki/Miracle Noodles
- [ ] Other: ___________
- [ ] Other: ___________
- [ ] Other: ___________

Calories: ___________

DINNER Time :

WAS AN ITEM EATEN AS A SNACK? WHICH?

Time:

Protein:

- [ ] Chicken
- [ ] Beef
- [ ] Veal
- [ ] Shrimp
- [ ] Lobster
- [ ] White fish: ___________
- [ ] Protein Shake
- [ ] Other: ___________

Serving Size:

- [ ] 100 grams
- [ ] Other: ___________

Calories: ___________

Vegetable:

- [ ] Asparagus
- [ ] Beet Greens
- [ ] Cabbage
- [ ] Celery
- [ ] Chard
- [ ] Cucumber
- [ ] Fennel
- [ ] Lettuce
- [ ] Onions
- [ ] Radishes
- [ ] Spinach
- [ ] Tomatoes
- [ ] Other: ___________
- [ ] Other: ___________
- [ ] Other: ___________

Calories: ___________

Fruit:

- [ ] Strawberries
- [ ] ½ Grapefruit
- [ ] Apple
- [ ] Orange
- [ ] Other: ___________

Starch:

- [ ] Grissini
- [ ] Melba
- [ ] Other: ___________

Calories: ___________

Other:

- [ ] TBS. Milk
- [ ] Juice of 1 Lemon
- [ ] Stevia
- [ ] Shirataki/Miracle Noodles
- [ ] Other: ___________
- [ ] Other: ___________
- [ ] Other: ___________

Calories: ___________

When OBSTACLES ARISE, you change your direction to reach your *goal*; you DO NOT CHANGE YOUR DECISION to get there.

- Zig Ziglar

VLCD 13 (Date): ______________

WEIGHT: ______________

HCG DOSAGE: ______________

HUNGER LEVEL: ______________

BEDTIME/WAKE TIME: ______________

HOURS SLEEP: ______________

TOTAL CALORIES: ______________

SUPPLEMENTS: ______________

☐ Multivitamin ☐ B12 Shot ☐ Lipo Shot

INJECTION LOCATION

TIME: ________

☐ Belly ☐ Deltoid ☐ Thigh ☐ Other: ____________

DROPS / PELLETS DOSE TIMING

1st Dose: ____________ 2nd Dose: ____________

3rd Dose: ____________ 4th Dose: ____________

LIQUIDS:

☐	4 LITERS
☐	3.5 LITERS
☐	3 LITERS
☐	2.5 LITERS
☐	2 LITERS
☐	1.5 LITERS
☐	1 LITER
☐	.5 LITERS

☐	128 oz = 1 GALLON
☐	120 oz
☐	112 oz
☐	104 oz
☐	96 oz = 3 QUARTS
☐	88 oz
☐	80 oz
☐	72 oz
☐	64 oz = 2 QUARTS
☐	56 oz
☐	48 oz
☐	40 oz
☐	32 oz = 1 QUART
☐	24 oz
☐	16 oz
☐	8 oz = 1 CUP

PERSONAL NOTES

BREAKFAST

Time:

☐ None ☐ Fruit: ____________ ☐ Protein: ____________ Calories: ____________

Serving Size: ____________ Serving Size: ____________

LUNCH Time:

WAS AN ITEM EATEN AS A SNACK? WHICH? Time:

Protein:

- [ ] Chicken breast
- [ ] Beef
- [ ] Veal
- [ ] Shrimp
- [ ] Lobster
- [ ] White fish: ___________
- [ ] Protein Shake
- [ ] Other: ___________

Serving Size:

- [ ] 100 grams/3.5 oz
- [ ] Other: ___________

Calories: ___________

Vegetable:

- [ ] Asparagus
- [ ] Beet Greens
- [ ] Cabbage
- [ ] Celery
- [ ] Chard
- [ ] Cucumber
- [ ] Fennel
- [ ] Lettuce
- [ ] Onions
- [ ] Radishes
- [ ] Spinach
- [ ] Tomatoes
- [ ] Other: ___________
- [ ] Other: ___________
- [ ] Other: ___________

Calories: ___________

Fruit:

- [ ] Strawberries
- [ ] ½ Grapefruit
- [ ] Apple
- [ ] Orange
- [ ] Other: ___________

Starch:

- [ ] Grissini
- [ ] Melba
- [ ] Other: ___________

Calories: ___________

Other:

- [ ] TBS. Milk
- [ ] Juice of 1 Lemon
- [ ] Stevia
- [ ] Shirataki/Miracle Noodles
- [ ] Other: ___________
- [ ] Other: ___________
- [ ] Other: ___________

Calories: ___________

DINNER Time:

WAS AN ITEM EATEN AS A SNACK? WHICH? Time:

Protein:

- [ ] Chicken
- [ ] Beef
- [ ] Veal
- [ ] Shrimp
- [ ] Lobster
- [ ] White fish: ___________
- [ ] Protein Shake
- [ ] Other: ___________

Serving Size:

- [ ] 100 grams
- [ ] Other: ___________

Calories: ___________

Vegetable:

- [ ] Asparagus
- [ ] Beet Greens
- [ ] Cabbage
- [ ] Celery
- [ ] Chard
- [ ] Cucumber
- [ ] Fennel
- [ ] Lettuce
- [ ] Onions
- [ ] Radishes
- [ ] Spinach
- [ ] Tomatoes
- [ ] Other: ___________
- [ ] Other: ___________
- [ ] Other: ___________

Calories: ___________

Fruit:

- [ ] Strawberries
- [ ] ½ Grapefruit
- [ ] Apple
- [ ] Orange
- [ ] Other: ___________

Starch:

- [ ] Grissini
- [ ] Melba
- [ ] Other: ___________

Calories: ___________

Other:

- [ ] TBS. Milk
- [ ] Juice of 1 Lemon
- [ ] Stevia
- [ ] Shirataki/Miracle Noodles
- [ ] Other: ___________
- [ ] Other: ___________
- [ ] Other: ___________

Calories: ___________

FELLOW HCGER TIP:

hCG Coffee Dessert

100 grams fat free cottage cheese mixed with a dollop of fat free greek yogurt, stevia, and 1-2 tsp. instant coffee.

Note: If you do this, the cottage cheese would replace 1 meat protein serving.

VLCD 14 (Date): ______________

WEIGHT: ______________

HCG DOSAGE: ______________

HUNGER LEVEL: ______________

BEDTIME/WAKE TIME: ______________

HOURS SLEEP: ______________

TOTAL CALORIES: ______________

SUPPLEMENTS: ______________

☐ Multivitamin ☐ B12 Shot ☐ Lipo Shot

INJECTION LOCATION

TIME: ________

☐ Belly ☐ Deltoid ☐ Thigh ☐ Other: ____________

DROPS / PELLETS DOSE TIMING

1st Dose: ____________ 2nd Dose: ____________

3rd Dose: ____________ 4th Dose: ____________

LIQUIDS:

	4 LITERS
	3.5 LITERS
	3 LITERS
	2.5 LITERS
	2 LITERS
	1.5 LITERS
	1 LITER
	.5 LITERS

	128 oz = 1 GALLON
	120 oz
	112 oz
	104 oz
	96 oz = 3 QUARTS
	88 oz
	80 oz
	72 oz
	64 oz = 2 QUARTS
	56 oz
	48 oz
	40 oz
	32 oz = 1 QUART
	24 oz
	16 oz
	8 oz = 1 CUP

PERSONAL NOTES

BREAKFAST

Time:

☐ None ☐ Fruit: ____________ ☐ Protein: ____________ Calories: ____________

Serving Size: ____________ Serving Size: ____________

LUNCH Time:

WAS AN ITEM EATEN AS A SNACK? WHICH?

Time:

Protein:

- ☐ Chicken breast
- ☐ Beef
- ☐ Veal
- ☐ Shrimp
- ☐ Lobster
- ☐ White fish: ___________
- ☐ Protein Shake
- ☐ Other: ___________

Serving Size:

- ☐ 100 grams/3.5 oz
- ☐ Other: ___________

Calories: ___________

Vegetable:

- ☐ Asparagus
- ☐ Beet Greens
- ☐ Cabbage
- ☐ Celery
- ☐ Chard
- ☐ Cucumber
- ☐ Fennel
- ☐ Lettuce
- ☐ Onions
- ☐ Radishes
- ☐ Spinach
- ☐ Tomatoes
- ☐ Other: ___________
- ☐ Other: ___________
- ☐ Other: ___________

Calories: ___________

Fruit:

- ☐ Strawberries
- ☐ ½ Grapefruit
- ☐ Apple
- ☐ Orange
- ☐ Other: ___________

Starch:

- ☐ Grissini
- ☐ Melba
- ☐ Other: ___________

Calories: ___________

Other:

- ☐ TBS. Milk
- ☐ Juice of 1 Lemon
- ☐ Stevia
- ☐ Shirataki/Miracle Noodles
- ☐ Other: ___________
- ☐ Other: ___________
- ☐ Other: ___________

Calories: ___________

DINNER Time:

WAS AN ITEM EATEN AS A SNACK? WHICH?

Time:

Protein:

- ☐ Chicken
- ☐ Beef
- ☐ Veal
- ☐ Shrimp
- ☐ Lobster
- ☐ White fish: ___________
- ☐ Protein Shake
- ☐ Other: ___________

Serving Size:

- ☐ 100 grams
- ☐ Other: ___________

Calories: ___________

Vegetable:

- ☐ Asparagus
- ☐ Beet Greens
- ☐ Cabbage
- ☐ Celery
- ☐ Chard
- ☐ Cucumber
- ☐ Fennel
- ☐ Lettuce
- ☐ Onions
- ☐ Radishes
- ☐ Spinach
- ☐ Tomatoes
- ☐ Other: ___________
- ☐ Other: ___________
- ☐ Other: ___________

Calories: ___________

Fruit:

- ☐ Strawberries
- ☐ ½ Grapefruit
- ☐ Apple
- ☐ Orange
- ☐ Other: ___________

Starch:

- ☐ Grissini
- ☐ Melba
- ☐ Other: ___________

Calories: ___________

Other:

- ☐ TBS. Milk
- ☐ Juice of 1 Lemon
- ☐ Stevia
- ☐ Shirataki/Miracle Noodles
- ☐ Other: ___________
- ☐ Other: ___________
- ☐ Other: ___________

Calories: ___________

Reflections ON WEEK 2

REMEMBER, THIS IS NOT JUST ABOUT LOSING WEIGHT. IT'S ABOUT CHANGING YOUR WHOLE MINDSET ABOUT FOOD AND YOUR BODY.

YOU ARE BREAKING OLD PATTERNS RIGHT NOW. YOU ARE CREATING NEW PATTERNS. TRY NOT TO FOCUS YOUR PROGESS SOLELY ON WEIGHT LOSS.

SO WITH THAT IN MIND, HOW DID THIS WEEK GO?

What are you proud of? Why are you proud of it? What did you struggle with? What would you like to work on changing? What specific logical ways can you think of to make those adjustments? Or maybe you're just burned out at the moment - it's okay to just make it a rant.

Prepping for **PHASE 3 – ALREADY?**

PHASE 3 NONCHALANCE = GAIN BACK WEIGHT.

I can honestly tell you that out of the many of emails I've received dealing specifically with **gaining back weight** that was lost with the hCG protocol, the number one cause that is shared with me for this happening is **not paying attention to Phase 3.**

Conversely, a do-over with subsequent strict attention to Phase 3 yielded much better, lasting results.

Your weight ***will*** be volatile at the start of Phase 3 and will go up easily if you don't have the knowledge and tools to know what to do or think it's not important.

This is not meant to scare you, but to iterate the importance of arming yourself with as much information for Phase 3 as you can, in advance, so you can have a plan when it arrives.

It might be easy to kind of freak out over Phase 3 a little, but as we've heard the saying go:

Worrying IS LIKE ROCKING IN A CHAIR. IT KEEPS YOU BUSY, BUT DOESN'T GET YOU ANYWHERE.

So let's **NOT** do that shall we?

INSTEAD, GET INFORMED and PLAN AHEAD. HOW?

I have 2 resources that can get you ready and prepared to face Phase 3 confidently. One is totally free and ready for you now, and the other costs less than a new top but as of this writing is not yet published.

The P3 & P4 resources page on my site is pretty detailed and will help you both plan and troubleshoot.

The P3 & P4 hCG Workbook, similar to this one (once I finish writing it!), will allow you to track these phases easily as well as contains more specific and detailed guidance for Phase 3 that is not on my blog.

You don't need to be afraid if you prepare and have the right tools.

FREE COMPREHENSIVE RESOURCE:

Simply: hcgchica.com/p3
hcgchica.com/p4

LESS THAN A NEW SHIRT RESOURCE:

My Phase 3 & Phase 4 hCG Workbook
(not yet published - stay tuned at link below for updates!)
find at: hcgchica.com/p3workbook
or
use this QR code:

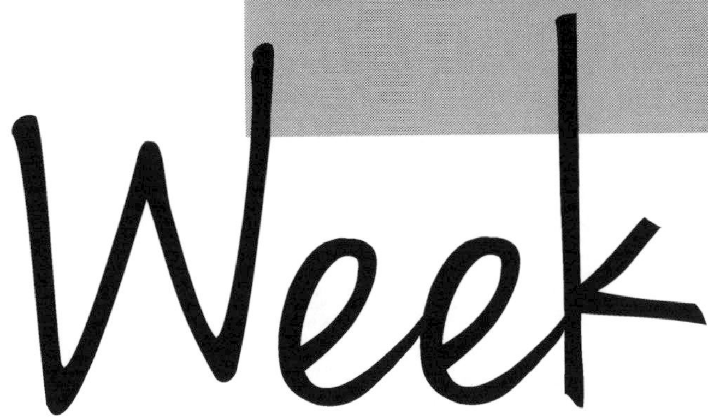

Week 3

"KNOWING TREES,
I understand the meaning of patience. Knowing grass, I understand the meaning of persistence."

- Hal Borland

Today is a new day. Hiding from your history only shackles you to it. WE CAN'T UNDO a single thing we have ever done, but WE CAN MAKE DECISIONS TODAY that propel us to the life we want and towards THE HEALING WE NEED.

- Steve Maraboli

VLCD 15 (Date): ______

WEIGHT: ______

HCG DOSAGE: ______

HUNGER LEVEL: ______

BEDTIME/WAKE TIME: ______

HOURS SLEEP: ______

TOTAL CALORIES: ______

SUPPLEMENTS: ______

☐ Multivitamin ☐ B12 Shot ☐ Lipo Shot

INJECTION LOCATION

TIME: ______

☐ Belly ☐ Deltoid ☐ Thigh ☐ Other: ______

DROPS / PELLETS DOSE TIMING

1st Dose: ______ 2nd Dose: ______

3rd Dose: ______ 4th Dose: ______

LIQUIDS:

Liters
4 LITERS
3.5 LITERS
3 LITERS
2.5 LITERS
2 LITERS
1.5 LITERS
1 LITER
.5 LITERS

Ounces
128 oz = 1 GALLON
120 oz
112 oz
104 oz
96 oz = 3 QUARTS
88 oz
80 oz
72 oz
64 oz = 2 QUARTS
56 oz
48 oz
40 oz
32 oz = 1 QUART
24 oz
16 oz
8 oz = 1 CUP

PERSONAL NOTES

BREAKFAST

Time :

☐ None ☐ Fruit: ______ ☐ Protein: ______ Calories: ______

Serving Size: ______ Serving Size: ______

LUNCH Time:

WAS AN ITEM EATEN AS A SNACK? WHICH? Time:

Protein:

- [ ] Chicken breast
- [ ] Beef
- [ ] Veal
- [ ] Shrimp
- [ ] Lobster
- [ ] White fish: ___________
- [ ] Protein Shake
- [ ] Other: ___________

Serving Size:

- [ ] 100 grams/3.5 oz
- [ ] Other: ___________

Calories: ___________

Vegetable:

- [ ] Asparagus
- [ ] Beet Greens
- [ ] Cabbage
- [ ] Celery
- [ ] Chard
- [ ] Cucumber
- [ ] Fennel
- [ ] Lettuce
- [ ] Onions
- [ ] Radishes
- [ ] Spinach
- [ ] Tomatoes
- [ ] Other: ___________
- [ ] Other: ___________
- [ ] Other: ___________

Calories: ___________

Fruit:

- [ ] Strawberries
- [ ] ½ Grapefruit
- [ ] Apple
- [ ] Orange
- [ ] Other: ___________

Starch:

- [ ] Grissini
- [ ] Melba
- [ ] Other: ___________

Calories: ___________

Other:

- [ ] TBS. Milk
- [ ] Juice of 1 Lemon
- [ ] Stevia
- [ ] Shirataki/Miracle Noodles
- [ ] Other: ___________
- [ ] Other: ___________
- [ ] Other: ___________

Calories: ___________

DINNER Time:

WAS AN ITEM EATEN AS A SNACK? WHICH? Time:

Protein:

- [ ] Chicken
- [ ] Beef
- [ ] Veal
- [ ] Shrimp
- [ ] Lobster
- [ ] White fish: ___________
- [ ] Protein Shake
- [ ] Other: ___________

Serving Size:

- [ ] 100 grams
- [ ] Other: ___________

Calories: ___________

Vegetable:

- [ ] Asparagus
- [ ] Beet Greens
- [ ] Cabbage
- [ ] Celery
- [ ] Chard
- [ ] Cucumber
- [ ] Fennel
- [ ] Lettuce
- [ ] Onions
- [ ] Radishes
- [ ] Spinach
- [ ] Tomatoes
- [ ] Other: ___________
- [ ] Other: ___________
- [ ] Other: ___________

Calories: ___________

Fruit:

- [ ] Strawberries
- [ ] ½ Grapefruit
- [ ] Apple
- [ ] Orange
- [ ] Other: ___________

Starch:

- [ ] Grissini
- [ ] Melba
- [ ] Other: ___________

Calories: ___________

Other:

- [ ] TBS. Milk
- [ ] Juice of 1 Lemon
- [ ] Stevia
- [ ] Shirataki/Miracle Noodles
- [ ] Other: ___________
- [ ] Other: ___________
- [ ] Other: ___________

Calories: ___________

HCGCHICA TIP:

You're Never Too Mature

Women in the 55-75 age bracket often email me, wondering if they are too, let's call it, mature, for this protocol to work for them. Let me just say this. The majority of my hCG success interviews are with women in this age bracket. Maturity has its benefits!

VLCD 16 (Date): ____________

WEIGHT: ____________

HCG DOSAGE: ____________

HUNGER LEVEL: ____________

BEDTIME/WAKE TIME: ____________

HOURS SLEEP: ____________

TOTAL CALORIES: ____________

SUPPLEMENTS: ____________

☐ Multivitamin ☐ B12 Shot ☐ Lipo Shot

INJECTION LOCATION

TIME: ________

☐ Belly ☐ Deltoid ☐ Thigh ☐ Other: ____________

DROPS / PELLETS DOSE TIMING

1st Dose: ____________ 2nd Dose: ____________

3rd Dose: ____________ 4th Dose: ____________

LIQUIDS:

4 LITERS
3.5 LITERS
3 LITERS
2.5 LITERS
2 LITERS
1.5 LITERS
1 LITER
.5 LITERS

128 oz = 1 GALLON
120 oz
112 oz
104 oz
96 oz = 3 QUARTS
88 oz
80 oz
72 oz
64 oz = 2 QUARTS
56 oz
48 oz
40 oz
32 oz = 1 QUART
24 oz
16 oz
8 oz = 1 CUP

PERSONAL NOTES

BREAKFAST

Time :

☐ None ☐ Fruit: ____________ ☐ Protein: ____________ Calories: ____________

Serving Size: ____________ Serving Size: ____________

LUNCH Time :

WAS AN ITEM EATEN AS A SNACK? WHICH? Time:

Protein:

- ☐ Chicken breast
- ☐ Beef
- ☐ Veal
- ☐ Shrimp
- ☐ Lobster
- ☐ White fish: ____________
- ☐ Protein Shake
- ☐ Other: ____________

Serving Size:

- ☐ 100 grams/3.5 oz
- ☐ Other: ____________

Calories: ____________

Vegetable:

- ☐ Asparagus
- ☐ Beet Greens
- ☐ Cabbage
- ☐ Celery
- ☐ Chard
- ☐ Cucumber
- ☐ Fennel
- ☐ Lettuce
- ☐ Onions
- ☐ Radishes
- ☐ Spinach
- ☐ Tomatoes
- ☐ Other: ____________
- ☐ Other: ____________
- ☐ Other: ____________

Calories: ____________

Fruit:

- ☐ Strawberries
- ☐ ½ Grapefruit
- ☐ Apple
- ☐ Orange
- ☐ Other: ____________

Starch:

- ☐ Grissini
- ☐ Melba
- ☐ Other: ____________

Calories: ____________

Other:

- ☐ TBS. Milk
- ☐ Juice of 1 Lemon
- ☐ Stevia
- ☐ Shirataki/Miracle Noodles
- ☐ Other: ____________
- ☐ Other: ____________
- ☐ Other: ____________

Calories: ____________

DINNER Time :

WAS AN ITEM EATEN AS A SNACK? WHICH? Time:

Protein:

- ☐ Chicken
- ☐ Beef
- ☐ Veal
- ☐ Shrimp
- ☐ Lobster
- ☐ White fish: ____________
- ☐ Protein Shake
- ☐ Other: ____________

Serving Size:

- ☐ 100 grams
- ☐ Other: ____________

Calories: ____________

Vegetable:

- ☐ Asparagus
- ☐ Beet Greens
- ☐ Cabbage
- ☐ Celery
- ☐ Chard
- ☐ Cucumber
- ☐ Fennel
- ☐ Lettuce
- ☐ Onions
- ☐ Radishes
- ☐ Spinach
- ☐ Tomatoes
- ☐ Other: ____________
- ☐ Other: ____________
- ☐ Other: ____________

Calories: ____________

Fruit:

- ☐ Strawberries
- ☐ ½ Grapefruit
- ☐ Apple
- ☐ Orange
- ☐ Other: ____________

Starch:

- ☐ Grissini
- ☐ Melba
- ☐ Other: ____________

Calories: ____________

Other:

- ☐ TBS. Milk
- ☐ Juice of 1 Lemon
- ☐ Stevia
- ☐ Shirataki/Miracle Noodles
- ☐ Other: ____________
- ☐ Other: ____________
- ☐ Other: ____________

Calories: ____________

FELLOW HCGER TIP:

Make it Fire Roasted

When it comes to canned tomatoes, the "fire roasted" kind have SO much more flavor than the regular kind.

Note: Be sure to check the ingredient label as some brands of canned tomatoes have added sugar.

VLCD 17 (Date): ____________

WEIGHT: ____________

HCG DOSAGE: ____________

HUNGER LEVEL: ____________

BEDTIME/WAKE TIME: ____________

HOURS SLEEP: ____________

TOTAL CALORIES: ____________

SUPPLEMENTS: ____________

☐ Multivitamin ☐ B12 Shot ☐ Lipo Shot

INJECTION LOCATION

TIME: ________

☐ Belly ☐ Deltoid ☐ Thigh ☐ Other: ____________

DROPS / PELLETS DOSE TIMING

1st Dose: ____________ 2nd Dose: ____________

3rd Dose: ____________ 4th Dose: ____________

LIQUIDS:

4 LITERS
3.5 LITERS
3 LITERS
2.5 LITERS
2 LITERS
1.5 LITERS
1 LITER
.5 LITERS

128 oz = 1 GALLON
120 oz
112 oz
104 oz
96 oz = 3 QUARTS
88 oz
80 oz
72 oz
64 oz = 2 QUARTS
56 oz
48 oz
40 oz
32 oz = 1 QUART
24 oz
16 oz
8 oz = 1 CUP

PERSONAL NOTES

BREAKFAST

Time:

☐ None ☐ Fruit: ____________ ☐ Protein: ____________ Calories: ____________

Serving Size: ____________ Serving Size: ____________

LUNCH Time:

WAS AN ITEM EATEN AS A SNACK? WHICH? Time:

Protein:

- [ ] Chicken breast
- [ ] Beef
- [ ] Veal
- [ ] Shrimp
- [ ] Lobster
- [ ] White fish: ____________
- [ ] Protein Shake
- [ ] Other: ____________

Serving Size:

- [ ] 100 grams/3.5 oz
- [ ] Other: ____________

Calories: ____________

Vegetable:

- [ ] Asparagus
- [ ] Beet Greens
- [ ] Cabbage
- [ ] Celery
- [ ] Chard
- [ ] Cucumber
- [ ] Fennel
- [ ] Lettuce
- [ ] Onions
- [ ] Radishes
- [ ] Spinach
- [ ] Tomatoes
- [ ] Other: ____________
- [ ] Other: ____________
- [ ] Other: ____________

Calories: ____________

Fruit:

- [ ] Strawberries
- [ ] ½ Grapefruit
- [ ] Apple
- [ ] Orange
- [ ] Other: ____________

Starch:

- [ ] Grissini
- [ ] Melba
- [ ] Other: ____________

Calories: ____________

Other:

- [ ] TBS. Milk
- [ ] Juice of 1 Lemon
- [ ] Stevia
- [ ] Shirataki/Miracle Noodles
- [ ] Other: ____________
- [ ] Other: ____________
- [ ] Other: ____________

Calories: ____________

DINNER Time:

WAS AN ITEM EATEN AS A SNACK? WHICH? Time:

Protein:

- [ ] Chicken
- [ ] Beef
- [ ] Veal
- [ ] Shrimp
- [ ] Lobster
- [ ] White fish: ____________
- [ ] Protein Shake
- [ ] Other: ____________

Serving Size:

- [ ] 100 grams
- [ ] Other: ____________

Calories: ____________

Vegetable:

- [ ] Asparagus
- [ ] Beet Greens
- [ ] Cabbage
- [ ] Celery
- [ ] Chard
- [ ] Cucumber
- [ ] Fennel
- [ ] Lettuce
- [ ] Onions
- [ ] Radishes
- [ ] Spinach
- [ ] Tomatoes
- [ ] Other: ____________
- [ ] Other: ____________
- [ ] Other: ____________

Calories: ____________

Fruit:

- [ ] Strawberries
- [ ] ½ Grapefruit
- [ ] Apple
- [ ] Orange
- [ ] Other: ____________

Starch:

- [ ] Grissini
- [ ] Melba
- [ ] Other: ____________

Calories: ____________

Other:

- [ ] TBS. Milk
- [ ] Juice of 1 Lemon
- [ ] Stevia
- [ ] Shirataki/Miracle Noodles
- [ ] Other: ____________
- [ ] Other: ____________
- [ ] Other: ____________

Calories: ____________

When we complain we are saying we do not have the POWER TO MAKE A DIFFERENCE in the situation and we make ourselves small... we become part of the problem instead of the solution! TAKE ACTION to make the situation better & live bigger!
- Jefroy Hanson

VLCD 18 (Date): ____________

WEIGHT: ____________

HCG DOSAGE: ____________

HUNGER LEVEL: ____________

BEDTIME/WAKE TIME: ____________

HOURS SLEEP: ____________

TOTAL CALORIES: ____________

SUPPLEMENTS: ______________________

☐ Multivitamin ☐ B12 Shot ☐ Lipo Shot

INJECTION LOCATION TIME: ________

☐ Belly ☐ Deltoid ☐ Thigh ☐ Other: ____________

DROPS / PELLETS DOSE TIMING

1st Dose: ____________ 2nd Dose: ____________

3rd Dose: ____________ 4th Dose: ____________

LIQUIDS:

4 LITERS
3.5 LITERS
3 LITERS
2.5 LITERS
2 LITERS
1.5 LITERS
1 LITER
.5 LITERS

128 oz = 1 GALLON
120 oz
112 oz
104 oz
96 oz = 3 QUARTS
88 oz
80 oz
72 oz
64 oz = 2 QUARTS
56 oz
48 oz
40 oz
32 oz = 1 QUART
24 oz
16 oz
8 oz = 1 CUP

PERSONAL NOTES

BREAKFAST

Time:

☐ None ☐ Fruit: ____________ ☐ Protein: ____________ Calories: ____________

Serving Size: ____________ Serving Size: ____________

LUNCH Time :

WAS AN ITEM EATEN AS A SNACK? WHICH? Time:

Protein:

- ☐ Chicken breast
- ☐ Beef
- ☐ Veal
- ☐ Shrimp
- ☐ Lobster
- ☐ White fish: ___________
- ☐ Protein Shake
- ☐ Other: ___________

Serving Size:

- ☐ 100 grams/3.5 oz
- ☐ Other: ___________

Calories: ___________

Vegetable:

- ☐ Asparagus
- ☐ Beet Greens
- ☐ Cabbage
- ☐ Celery
- ☐ Chard
- ☐ Cucumber
- ☐ Fennel
- ☐ Lettuce
- ☐ Onions
- ☐ Radishes
- ☐ Spinach
- ☐ Tomatoes
- ☐ Other: ___________
- ☐ Other: ___________
- ☐ Other: ___________

Calories: ___________

Fruit:

- ☐ Strawberries
- ☐ ½ Grapefruit
- ☐ Apple
- ☐ Orange
- ☐ Other: ___________

Starch:

- ☐ Grissini
- ☐ Melba
- ☐ Other: ___________

Calories: ___________

Other:

- ☐ TBS. Milk
- ☐ Juice of 1 Lemon
- ☐ Stevia
- ☐ Shirataki/Miracle Noodles
- ☐ Other: ___________
- ☐ Other: ___________
- ☐ Other: ___________

Calories: ___________

DINNER Time :

WAS AN ITEM EATEN AS A SNACK? WHICH? Time:

Protein:

- ☐ Chicken
- ☐ Beef
- ☐ Veal
- ☐ Shrimp
- ☐ Lobster
- ☐ White fish: ___________
- ☐ Protein Shake
- ☐ Other: ___________

Serving Size:

- ☐ 100 grams
- ☐ Other: ___________

Calories: ___________

Vegetable:

- ☐ Asparagus
- ☐ Beet Greens
- ☐ Cabbage
- ☐ Celery
- ☐ Chard
- ☐ Cucumber
- ☐ Fennel
- ☐ Lettuce
- ☐ Onions
- ☐ Radishes
- ☐ Spinach
- ☐ Tomatoes
- ☐ Other: ___________
- ☐ Other: ___________
- ☐ Other: ___________

Calories: ___________

Fruit:

- ☐ Strawberries
- ☐ ½ Grapefruit
- ☐ Apple
- ☐ Orange
- ☐ Other: ___________

Starch:

- ☐ Grissini
- ☐ Melba
- ☐ Other: ___________

Calories: ___________

Other:

- ☐ TBS. Milk
- ☐ Juice of 1 Lemon
- ☐ Stevia
- ☐ Shirataki/Miracle Noodles
- ☐ Other: ___________
- ☐ Other: ___________
- ☐ Other: ___________

Calories: ___________

FELLOW HCGER TIP:

When You Need Quick

Keep a container in the fridge with chopped hCG veggies so you can quickly prepare a meal when in a hurry.

VLCD 19 (Date): ____________

WEIGHT: ____________

HCG DOSAGE: ____________

HUNGER LEVEL: ____________

BEDTIME/WAKE TIME: ____________

HOURS SLEEP: ____________

TOTAL CALORIES: ____________

SUPPLEMENTS: ____________

☐ Multivitamin ☐ B12 Shot ☐ Lipo Shot

INJECTION LOCATION

TIME: ________

☐ Belly ☐ Deltoid ☐ Thigh ☐ Other: ____________

DROPS / PELLETS DOSE TIMING

1st Dose: ____________ 2nd Dose: ____________

3rd Dose: ____________ 4th Dose: ____________

LIQUIDS:

	4 LITERS
	3.5 LITERS
	3 LITERS
	2.5 LITERS
	2 LITERS
	1.5 LITERS
	1 LITER
	.5 LITERS

	128 oz = 1 GALLON
	120 oz
	112 oz
	104 oz
	96 oz = 3 QUARTS
	88 oz
	80 oz
	72 oz
	64 oz = 2 QUARTS
	56 oz
	48 oz
	40 oz
	32 oz = 1 QUART
	24 oz
	16 oz
	8 oz = 1 CUP

PERSONAL NOTES

BREAKFAST

Time:

☐ None ☐ Fruit: ____________ ☐ Protein: ____________ Calories: ____________

Serving Size: ____________ Serving Size: ____________

LUNCH Time:

WAS AN ITEM EATEN AS A SNACK? WHICH? Time:

Protein:

- [ ] Chicken breast
- [ ] Beef
- [ ] Veal
- [ ] Shrimp
- [ ] Lobster
- [ ] White fish: ____________
- [ ] Protein Shake
- [ ] Other: ____________

Serving Size:

- [ ] 100 grams/3.5 oz
- [ ] Other: ____________

Calories: ____________

Vegetable:

- [ ] Asparagus
- [ ] Beet Greens
- [ ] Cabbage
- [ ] Celery
- [ ] Chard
- [ ] Cucumber
- [ ] Fennel
- [ ] Lettuce
- [ ] Onions
- [ ] Radishes
- [ ] Spinach
- [ ] Tomatoes
- [ ] Other: ____________
- [ ] Other: ____________
- [ ] Other: ____________

Calories: ____________

Fruit:

- [ ] Strawberries
- [ ] ½ Grapefruit
- [ ] Apple
- [ ] Orange
- [ ] Other: ____________

Starch:

- [ ] Grissini
- [ ] Melba
- [ ] Other: ____________

Calories: ____________

Other:

- [ ] TBS. Milk
- [ ] Juice of 1 Lemon
- [ ] Stevia
- [ ] Shirataki/Miracle Noodles
- [ ] Other: ____________
- [ ] Other: ____________
- [ ] Other: ____________

Calories: ____________

DINNER Time:

WAS AN ITEM EATEN AS A SNACK? WHICH? Time:

Protein:

- [ ] Chicken
- [ ] Beef
- [ ] Veal
- [ ] Shrimp
- [ ] Lobster
- [ ] White fish: ____________
- [ ] Protein Shake
- [ ] Other: ____________

Serving Size:

- [ ] 100 grams
- [ ] Other: ____________

Calories: ____________

Vegetable:

- [ ] Asparagus
- [ ] Beet Greens
- [ ] Cabbage
- [ ] Celery
- [ ] Chard
- [ ] Cucumber
- [ ] Fennel
- [ ] Lettuce
- [ ] Onions
- [ ] Radishes
- [ ] Spinach
- [ ] Tomatoes
- [ ] Other: ____________
- [ ] Other: ____________
- [ ] Other: ____________

Calories: ____________

Fruit:

- [ ] Strawberries
- [ ] ½ Grapefruit
- [ ] Apple
- [ ] Orange
- [ ] Other: ____________

Starch:

- [ ] Grissini
- [ ] Melba
- [ ] Other: ____________

Calories: ____________

Other:

- [ ] TBS. Milk
- [ ] Juice of 1 Lemon
- [ ] Stevia
- [ ] Shirataki/Miracle Noodles
- [ ] Other: ____________
- [ ] Other: ____________
- [ ] Other: ____________

Calories: ____________

Courage doesn't always roar. Sometimes courage is THE QUIET VOICE at the end of the day saying, 'I will try again tomorrow.

- Mary Anne Radmacher

VLCD 20 (Date): ____________

WEIGHT: ____________

HCG DOSAGE: ____________

HUNGER LEVEL: ____________

BEDTIME/WAKE TIME: ____________

HOURS SLEEP: ____________

TOTAL CALORIES: ____________

SUPPLEMENTS: ____________

☐ Multivitamin ☐ B12 Shot ☐ Lipo Shot

INJECTION LOCATION

TIME: ________

☐ Belly ☐ Deltoid ☐ Thigh ☐ Other: ____________

DROPS / PELLETS DOSE TIMING

1st Dose: ____________ 2nd Dose: ____________

3rd Dose: ____________ 4th Dose: ____________

LIQUIDS:

4 LITERS
3.5 LITERS
3 LITERS
2.5 LITERS
2 LITERS
1.5 LITERS
1 LITER
.5 LITERS

128 oz = 1 GALLON
120 oz
112 oz
104 oz
96 oz = 3 QUARTS
88 oz
80 oz
72 oz
64 oz = 2 QUARTS
56 oz
48 oz
40 oz
32 oz = 1 QUART
24 oz
16 oz
8 oz = 1 CUP

PERSONAL NOTES

BREAKFAST

Time:

☐ None ☐ Fruit: ____________ ☐ Protein: ____________ Calories: ____________

Serving Size: ____________ Serving Size: ____________

LUNCH Time:

WAS AN ITEM EATEN AS A SNACK? WHICH? Time:

Protein:

- ☐ Chicken breast
- ☐ Beef
- ☐ Veal
- ☐ Shrimp
- ☐ Lobster
- ☐ White fish: ___________
- ☐ Protein Shake
- ☐ Other: ___________

Serving Size:

- ☐ 100 grams/3.5 oz
- ☐ Other: ___________

Calories: ___________

Vegetable:

- ☐ Asparagus
- ☐ Beet Greens
- ☐ Cabbage
- ☐ Celery
- ☐ Chard
- ☐ Cucumber
- ☐ Fennel
- ☐ Lettuce
- ☐ Onions
- ☐ Radishes
- ☐ Spinach
- ☐ Tomatoes
- ☐ Other: ___________
- ☐ Other: ___________
- ☐ Other: ___________

Calories: ___________

Fruit:

- ☐ Strawberries
- ☐ ½ Grapefruit
- ☐ Apple
- ☐ Orange
- ☐ Other: ___________

Starch:

- ☐ Grissini
- ☐ Melba
- ☐ Other: ___________

Calories: ___________

Other:

- ☐ TBS. Milk
- ☐ Juice of 1 Lemon
- ☐ Stevia
- ☐ Shirataki/Miracle Noodles
- ☐ Other: ___________
- ☐ Other: ___________
- ☐ Other: ___________

Calories: ___________

DINNER Time:

WAS AN ITEM EATEN AS A SNACK? WHICH? Time:

Protein:

- ☐ Chicken
- ☐ Beef
- ☐ Veal
- ☐ Shrimp
- ☐ Lobster
- ☐ White fish: ___________
- ☐ Protein Shake
- ☐ Other: ___________

Serving Size:

- ☐ 100 grams
- ☐ Other: ___________

Calories: ___________

Vegetable:

- ☐ Asparagus
- ☐ Beet Greens
- ☐ Cabbage
- ☐ Celery
- ☐ Chard
- ☐ Cucumber
- ☐ Fennel
- ☐ Lettuce
- ☐ Onions
- ☐ Radishes
- ☐ Spinach
- ☐ Tomatoes
- ☐ Other: ___________
- ☐ Other: ___________
- ☐ Other: ___________

Calories: ___________

Fruit:

- ☐ Strawberries
- ☐ ½ Grapefruit
- ☐ Apple
- ☐ Orange
- ☐ Other: ___________

Starch:

- ☐ Grissini
- ☐ Melba
- ☐ Other: ___________

Calories: ___________

Other:

- ☐ TBS. Milk
- ☐ Juice of 1 Lemon
- ☐ Stevia
- ☐ Shirataki/Miracle Noodles
- ☐ Other: ___________
- ☐ Other: ___________
- ☐ Other: ___________

Calories: ___________

VLCD 21 (Date): ____________

HCGCHICA TIP:

P2 Tea Smoothies

Eating without calories. Make batches of flavored tea - hibiscus tea is my favorite - and cold brew retains the most flavor. Add stevia to taste. Make ice cubes with them. Blend several tea-ice-cubes with water for a smoothie.

WEIGHT: ____________

HCG DOSAGE: ____________

HUNGER LEVEL: ____________

BEDTIME/WAKE TIME: ____________

HOURS SLEEP: ____________

TOTAL CALORIES: ____________

SUPPLEMENTS: ____________

☐ Multivitamin ☐ B12 Shot ☐ Lipo Shot

INJECTION LOCATION

TIME: ________

☐ Belly ☐ Deltoid ☐ Thigh ☐ Other: ____________

DROPS / PELLETS DOSE TIMING

1st Dose: ____________ 2nd Dose: ____________

3rd Dose: ____________ 4th Dose: ____________

LIQUIDS:

	4 LITERS
	3.5 LITERS
	3 LITERS
	2.5 LITERS
	2 LITERS
	1.5 LITERS
	1 LITER
	.5 LITERS

	128 oz = 1 GALLON
	120 oz
	112 oz
	104 oz
	96 oz = 3 QUARTS
	88 oz
	80 oz
	72 oz
	64 oz = 2 QUARTS
	56 oz
	48 oz
	40 oz
	32 oz = 1 QUART
	24 oz
	16 oz
	8 oz = 1 CUP

PERSONAL NOTES

BREAKFAST

Time:

☐ None ☐ Fruit: ____________ ☐ Protein: ____________ Calories: ____________

Serving Size: ____________ Serving Size: ____________

LUNCH Time:

WAS AN ITEM EATEN AS A SNACK? WHICH? Time:

Protein:

- ☐ Chicken breast
- ☐ Beef
- ☐ Veal
- ☐ Shrimp
- ☐ Lobster
- ☐ White fish: ____________
- ☐ Protein Shake
- ☐ Other: ____________

Serving Size:

- ☐ 100 grams/3.5 oz
- ☐ Other: ____________

Calories: ____________

Vegetable:

- ☐ Asparagus
- ☐ Beet Greens
- ☐ Cabbage
- ☐ Celery
- ☐ Chard
- ☐ Cucumber
- ☐ Fennel
- ☐ Lettuce
- ☐ Onions
- ☐ Radishes
- ☐ Spinach
- ☐ Tomatoes
- ☐ Other: ____________
- ☐ Other: ____________
- ☐ Other: ____________

Calories: ____________

Fruit:

- ☐ Strawberries
- ☐ ½ Grapefruit
- ☐ Apple
- ☐ Orange
- ☐ Other: ____________

Starch:

- ☐ Grissini
- ☐ Melba
- ☐ Other: ____________

Calories: ____________

Other:

- ☐ TBS. Milk
- ☐ Juice of 1 Lemon
- ☐ Stevia
- ☐ Shirataki/Miracle Noodles
- ☐ Other: ____________
- ☐ Other: ____________
- ☐ Other: ____________

Calories: ____________

DINNER Time:

WAS AN ITEM EATEN AS A SNACK? WHICH? Time:

Protein:

- ☐ Chicken
- ☐ Beef
- ☐ Veal
- ☐ Shrimp
- ☐ Lobster
- ☐ White fish: ____________
- ☐ Protein Shake
- ☐ Other: ____________

Serving Size:

- ☐ 100 grams
- ☐ Other: ____________

Calories: ____________

Vegetable:

- ☐ Asparagus
- ☐ Beet Greens
- ☐ Cabbage
- ☐ Celery
- ☐ Chard
- ☐ Cucumber
- ☐ Fennel
- ☐ Lettuce
- ☐ Onions
- ☐ Radishes
- ☐ Spinach
- ☐ Tomatoes
- ☐ Other: ____________
- ☐ Other: ____________
- ☐ Other: ____________

Calories: ____________

Fruit:

- ☐ Strawberries
- ☐ ½ Grapefruit
- ☐ Apple
- ☐ Orange
- ☐ Other: ____________

Starch:

- ☐ Grissini
- ☐ Melba
- ☐ Other: ____________

Calories: ____________

Other:

- ☐ TBS. Milk
- ☐ Juice of 1 Lemon
- ☐ Stevia
- ☐ Shirataki/Miracle Noodles
- ☐ Other: ____________
- ☐ Other: ____________
- ☐ Other: ____________

Calories: ____________

Reflections ON WEEK 3

REMEMBER, THIS IS NOT JUST ABOUT LOSING WEIGHT. IT'S ABOUT CHANGING YOUR WHOLE MINDSET ABOUT FOOD AND YOUR BODY.

YOU ARE BREAKING OLD PATTERNS RIGHT NOW. YOU ARE CREATING NEW PATTERNS. TRY NOT TO FOCUS YOUR PROGESS SOLELY ON WEIGHT LOSS.

SO WITH THAT IN MIND, HOW DID THIS WEEK GO?

What are you proud of? Why are you proud of it? What did you struggle with? What would you like to work on changing? What specific logical ways can you think of to make those adjustments? Or maybe you're just burned out at the moment - it's okay to just make it a rant.

Week 4

"IT MAY TAKE A LITTLE TIME to get where you want to be, but if you pause and think for a moment, you will notice that you are no longer where you were. Do not stop - keep going."

- Rodolfo Costa

And the day came when the RISK TO REMAIN tight in a bud was more painful than the RISK it took to blossom.

- Anais Nin

VLCD 22 (Date): ____________

WEIGHT: ____________

HCG DOSAGE: ____________

HUNGER LEVEL: ____________

BEDTIME/WAKE TIME: ____________

HOURS SLEEP: ____________

TOTAL CALORIES: ____________

SUPPLEMENTS: ____________

☐ Multivitamin ☐ B12 Shot ☐ Lipo Shot

INJECTION LOCATION

TIME: ________

☐ Belly ☐ Deltoid ☐ Thigh ☐ Other: ____________

DROPS / PELLETS DOSE TIMING

1st Dose: ____________ 2nd Dose: ____________

3rd Dose: ____________ 4th Dose: ____________

LIQUIDS:

4 LITERS
3.5 LITERS
3 LITERS
2.5 LITERS
2 LITERS
1.5 LITERS
1 LITER
.5 LITERS

128 oz = 1 GALLON
120 oz
112 oz
104 oz
96 oz = 3 QUARTS
88 oz
80 oz
72 oz
64 oz = 2 QUARTS
56 oz
48 oz
40 oz
32 oz = 1 QUART
24 oz
16 oz
8 oz = 1 CUP

PERSONAL NOTES

BREAKFAST

Time:

☐ None ☐ Fruit: ____________ ☐ Protein: ____________ Calories: ____________

Serving Size: ____________ Serving Size: ____________

LUNCH Time:

WAS AN ITEM EATEN AS A SNACK? WHICH? Time:

Protein:

- ☐ Chicken breast
- ☐ Beef
- ☐ Veal
- ☐ Shrimp
- ☐ Lobster
- ☐ White fish: ___________
- ☐ Protein Shake
- ☐ Other: ___________

Serving Size:

- ☐ 100 grams/3.5 oz
- ☐ Other: ___________

Calories: ___________

Vegetable:

- ☐ Asparagus
- ☐ Beet Greens
- ☐ Cabbage
- ☐ Celery
- ☐ Chard
- ☐ Cucumber
- ☐ Fennel
- ☐ Lettuce
- ☐ Onions
- ☐ Radishes
- ☐ Spinach
- ☐ Tomatoes
- ☐ Other: ___________
- ☐ Other: ___________
- ☐ Other: ___________

Calories: ___________

Fruit:

- ☐ Strawberries
- ☐ ½ Grapefruit
- ☐ Apple
- ☐ Orange
- ☐ Other: ___________

Starch:

- ☐ Grissini
- ☐ Melba
- ☐ Other: ___________

Calories: ___________

Other:

- ☐ TBS. Milk
- ☐ Juice of 1 Lemon
- ☐ Stevia
- ☐ Shirataki/Miracle Noodles
- ☐ Other: ___________
- ☐ Other: ___________
- ☐ Other: ___________

Calories: ___________

DINNER Time:

WAS AN ITEM EATEN AS A SNACK? WHICH? Time:

Protein:

- ☐ Chicken
- ☐ Beef
- ☐ Veal
- ☐ Shrimp
- ☐ Lobster
- ☐ White fish: ___________
- ☐ Protein Shake
- ☐ Other: ___________

Serving Size:

- ☐ 100 grams
- ☐ Other: ___________

Calories: ___________

Vegetable:

- ☐ Asparagus
- ☐ Beet Greens
- ☐ Cabbage
- ☐ Celery
- ☐ Chard
- ☐ Cucumber
- ☐ Fennel
- ☐ Lettuce
- ☐ Onions
- ☐ Radishes
- ☐ Spinach
- ☐ Tomatoes
- ☐ Other: ___________
- ☐ Other: ___________
- ☐ Other: ___________

Calories: ___________

Fruit:

- ☐ Strawberries
- ☐ ½ Grapefruit
- ☐ Apple
- ☐ Orange
- ☐ Other: ___________

Starch:

- ☐ Grissini
- ☐ Melba
- ☐ Other: ___________

Calories: ___________

Other:

- ☐ TBS. Milk
- ☐ Juice of 1 Lemon
- ☐ Stevia
- ☐ Shirataki/Miracle Noodles
- ☐ Other: ___________
- ☐ Other: ___________
- ☐ Other: ___________

Calories: ___________

VLCD 23 (Date): ____________

FELLOW HCGER TIP:

Being Real

"Between having a crazy-busy life and having to prepare non-hCG food for my family, I find that preparing meals or at least meal components ahead of a time is a lifesaver and makes it easy to make the right choices."

WEIGHT: ____________

HCG DOSAGE: ____________

HUNGER LEVEL: ____________

BEDTIME/WAKE TIME: ____________

HOURS SLEEP: ____________

TOTAL CALORIES: ____________

SUPPLEMENTS: ____________

☐ Multivitamin ☐ B12 Shot ☐ Lipo Shot

INJECTION LOCATION

TIME: ________

☐ Belly ☐ Deltoid ☐ Thigh ☐ Other: ____________

DROPS / PELLETS DOSE TIMING

1st Dose: ____________ 2nd Dose: ____________

3rd Dose: ____________ 4th Dose: ____________

LIQUIDS:

Liters
4 LITERS
3.5 LITERS
3 LITERS
2.5 LITERS
2 LITERS
1.5 LITERS
1 LITER
.5 LITERS

Ounces
128 OZ = 1 GALLON
120 OZ
112 OZ
104 OZ
96 OZ = 3 QUARTS
88 OZ
80 OZ
72 OZ
64 OZ = 2 QUARTS
56 OZ
48 OZ
40 OZ
32 OZ = 1 QUART
24 OZ
16 OZ
8 OZ = 1 CUP

PERSONAL NOTES

BREAKFAST

Time:

☐ None ☐ Fruit: ____________ ☐ Protein: ____________ Calories: ____________

Serving Size: ____________ Serving Size: ____________

LUNCH Time:

WAS AN ITEM EATEN AS A SNACK? WHICH? Time:

Protein:

- ☐ Chicken breast
- ☐ Beef
- ☐ Veal
- ☐ Shrimp
- ☐ Lobster
- ☐ White fish: ____________
- ☐ Protein Shake
- ☐ Other: ____________

Serving Size:

- ☐ 100 grams/3.5 oz
- ☐ Other: ____________

Calories: ____________

Vegetable:

- ☐ Asparagus
- ☐ Beet Greens
- ☐ Cabbage
- ☐ Celery
- ☐ Chard
- ☐ Cucumber
- ☐ Fennel
- ☐ Lettuce
- ☐ Onions
- ☐ Radishes
- ☐ Spinach
- ☐ Tomatoes
- ☐ Other: ____________
- ☐ Other: ____________
- ☐ Other: ____________

Calories: ____________

Fruit:

- ☐ Strawberries
- ☐ ½ Grapefruit
- ☐ Apple
- ☐ Orange
- ☐ Other: ____________

Starch:

- ☐ Grissini
- ☐ Melba
- ☐ Other: ____________

Calories: ____________

Other:

- ☐ TBS. Milk
- ☐ Juice of 1 Lemon
- ☐ Stevia
- ☐ Shirataki/Miracle Noodles
- ☐ Other: ____________
- ☐ Other: ____________
- ☐ Other: ____________

Calories: ____________

DINNER Time:

WAS AN ITEM EATEN AS A SNACK? WHICH? Time:

Protein:

- ☐ Chicken
- ☐ Beef
- ☐ Veal
- ☐ Shrimp
- ☐ Lobster
- ☐ White fish: ____________
- ☐ Protein Shake
- ☐ Other: ____________

Serving Size:

- ☐ 100 grams
- ☐ Other: ____________

Calories: ____________

Vegetable:

- ☐ Asparagus
- ☐ Beet Greens
- ☐ Cabbage
- ☐ Celery
- ☐ Chard
- ☐ Cucumber
- ☐ Fennel
- ☐ Lettuce
- ☐ Onions
- ☐ Radishes
- ☐ Spinach
- ☐ Tomatoes
- ☐ Other: ____________
- ☐ Other: ____________
- ☐ Other: ____________

Calories: ____________

Fruit:

- ☐ Strawberries
- ☐ ½ Grapefruit
- ☐ Apple
- ☐ Orange
- ☐ Other: ____________

Starch:

- ☐ Grissini
- ☐ Melba
- ☐ Other: ____________

Calories: ____________

Other:

- ☐ TBS. Milk
- ☐ Juice of 1 Lemon
- ☐ Stevia
- ☐ Shirataki/Miracle Noodles
- ☐ Other: ____________
- ☐ Other: ____________
- ☐ Other: ____________

Calories: ____________

Most **GOOD DECISIONS** that a person makes are a result of *reflection* and the **WILL TO CHANGE.**

- *Innocent Mwatsikesimbe*

VLCD 24

(Date): ____________

WEIGHT: ____________

HCG DOSAGE: ____________

HUNGER LEVEL: ____________

BEDTIME/WAKE TIME: ____________

HOURS SLEEP: ____________

TOTAL CALORIES: ____________

SUPPLEMENTS: ____________

☐ Multivitamin ☐ B12 Shot ☐ Lipo Shot

INJECTION LOCATION

TIME: ________

☐ Belly ☐ Deltoid ☐ Thigh ☐ Other: ____________

DROPS / PELLETS DOSE TIMING

1st Dose: ____________ 2nd Dose: ____________

3rd Dose: ____________ 4th Dose: ____________

LIQUIDS:

4 LITERS
3.5 LITERS
3 LITERS
2.5 LITERS
2 LITERS
1.5 LITERS
1 LITER
.5 LITERS

128 oz = 1 GALLON
120 oz
112 oz
104 oz
96 oz = 3 QUARTS
88 oz
80 oz
72 oz
64 oz = 2 QUARTS
56 oz
48 oz
40 oz
32 oz = 1 QUART
24 oz
16 oz
8 oz = 1 CUP

PERSONAL NOTES

BREAKFAST

Time:

☐ None ☐ Fruit: ____________ ☐ Protein: ____________ *Calories:* ____________

Serving Size: ____________ *Serving Size:* ____________

LUNCH Time:

WAS AN ITEM EATEN AS A SNACK? WHICH? Time:

Protein:

- ☐ Chicken breast
- ☐ Beef
- ☐ Veal
- ☐ Shrimp
- ☐ Lobster
- ☐ White fish: ____________
- ☐ Protein Shake
- ☐ Other: ____________

Serving Size:

- ☐ 100 grams/3.5 oz
- ☐ Other: ____________

Calories: ____________

Vegetable:

- ☐ Asparagus
- ☐ Beet Greens
- ☐ Cabbage
- ☐ Celery
- ☐ Chard
- ☐ Cucumber
- ☐ Fennel
- ☐ Lettuce
- ☐ Onions
- ☐ Radishes
- ☐ Spinach
- ☐ Tomatoes
- ☐ Other: ____________
- ☐ Other: ____________
- ☐ Other: ____________

Calories: ____________

Fruit:

- ☐ Strawberries
- ☐ ½ Grapefruit
- ☐ Apple
- ☐ Orange
- ☐ Other: ____________

Starch:

- ☐ Grissini
- ☐ Melba
- ☐ Other: ____________

Calories: ____________

Other:

- ☐ TBS. Milk
- ☐ Juice of 1 Lemon
- ☐ Stevia
- ☐ Shirataki/Miracle Noodles
- ☐ Other: ____________
- ☐ Other: ____________
- ☐ Other: ____________

Calories: ____________

DINNER Time:

WAS AN ITEM EATEN AS A SNACK? WHICH? Time:

Protein:

- ☐ Chicken
- ☐ Beef
- ☐ Veal
- ☐ Shrimp
- ☐ Lobster
- ☐ White fish: ____________
- ☐ Protein Shake
- ☐ Other: ____________

Serving Size:

- ☐ 100 grams
- ☐ Other: ____________

Calories: ____________

Vegetable:

- ☐ Asparagus
- ☐ Beet Greens
- ☐ Cabbage
- ☐ Celery
- ☐ Chard
- ☐ Cucumber
- ☐ Fennel
- ☐ Lettuce
- ☐ Onions
- ☐ Radishes
- ☐ Spinach
- ☐ Tomatoes
- ☐ Other: ____________
- ☐ Other: ____________
- ☐ Other: ____________

Calories: ____________

Fruit:

- ☐ Strawberries
- ☐ ½ Grapefruit
- ☐ Apple
- ☐ Orange
- ☐ Other: ____________

Starch:

- ☐ Grissini
- ☐ Melba
- ☐ Other: ____________

Calories: ____________

Other:

- ☐ TBS. Milk
- ☐ Juice of 1 Lemon
- ☐ Stevia
- ☐ Shirataki/Miracle Noodles
- ☐ Other: ____________
- ☐ Other: ____________
- ☐ Other: ____________

Calories: ____________

VLCD 25 (Date): ____________

HCGCHICA TIP:

Hard Days = Worth It

Frequently hCGers find that on the hardest days, when they crave the most, they will often have a larger loss than usual on the scale the following day.

WEIGHT: ____________

HCG DOSAGE: ____________

HUNGER LEVEL: ____________

BEDTIME/WAKE TIME: ____________

HOURS SLEEP: ____________

TOTAL CALORIES: ____________

SUPPLEMENTS: ____________

☐ Multivitamin ☐ B12 Shot ☐ Lipo Shot

INJECTION LOCATION

TIME: ________

☐ Belly ☐ Deltoid ☐ Thigh ☐ Other: ____________

DROPS / PELLETS DOSE TIMING

1st Dose: ____________ 2nd Dose: ____________

3rd Dose: ____________ 4th Dose: ____________

LIQUIDS:

4 LITERS
3.5 LITERS
3 LITERS
2.5 LITERS
2 LITERS
1.5 LITERS
1 LITER
.5 LITERS

128 oz = 1 GALLON
120 oz
112 oz
104 oz
96 oz = 3 QUARTS
88 oz
80 oz
72 oz
64 oz = 2 QUARTS
56 oz
48 oz
40 oz
32 oz = 1 QUART
24 oz
16 oz
8 oz = 1 CUP

PERSONAL NOTES

BREAKFAST

Time:

☐ None ☐ Fruit: ____________ ☐ Protein: ____________ Calories: ____________

Serving Size: ____________ Serving Size: ____________

LUNCH Time:

WAS AN ITEM EATEN AS A SNACK? WHICH? Time:

Protein:

- ☐ Chicken breast
- ☐ Beef
- ☐ Veal
- ☐ Shrimp
- ☐ Lobster
- ☐ White fish: ___________
- ☐ Protein Shake
- ☐ Other: ___________

Serving Size:

- ☐ 100 grams/3.5 oz
- ☐ Other: ___________

Calories: ___________

Vegetable:

- ☐ Asparagus
- ☐ Beet Greens
- ☐ Cabbage
- ☐ Celery
- ☐ Chard
- ☐ Cucumber
- ☐ Fennel
- ☐ Lettuce
- ☐ Onions
- ☐ Radishes
- ☐ Spinach
- ☐ Tomatoes
- ☐ Other: ___________
- ☐ Other: ___________
- ☐ Other: ___________

Calories: ___________

Fruit:

- ☐ Strawberries
- ☐ ½ Grapefruit
- ☐ Apple
- ☐ Orange
- ☐ Other: ___________

Starch:

- ☐ Grissini
- ☐ Melba
- ☐ Other: ___________

Calories: ___________

Other:

- ☐ TBS. Milk
- ☐ Juice of 1 Lemon
- ☐ Stevia
- ☐ Shirataki/Miracle Noodles
- ☐ Other: ___________
- ☐ Other: ___________
- ☐ Other: ___________

Calories: ___________

DINNER Time:

WAS AN ITEM EATEN AS A SNACK? WHICH? Time:

Protein:

- ☐ Chicken
- ☐ Beef
- ☐ Veal
- ☐ Shrimp
- ☐ Lobster
- ☐ White fish: ___________
- ☐ Protein Shake
- ☐ Other: ___________

Serving Size:

- ☐ 100 grams
- ☐ Other: ___________

Calories: ___________

Vegetable:

- ☐ Asparagus
- ☐ Beet Greens
- ☐ Cabbage
- ☐ Celery
- ☐ Chard
- ☐ Cucumber
- ☐ Fennel
- ☐ Lettuce
- ☐ Onions
- ☐ Radishes
- ☐ Spinach
- ☐ Tomatoes
- ☐ Other: ___________
- ☐ Other: ___________
- ☐ Other: ___________

Calories: ___________

Fruit:

- ☐ Strawberries
- ☐ ½ Grapefruit
- ☐ Apple
- ☐ Orange
- ☐ Other: ___________

Starch:

- ☐ Grissini
- ☐ Melba
- ☐ Other: ___________

Calories: ___________

Other:

- ☐ TBS. Milk
- ☐ Juice of 1 Lemon
- ☐ Stevia
- ☐ Shirataki/Miracle Noodles
- ☐ Other: ___________
- ☐ Other: ___________
- ☐ Other: ___________

Calories: ___________

FELLOW HCGER TIP:

Pickle Fetish

Keep some pickles around! Multiple hCGers reference pickles as just the thing when you want something salty, juicy, and crunchy.

Note: Be sure to check the ingredient label for added sugars.

VLCD 26 (Date): ____________

WEIGHT: ____________

HCG DOSAGE: ____________

HUNGER LEVEL: ____________

BEDTIME/WAKE TIME: ____________

HOURS SLEEP: ____________

TOTAL CALORIES: ____________

SUPPLEMENTS: ____________

☐ Multivitamin ☐ B12 Shot ☐ Lipo Shot

INJECTION LOCATION

TIME: ________

☐ Belly ☐ Deltoid ☐ Thigh ☐ Other: ____________

DROPS / PELLETS DOSE TIMING

1st Dose: ____________ 2nd Dose: ____________

3rd Dose: ____________ 4th Dose: ____________

LIQUIDS:

4 LITERS
3.5 LITERS
3 LITERS
2.5 LITERS
2 LITERS
1.5 LITERS
1 LITER
.5 LITERS

128 oz = 1 GALLON
120 oz
112 oz
104 oz
96 oz = 3 QUARTS
88 oz
80 oz
72 oz
64 oz = 2 QUARTS
56 oz
48 oz
40 oz
32 oz = 1 QUART
24 oz
16 oz
8 oz = 1 CUP

PERSONAL NOTES

BREAKFAST

Time:

☐ None ☐ Fruit: ____________ ☐ Protein: ____________ Calories: ____________

Serving Size: ____________ Serving Size: ____________

LUNCH Time :

WAS AN ITEM EATEN AS A SNACK? WHICH? Time:

Protein:

- ☐ Chicken breast
- ☐ Beef
- ☐ Veal
- ☐ Shrimp
- ☐ Lobster
- ☐ White fish: ___________
- ☐ Protein Shake
- ☐ Other: ___________

Serving Size:

- ☐ 100 grams/3.5 oz
- ☐ Other: ___________

Calories: ___________

Vegetable:

- ☐ Asparagus
- ☐ Beet Greens
- ☐ Cabbage
- ☐ Celery
- ☐ Chard
- ☐ Cucumber
- ☐ Fennel
- ☐ Lettuce
- ☐ Onions
- ☐ Radishes
- ☐ Spinach
- ☐ Tomatoes
- ☐ Other: ___________
- ☐ Other: ___________
- ☐ Other: ___________

Calories: ___________

Fruit:

- ☐ Strawberries
- ☐ ½ Grapefruit
- ☐ Apple
- ☐ Orange
- ☐ Other: ___________

Starch:

- ☐ Grissini
- ☐ Melba
- ☐ Other: ___________

Calories: ___________

Other:

- ☐ TBS. Milk
- ☐ Juice of 1 Lemon
- ☐ Stevia
- ☐ Shirataki/Miracle Noodles
- ☐ Other: ___________
- ☐ Other: ___________
- ☐ Other: ___________

Calories: ___________

DINNER Time :

WAS AN ITEM EATEN AS A SNACK? WHICH? Time:

Protein:

- ☐ Chicken
- ☐ Beef
- ☐ Veal
- ☐ Shrimp
- ☐ Lobster
- ☐ White fish: ___________
- ☐ Protein Shake
- ☐ Other: ___________

Serving Size:

- ☐ 100 grams
- ☐ Other: ___________

Calories: ___________

Vegetable:

- ☐ Asparagus
- ☐ Beet Greens
- ☐ Cabbage
- ☐ Celery
- ☐ Chard
- ☐ Cucumber
- ☐ Fennel
- ☐ Lettuce
- ☐ Onions
- ☐ Radishes
- ☐ Spinach
- ☐ Tomatoes
- ☐ Other: ___________
- ☐ Other: ___________
- ☐ Other: ___________

Calories: ___________

Fruit:

- ☐ Strawberries
- ☐ ½ Grapefruit
- ☐ Apple
- ☐ Orange
- ☐ Other: ___________

Starch:

- ☐ Grissini
- ☐ Melba
- ☐ Other: ___________

Calories: ___________

Other:

- ☐ TBS. Milk
- ☐ Juice of 1 Lemon
- ☐ Stevia
- ☐ Shirataki/Miracle Noodles
- ☐ Other: ___________
- ☐ Other: ___________
- ☐ Other: ___________

Calories: ___________

Often,
it's not about becoming
a new person, but becoming
THE PERSON YOU were meant to be,
and ALREADY ARE,
but don't know how to be.
- Heath L. Buckmaster

VLCD 27 (Date): ____________

WEIGHT: ____________

HCG DOSAGE: ____________

HUNGER LEVEL: ____________

BEDTIME/WAKE TIME: ____________

HOURS SLEEP: ____________

TOTAL CALORIES: ____________

SUPPLEMENTS: ____________

☐ Multivitamin ☐ B12 Shot ☐ Lipo Shot

INJECTION LOCATION

TIME: ________

☐ Belly ☐ Deltoid ☐ Thigh ☐ Other: ____________

DROPS / PELLETS DOSE TIMING

1st Dose: ____________ 2nd Dose: ____________

3rd Dose: ____________ 4th Dose: ____________

LIQUIDS:

4 LITERS
3.5 LITERS
3 LITERS
2.5 LITERS
2 LITERS
1.5 LITERS
1 LITER
.5 LITERS

128 oz = 1 GALLON
120 oz
112 oz
104 oz
96 oz = 3 QUARTS
88 oz
80 oz
72 oz
64 oz = 2 QUARTS
56 oz
48 oz
40 oz
32 oz = 1 QUART
24 oz
16 oz
8 oz = 1 CUP

PERSONAL NOTES

BREAKFAST

Time:

☐ None ☐ Fruit: ____________ ☐ Protein: ____________ Calories: ____________

Serving Size: ____________ Serving Size: ____________

LUNCH Time:

WAS AN ITEM EATEN AS A SNACK? WHICH? Time:

Protein:

- [ ] Chicken breast
- [ ] Beef
- [ ] Veal
- [ ] Shrimp
- [ ] Lobster
- [ ] White fish: ___________
- [ ] Protein Shake
- [ ] Other: ___________

Serving Size:

- [ ] 100 grams/3.5 oz
- [ ] Other: ___________

Calories: ___________

Vegetable:

- [ ] Asparagus
- [ ] Beet Greens
- [ ] Cabbage
- [ ] Celery
- [ ] Chard
- [ ] Cucumber
- [ ] Fennel
- [ ] Lettuce
- [ ] Onions
- [ ] Radishes
- [ ] Spinach
- [ ] Tomatoes
- [ ] Other: ___________
- [ ] Other: ___________
- [ ] Other: ___________

Calories: ___________

Fruit:

- [ ] Strawberries
- [ ] ½ Grapefruit
- [ ] Apple
- [ ] Orange
- [ ] Other: ___________

Starch:

- [ ] Grissini
- [ ] Melba
- [ ] Other: ___________

Calories: ___________

Other:

- [ ] TBS. Milk
- [ ] Juice of 1 Lemon
- [ ] Stevia
- [ ] Shirataki/Miracle Noodles
- [ ] Other: ___________
- [ ] Other: ___________
- [ ] Other: ___________

Calories: ___________

DINNER Time:

WAS AN ITEM EATEN AS A SNACK? WHICH? Time:

Protein:

- [ ] Chicken
- [ ] Beef
- [ ] Veal
- [ ] Shrimp
- [ ] Lobster
- [ ] White fish: ___________
- [ ] Protein Shake
- [ ] Other: ___________

Serving Size:

- [ ] 100 grams
- [ ] Other: ___________

Calories: ___________

Vegetable:

- [ ] Asparagus
- [ ] Beet Greens
- [ ] Cabbage
- [ ] Celery
- [ ] Chard
- [ ] Cucumber
- [ ] Fennel
- [ ] Lettuce
- [ ] Onions
- [ ] Radishes
- [ ] Spinach
- [ ] Tomatoes
- [ ] Other: ___________
- [ ] Other: ___________
- [ ] Other: ___________

Calories: ___________

Fruit:

- [ ] Strawberries
- [ ] ½ Grapefruit
- [ ] Apple
- [ ] Orange
- [ ] Other: ___________

Starch:

- [ ] Grissini
- [ ] Melba
- [ ] Other: ___________

Calories: ___________

Other:

- [ ] TBS. Milk
- [ ] Juice of 1 Lemon
- [ ] Stevia
- [ ] Shirataki/Miracle Noodles
- [ ] Other: ___________
- [ ] Other: ___________
- [ ] Other: ___________

Calories: ___________

HCGCHICA TIP:

Break It Up

Some hCGers have jobs with long or odd hours. It can be helpful to spread your food out - even splitting your 100 gram protein into two 50 gram servings.

VLCD 28 (Date): ____________

WEIGHT: ____________

HCG DOSAGE: ____________

HUNGER LEVEL: ____________

BEDTIME/WAKE TIME: ____________

HOURS SLEEP: ____________

TOTAL CALORIES: ____________

SUPPLEMENTS: ____________

☐ Multivitamin ☐ B12 Shot ☐ Lipo Shot

INJECTION LOCATION

TIME: ________

☐ Belly ☐ Deltoid ☐ Thigh ☐ Other: ____________

LIQUIDS:

4 LITERS
3.5 LITERS
3 LITERS
2.5 LITERS
2 LITERS
1.5 LITERS
1 LITER
.5 LITERS

128 oz = 1 GALLON
120 oz
112 oz
104 oz
96 oz = 3 QUARTS
88 oz
80 oz
72 oz
64 oz = 2 QUARTS
56 oz
48 oz
40 oz
32 oz = 1 QUART
24 oz
16 oz
8 oz = 1 CUP

DROPS / PELLETS DOSE TIMING

1st Dose: ____________ 2nd Dose: ____________

3rd Dose: ____________ 4th Dose: ____________

PERSONAL NOTES

BREAKFAST

Time :

☐ None ☐ Fruit: ____________ ☐ Protein: ____________ Calories: ____________

Serving Size: ____________ Serving Size: ____________

LUNCH Time:

WAS AN ITEM EATEN AS A SNACK? WHICH? Time:

Protein:

- ☐ Chicken breast
- ☐ Beef
- ☐ Veal
- ☐ Shrimp
- ☐ Lobster
- ☐ White fish: ____________
- ☐ Protein Shake
- ☐ Other: ____________

Serving Size:

- ☐ 100 grams/3.5 oz
- ☐ Other: ____________

Calories: ____________

Vegetable:

- ☐ Asparagus
- ☐ Beet Greens
- ☐ Cabbage
- ☐ Celery
- ☐ Chard
- ☐ Cucumber
- ☐ Fennel
- ☐ Lettuce
- ☐ Onions
- ☐ Radishes
- ☐ Spinach
- ☐ Tomatoes
- ☐ Other: ____________
- ☐ Other: ____________
- ☐ Other: ____________

Calories: ____________

Fruit:

- ☐ Strawberries
- ☐ ½ Grapefruit
- ☐ Apple
- ☐ Orange
- ☐ Other: ____________

Starch:

- ☐ Grissini
- ☐ Melba
- ☐ Other: ____________

Calories: ____________

Other:

- ☐ TBS. Milk
- ☐ Juice of 1 Lemon
- ☐ Stevia
- ☐ Shirataki/Miracle Noodles
- ☐ Other: ____________
- ☐ Other: ____________
- ☐ Other: ____________

Calories: ____________

DINNER Time:

WAS AN ITEM EATEN AS A SNACK? WHICH? Time:

Protein:

- ☐ Chicken
- ☐ Beef
- ☐ Veal
- ☐ Shrimp
- ☐ Lobster
- ☐ White fish: ____________
- ☐ Protein Shake
- ☐ Other: ____________

Serving Size:

- ☐ 100 grams
- ☐ Other: ____________

Calories: ____________

Vegetable:

- ☐ Asparagus
- ☐ Beet Greens
- ☐ Cabbage
- ☐ Celery
- ☐ Chard
- ☐ Cucumber
- ☐ Fennel
- ☐ Lettuce
- ☐ Onions
- ☐ Radishes
- ☐ Spinach
- ☐ Tomatoes
- ☐ Other: ____________
- ☐ Other: ____________
- ☐ Other: ____________

Calories: ____________

Fruit:

- ☐ Strawberries
- ☐ ½ Grapefruit
- ☐ Apple
- ☐ Orange
- ☐ Other: ____________

Starch:

- ☐ Grissini
- ☐ Melba
- ☐ Other: ____________

Calories: ____________

Other:

- ☐ TBS. Milk
- ☐ Juice of 1 Lemon
- ☐ Stevia
- ☐ Shirataki/Miracle Noodles
- ☐ Other: ____________
- ☐ Other: ____________
- ☐ Other: ____________

Calories: ____________

Reflections ON WEEK 4

REMEMBER, THIS IS NOT JUST ABOUT LOSING WEIGHT. IT'S ABOUT CHANGING YOUR WHOLE MINDSET ABOUT FOOD AND YOUR BODY.

YOU ARE BREAKING OLD PAT-TERNS RIGHT NOW. YOU ARE CREATING NEW PATTERNS. TRY NOT TO FOCUS YOUR PROGESS SOLELY ON WEIGHT LOSS.

SO WITH THAT IN MIND, HOW DID THIS WEEK GO?

What are you proud of? Why are you proud of it? What did you struggle with? What would you like to work on changing? What specific logical ways can you think of to make those adjustments? Or maybe you're just burned out at the moment - it's okay to just make it a rant.

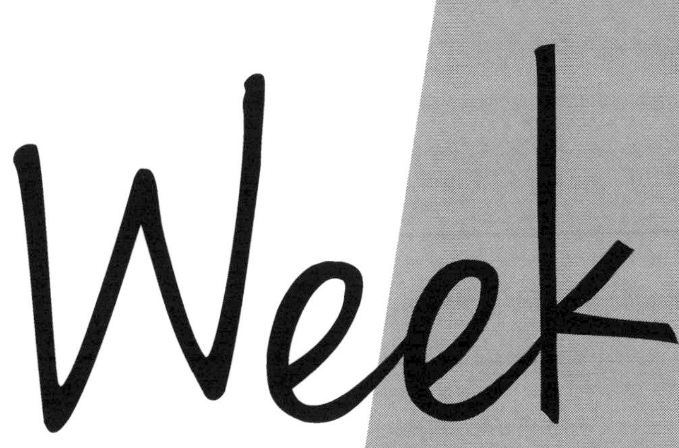

Week 5

"WE HAVE TO ARTICULATE what we mean by change, define what we perceive as essential to our way of life. We have to refuse to accept blindly other's perceptions of progress."

- Patricia Locke, Lakota Indian

FELLOW HCGER TIP:

Remember

Remember that you are putting a hormone into your body. You are creating an environment in which your body is both ready for incredible fat releases but also vulnerable to incredible fat gains. Cheats can set you back. As yourself, is it worth it?

VLCD 29 (Date): ______

WEIGHT: ______

HCG DOSAGE: ______

HUNGER LEVEL: ______

BEDTIME/WAKE TIME: ______

HOURS SLEEP: ______

TOTAL CALORIES: ______

SUPPLEMENTS: ______

☐ Multivitamin ☐ B12 Shot ☐ Lipo Shot

INJECTION LOCATION

TIME: ______

☐ Belly ☐ Deltoid ☐ Thigh ☐ Other: ______

LIQUIDS:

	4 LITERS
	3.5 LITERS
	3 LITERS
	2.5 LITERS
	2 LITERS
	1.5 LITERS
	1 LITER
	.5 LITERS

	128 oz = 1 GALLON
	120 oz
	112 oz
	104 oz
	96 oz = 3 QUARTS
	88 oz
	80 oz
	72 oz
	64 oz = 2 QUARTS
	56 oz
	48 oz
	40 oz
	32 oz = 1 QUART
	24 oz
	16 oz
	8 oz = 1 CUP

DROPS / PELLETS DOSE TIMING

1st Dose: ______ 2nd Dose: ______

3rd Dose: ______ 4th Dose: ______

PERSONAL NOTES

BREAKFAST

Time:

☐ None ☐ Fruit: ______ ☐ Protein: ______ Calories: ______

Serving Size: ______ Serving Size: ______

LUNCH Time :

WAS AN ITEM EATEN AS A SNACK? WHICH? Time:

Protein:

- [ ] Chicken breast
- [ ] Beef
- [ ] Veal
- [ ] Shrimp
- [ ] Lobster
- [ ] White fish: ___________
- [ ] Protein Shake
- [ ] Other: ___________

Serving Size:

- [ ] 100 grams/3.5 oz
- [ ] Other: ___________

Calories: ___________

Vegetable:

- [ ] Asparagus
- [ ] Beet Greens
- [ ] Cabbage
- [ ] Celery
- [ ] Chard
- [ ] Cucumber
- [ ] Fennel
- [ ] Lettuce
- [ ] Onions
- [ ] Radishes
- [ ] Spinach
- [ ] Tomatoes
- [ ] Other: ___________
- [ ] Other: ___________
- [ ] Other: ___________

Calories: ___________

Fruit:

- [ ] Strawberries
- [ ] ½ Grapefruit
- [ ] Apple
- [ ] Orange
- [ ] Other: ___________

Starch:

- [ ] Grissini
- [ ] Melba
- [ ] Other: ___________

Calories: ___________

Other:

- [ ] TBS. Milk
- [ ] Juice of 1 Lemon
- [ ] Stevia
- [ ] Shirataki/Miracle Noodles
- [ ] Other: ___________
- [ ] Other: ___________
- [ ] Other: ___________

Calories: ___________

DINNER Time :

WAS AN ITEM EATEN AS A SNACK? WHICH? Time:

Protein:

- [ ] Chicken
- [ ] Beef
- [ ] Veal
- [ ] Shrimp
- [ ] Lobster
- [ ] White fish: ___________
- [ ] Protein Shake
- [ ] Other: ___________

Serving Size:

- [ ] 100 grams
- [ ] Other: ___________

Calories: ___________

Vegetable:

- [ ] Asparagus
- [ ] Beet Greens
- [ ] Cabbage
- [ ] Celery
- [ ] Chard
- [ ] Cucumber
- [ ] Fennel
- [ ] Lettuce
- [ ] Onions
- [ ] Radishes
- [ ] Spinach
- [ ] Tomatoes
- [ ] Other: ___________
- [ ] Other: ___________
- [ ] Other: ___________

Calories: ___________

Fruit:

- [ ] Strawberries
- [ ] ½ Grapefruit
- [ ] Apple
- [ ] Orange
- [ ] Other: ___________

Starch:

- [ ] Grissini
- [ ] Melba
- [ ] Other: ___________

Calories: ___________

Other:

- [ ] TBS. Milk
- [ ] Juice of 1 Lemon
- [ ] Stevia
- [ ] Shirataki/Miracle Noodles
- [ ] Other: ___________
- [ ] Other: ___________
- [ ] Other: ___________

Calories: ___________

Bad habits

are like having a SUMO WRESTLER

in the back of your canoe

ROWING THE OPPOSITE DIRECTION.

- J Loren Norris

VLCD **30** (Date): ____________

WEIGHT: ____________

HCG DOSAGE: ____________

HUNGER LEVEL: ____________

BEDTIME/WAKE TIME: ____________

HOURS SLEEP: ____________

TOTAL CALORIES: ____________

SUPPLEMENTS: ____________

☐ Multivitamin ☐ B12 Shot ☐ Lipo Shot

INJECTION LOCATION **TIME:** ________

☐ Belly ☐ Deltoid ☐ Thigh ☐ Other: ____________

LIQUIDS:

	4 LITERS
	3.5 LITERS
	3 LITERS
	2.5 LITERS
	2 LITERS
	1.5 LITERS
	1 LITER
	.5 LITERS

	128 oz = 1 GALLON
	120 oz
	112 oz
	104 oz
	96 oz = 3 QUARTS
	88 oz
	80 oz
	72 oz
	64 oz = 2 QUARTS
	56 oz
	48 oz
	40 oz
	32 oz = 1 QUART
	24 oz
	16 oz
	8 oz = 1 CUP

DROPS / PELLETS DOSE TIMING

1st Dose: ____________ 2nd Dose: ____________

3rd Dose: ____________ 4th Dose: ____________

PERSONAL NOTES

BREAKFAST

Time:

☐ None ☐ Fruit: ____________ ☐ Protein: ____________ Calories: ____________

Serving Size: ____________ Serving Size: ____________

LUNCH Time:

WAS AN ITEM EATEN AS A SNACK? WHICH? Time:

Protein:

- ☐ Chicken breast
- ☐ Beef
- ☐ Veal
- ☐ Shrimp
- ☐ Lobster
- ☐ White fish: ___________
- ☐ Protein Shake
- ☐ Other: ___________

Serving Size:

- ☐ 100 grams/3.5 oz
- ☐ Other: ___________

Calories: ___________

Vegetable:

- ☐ Asparagus
- ☐ Beet Greens
- ☐ Cabbage
- ☐ Celery
- ☐ Chard
- ☐ Cucumber
- ☐ Fennel
- ☐ Lettuce
- ☐ Onions
- ☐ Radishes
- ☐ Spinach
- ☐ Tomatoes
- ☐ Other: ___________
- ☐ Other: ___________
- ☐ Other: ___________

Calories: ___________

Fruit:

- ☐ Strawberries
- ☐ ½ Grapefruit
- ☐ Apple
- ☐ Orange
- ☐ Other: ___________

Starch:

- ☐ Grissini
- ☐ Melba
- ☐ Other: ___________

Calories: ___________

Other:

- ☐ TBS. Milk
- ☐ Juice of 1 Lemon
- ☐ Stevia
- ☐ Shirataki/Miracle Noodles
- ☐ Other: ___________
- ☐ Other: ___________
- ☐ Other: ___________

Calories: ___________

DINNER Time:

WAS AN ITEM EATEN AS A SNACK? WHICH? Time:

Protein:

- ☐ Chicken
- ☐ Beef
- ☐ Veal
- ☐ Shrimp
- ☐ Lobster
- ☐ White fish: ___________
- ☐ Protein Shake
- ☐ Other: ___________

Serving Size:

- ☐ 100 grams
- ☐ Other: ___________

Calories: ___________

Vegetable:

- ☐ Asparagus
- ☐ Beet Greens
- ☐ Cabbage
- ☐ Celery
- ☐ Chard
- ☐ Cucumber
- ☐ Fennel
- ☐ Lettuce
- ☐ Onions
- ☐ Radishes
- ☐ Spinach
- ☐ Tomatoes
- ☐ Other: ___________
- ☐ Other: ___________
- ☐ Other: ___________

Calories: ___________

Fruit:

- ☐ Strawberries
- ☐ ½ Grapefruit
- ☐ Apple
- ☐ Orange
- ☐ Other: ___________

Starch:

- ☐ Grissini
- ☐ Melba
- ☐ Other: ___________

Calories: ___________

Other:

- ☐ TBS. Milk
- ☐ Juice of 1 Lemon
- ☐ Stevia
- ☐ Shirataki/Miracle Noodles
- ☐ Other: ___________
- ☐ Other: ___________
- ☐ Other: ___________

Calories: ___________

VLCD 31 (Date): ____________

HCGCHICA TIP:

Start Looking Ahead

Towards the end of my rounds, I found it helpful and exciting to research recipes for Phase 3 on Pinterest that would replace my previous unhealthy stand-bys.

WEIGHT: ____________

HCG DOSAGE: ____________

HUNGER LEVEL: ____________

BEDTIME/WAKE TIME: ____________

HOURS SLEEP: ____________

TOTAL CALORIES: ____________

SUPPLEMENTS: ____________

☐ Multivitamin ☐ B12 Shot ☐ Lipo Shot

INJECTION LOCATION

TIME: ________

☐ Belly ☐ Deltoid ☐ Thigh ☐ Other: ____________

DROPS / PELLETS DOSE TIMING

1st Dose: ____________ 2nd Dose: ____________

3rd Dose: ____________ 4th Dose: ____________

LIQUIDS:

☐	4 LITERS
☐	3.5 LITERS
☐	3 LITERS
☐	2.5 LITERS
☐	2 LITERS
☐	1.5 LITERS
☐	1 LITER
☐	.5 LITERS

☐	128 OZ = 1 GALLON
☐	120 OZ
☐	112 OZ
☐	104 OZ
☐	96 OZ = 3 QUARTS
☐	88 OZ
☐	80 OZ
☐	72 OZ
☐	64 OZ = 2 QUARTS
☐	56 OZ
☐	48 OZ
☐	40 OZ
☐	32 OZ = 1 QUART
☐	24 OZ
☐	16 OZ
☐	8 OZ = 1 CUP

PERSONAL NOTES

BREAKFAST

Time:

☐ None ☐ Fruit: ____________ ☐ Protein: ____________ Calories: ____________

Serving Size: ____________ Serving Size: ____________

LUNCH Time:

WAS AN ITEM EATEN AS A SNACK? WHICH? Time:

Protein:

- ☐ Chicken breast
- ☐ Beef
- ☐ Veal
- ☐ Shrimp
- ☐ Lobster
- ☐ White fish: ___________
- ☐ Protein Shake
- ☐ Other: ___________

Serving Size:

- ☐ 100 grams/3.5 oz
- ☐ Other: ___________

Calories: ___________

Vegetable:

- ☐ Asparagus
- ☐ Beet Greens
- ☐ Cabbage
- ☐ Celery
- ☐ Chard
- ☐ Cucumber
- ☐ Fennel
- ☐ Lettuce
- ☐ Onions
- ☐ Radishes
- ☐ Spinach
- ☐ Tomatoes
- ☐ Other: ___________
- ☐ Other: ___________
- ☐ Other: ___________

Calories: ___________

Fruit:

- ☐ Strawberries
- ☐ ½ Grapefruit
- ☐ Apple
- ☐ Orange
- ☐ Other: ___________

Starch:

- ☐ Grissini
- ☐ Melba
- ☐ Other: ___________

Calories: ___________

Other:

- ☐ TBS. Milk
- ☐ Juice of 1 Lemon
- ☐ Stevia
- ☐ Shirataki/Miracle Noodles
- ☐ Other: ___________
- ☐ Other: ___________
- ☐ Other: ___________

Calories: ___________

DINNER Time:

WAS AN ITEM EATEN AS A SNACK? WHICH? Time:

Protein:

- ☐ Chicken
- ☐ Beef
- ☐ Veal
- ☐ Shrimp
- ☐ Lobster
- ☐ White fish: ___________
- ☐ Protein Shake
- ☐ Other: ___________

Serving Size:

- ☐ 100 grams
- ☐ Other: ___________

Calories: ___________

Vegetable:

- ☐ Asparagus
- ☐ Beet Greens
- ☐ Cabbage
- ☐ Celery
- ☐ Chard
- ☐ Cucumber
- ☐ Fennel
- ☐ Lettuce
- ☐ Onions
- ☐ Radishes
- ☐ Spinach
- ☐ Tomatoes
- ☐ Other: ___________
- ☐ Other: ___________
- ☐ Other: ___________

Calories: ___________

Fruit:

- ☐ Strawberries
- ☐ ½ Grapefruit
- ☐ Apple
- ☐ Orange
- ☐ Other: ___________

Starch:

- ☐ Grissini
- ☐ Melba
- ☐ Other: ___________

Calories: ___________

Other:

- ☐ TBS. Milk
- ☐ Juice of 1 Lemon
- ☐ Stevia
- ☐ Shirataki/Miracle Noodles
- ☐ Other: ___________
- ☐ Other: ___________
- ☐ Other: ___________

Calories: ___________

Sometimes,
BEING TRUE to yourself
means changing your mind.
SELF CHANGES,
and you follow.
- Vera Nazarian

VLCD 32 (Date): ____

WEIGHT: ____

HCG DOSAGE: ____

HUNGER LEVEL: ____

BEDTIME/WAKE TIME: ____

HOURS SLEEP: ____

TOTAL CALORIES: ____

SUPPLEMENTS: ____

☐ Multivitamin ☐ B12 Shot ☐ Lipo Shot

INJECTION LOCATION

TIME: ____

☐ Belly ☐ Deltoid ☐ Thigh ☐ Other: ____

DROPS / PELLETS DOSE TIMING

1st Dose: ____ 2nd Dose: ____
3rd Dose: ____ 4th Dose: ____

LIQUIDS:

4 LITERS
3.5 LITERS
3 LITERS
2.5 LITERS
2 LITERS
1.5 LITERS
1 LITER
.5 LITERS

128 oz = 1 GALLON
120 oz
112 oz
104 oz
96 oz = 3 QUARTS
88 oz
80 oz
72 oz
64 oz = 2 QUARTS
56 oz
48 oz
40 oz
32 oz = 1 QUART
24 oz
16 oz
8 oz = 1 CUP

PERSONAL NOTES

BREAKFAST

Time:

☐ None ☐ Fruit: ____ ☐ Protein: ____ Calories: ____

Serving Size: ____ Serving Size: ____

LUNCH Time:

WAS AN ITEM EATEN AS A SNACK? WHICH? Time:

Protein:

- ☐ Chicken breast
- ☐ Beef
- ☐ Veal
- ☐ Shrimp
- ☐ Lobster
- ☐ White fish: ____________
- ☐ Protein Shake
- ☐ Other: ____________

Serving Size:

- ☐ 100 grams/3.5 oz
- ☐ Other: ____________

Calories: ____________

Vegetable:

- ☐ Asparagus
- ☐ Beet Greens
- ☐ Cabbage
- ☐ Celery
- ☐ Chard
- ☐ Cucumber
- ☐ Fennel
- ☐ Lettuce
- ☐ Onions
- ☐ Radishes
- ☐ Spinach
- ☐ Tomatoes
- ☐ Other: ____________
- ☐ Other: ____________
- ☐ Other: ____________

Calories: ____________

Fruit:

- ☐ Strawberries
- ☐ ½ Grapefruit
- ☐ Apple
- ☐ Orange
- ☐ Other: ____________

Starch:

- ☐ Grissini
- ☐ Melba
- ☐ Other: ____________

Calories: ____________

Other:

- ☐ TBS. Milk
- ☐ Juice of 1 Lemon
- ☐ Stevia
- ☐ Shirataki/Miracle Noodles
- ☐ Other: ____________
- ☐ Other: ____________
- ☐ Other: ____________

Calories: ____________

DINNER Time:

WAS AN ITEM EATEN AS A SNACK? WHICH? Time:

Protein:

- ☐ Chicken
- ☐ Beef
- ☐ Veal
- ☐ Shrimp
- ☐ Lobster
- ☐ White fish: ____________
- ☐ Protein Shake
- ☐ Other: ____________

Serving Size:

- ☐ 100 grams
- ☐ Other: ____________

Calories: ____________

Vegetable:

- ☐ Asparagus
- ☐ Beet Greens
- ☐ Cabbage
- ☐ Celery
- ☐ Chard
- ☐ Cucumber
- ☐ Fennel
- ☐ Lettuce
- ☐ Onions
- ☐ Radishes
- ☐ Spinach
- ☐ Tomatoes
- ☐ Other: ____________
- ☐ Other: ____________
- ☐ Other: ____________

Calories: ____________

Fruit:

- ☐ Strawberries
- ☐ ½ Grapefruit
- ☐ Apple
- ☐ Orange
- ☐ Other: ____________

Starch:

- ☐ Grissini
- ☐ Melba
- ☐ Other: ____________

Calories: ____________

Other:

- ☐ TBS. Milk
- ☐ Juice of 1 Lemon
- ☐ Stevia
- ☐ Shirataki/Miracle Noodles
- ☐ Other: ____________
- ☐ Other: ____________
- ☐ Other: ____________

Calories: ____________

VLCD 33 (Date): ____________

HCGCHICA TIP:

Get Motivation by Email

If you're not already on my email list, you might consider joining. I send out something motivational or my latest blogpost once a week. You can join free at:

hcgchica.com/help

WEIGHT: ____________

HCG DOSAGE: ____________

HUNGER LEVEL: ____________

BEDTIME/WAKE TIME: ____________

HOURS SLEEP: ____________

TOTAL CALORIES: ____________

SUPPLEMENTS: ____________

☐ Multivitamin ☐ B12 Shot ☐ Lipo Shot

INJECTION LOCATION

TIME: ________

☐ Belly ☐ Deltoid ☐ Thigh ☐ Other: ____________

DROPS / PELLETS DOSE TIMING

1st Dose: ____________ 2nd Dose: ____________

3rd Dose: ____________ 4th Dose: ____________

LIQUIDS:

4 LITERS
3.5 LITERS
3 LITERS
2.5 LITERS
2 LITERS
1.5 LITERS
1 LITER
.5 LITERS

128 oz = 1 GALLON
120 oz
112 oz
104 oz
96 oz = 3 QUARTS
88 oz
80 oz
72 oz
64 oz = 2 QUARTS
56 oz
48 oz
40 oz
32 oz = 1 QUART
24 oz
16 oz
8 oz = 1 CUP

PERSONAL NOTES

BREAKFAST

Time:

☐ None ☐ Fruit: ____________ ☐ Protein: ____________ Calories: ____________

Serving Size: ____________ Serving Size: ____________

LUNCH Time:

WAS AN ITEM EATEN AS A SNACK? WHICH? Time:

Protein:

- ☐ Chicken breast
- ☐ Beef
- ☐ Veal
- ☐ Shrimp
- ☐ Lobster
- ☐ White fish: ___________
- ☐ Protein Shake
- ☐ Other: ___________

Serving Size:

- ☐ 100 grams/3.5 oz
- ☐ Other: ___________

Calories: ___________

Vegetable:

- ☐ Asparagus
- ☐ Beet Greens
- ☐ Cabbage
- ☐ Celery
- ☐ Chard
- ☐ Cucumber
- ☐ Fennel
- ☐ Lettuce
- ☐ Onions
- ☐ Radishes
- ☐ Spinach
- ☐ Tomatoes
- ☐ Other: ___________
- ☐ Other: ___________
- ☐ Other: ___________

Calories: ___________

Fruit:

- ☐ Strawberries
- ☐ ½ Grapefruit
- ☐ Apple
- ☐ Orange
- ☐ Other: ___________

Starch:

- ☐ Grissini
- ☐ Melba
- ☐ Other: ___________

Calories: ___________

Other:

- ☐ TBS. Milk
- ☐ Juice of 1 Lemon
- ☐ Stevia
- ☐ Shirataki/Miracle Noodles
- ☐ Other: ___________
- ☐ Other: ___________
- ☐ Other: ___________

Calories: ___________

DINNER Time:

WAS AN ITEM EATEN AS A SNACK? WHICH? Time:

Protein:

- ☐ Chicken
- ☐ Beef
- ☐ Veal
- ☐ Shrimp
- ☐ Lobster
- ☐ White fish: ___________
- ☐ Protein Shake
- ☐ Other: ___________

Serving Size:

- ☐ 100 grams
- ☐ Other: ___________

Calories: ___________

Vegetable:

- ☐ Asparagus
- ☐ Beet Greens
- ☐ Cabbage
- ☐ Celery
- ☐ Chard
- ☐ Cucumber
- ☐ Fennel
- ☐ Lettuce
- ☐ Onions
- ☐ Radishes
- ☐ Spinach
- ☐ Tomatoes
- ☐ Other: ___________
- ☐ Other: ___________
- ☐ Other: ___________

Calories: ___________

Fruit:

- ☐ Strawberries
- ☐ ½ Grapefruit
- ☐ Apple
- ☐ Orange
- ☐ Other: ___________

Starch:

- ☐ Grissini
- ☐ Melba
- ☐ Other: ___________

Calories: ___________

Other:

- ☐ TBS. Milk
- ☐ Juice of 1 Lemon
- ☐ Stevia
- ☐ Shirataki/Miracle Noodles
- ☐ Other: ___________
- ☐ Other: ___________
- ☐ Other: ___________

Calories: ___________

To **PERSIST** with a *goal*, you must **TREASURE** the dream more than the *costs of sacrifice* to **ATTAIN** it.

- Richelle E. Goodrich

VLCD 34 (Date): ____________

WEIGHT: ____________

HCG DOSAGE: ____________

HUNGER LEVEL: ____________

BEDTIME/WAKE TIME: ____________

HOURS SLEEP: ____________

TOTAL CALORIES: ____________

SUPPLEMENTS: ____________

☐ Multivitamin ☐ B12 Shot ☐ Lipo Shot

INJECTION LOCATION

TIME: ________

☐ Belly ☐ Deltoid ☐ Thigh ☐ Other: ____________

DROPS / PELLETS DOSE TIMING

1st Dose: ____________ 2nd Dose: ____________

3rd Dose: ____________ 4th Dose: ____________

LIQUIDS:

4 LITERS
3.5 LITERS
3 LITERS
2.5 LITERS
2 LITERS
1.5 LITERS
1 LITER
.5 LITERS

128 oz = 1 GALLON
120 oz
112 oz
104 oz
96 oz = 3 QUARTS
88 oz
80 oz
72 oz
64 oz = 2 QUARTS
56 oz
48 oz
40 oz
32 oz = 1 QUART
24 oz
16 oz
8 oz = 1 CUP

PERSONAL NOTES

BREAKFAST

Time:

☐ None ☐ Fruit: ____________ ☐ Protein: ____________ *Calories:* ____________

Serving Size: ____________ *Serving Size:* ____________

LUNCH Time:

WAS AN ITEM EATEN AS A SNACK? WHICH? Time:

Protein:

- ☐ Chicken breast
- ☐ Beef
- ☐ Veal
- ☐ Shrimp
- ☐ Lobster
- ☐ White fish: ___________
- ☐ Protein Shake
- ☐ Other: ___________

Serving Size:

- ☐ 100 grams/3.5 oz
- ☐ Other: ___________

Calories: ___________

Vegetable:

- ☐ Asparagus
- ☐ Beet Greens
- ☐ Cabbage
- ☐ Celery
- ☐ Chard
- ☐ Cucumber
- ☐ Fennel
- ☐ Lettuce
- ☐ Onions
- ☐ Radishes
- ☐ Spinach
- ☐ Tomatoes
- ☐ Other: ___________
- ☐ Other: ___________
- ☐ Other: ___________

Calories: ___________

Fruit:

- ☐ Strawberries
- ☐ ½ Grapefruit
- ☐ Apple
- ☐ Orange
- ☐ Other: ___________

Starch:

- ☐ Grissini
- ☐ Melba
- ☐ Other: ___________

Calories: ___________

Other:

- ☐ TBS. Milk
- ☐ Juice of 1 Lemon
- ☐ Stevia
- ☐ Shirataki/Miracle Noodles
- ☐ Other: ___________
- ☐ Other: ___________
- ☐ Other: ___________

Calories: ___________

DINNER Time:

WAS AN ITEM EATEN AS A SNACK? WHICH? Time:

Protein:

- ☐ Chicken
- ☐ Beef
- ☐ Veal
- ☐ Shrimp
- ☐ Lobster
- ☐ White fish: ___________
- ☐ Protein Shake
- ☐ Other: ___________

Serving Size:

- ☐ 100 grams
- ☐ Other: ___________

Calories: ___________

Vegetable:

- ☐ Asparagus
- ☐ Beet Greens
- ☐ Cabbage
- ☐ Celery
- ☐ Chard
- ☐ Cucumber
- ☐ Fennel
- ☐ Lettuce
- ☐ Onions
- ☐ Radishes
- ☐ Spinach
- ☐ Tomatoes
- ☐ Other: ___________
- ☐ Other: ___________
- ☐ Other: ___________

Calories: ___________

Fruit:

- ☐ Strawberries
- ☐ ½ Grapefruit
- ☐ Apple
- ☐ Orange
- ☐ Other: ___________

Starch:

- ☐ Grissini
- ☐ Melba
- ☐ Other: ___________

Calories: ___________

Other:

- ☐ TBS. Milk
- ☐ Juice of 1 Lemon
- ☐ Stevia
- ☐ Shirataki/Miracle Noodles
- ☐ Other: ___________
- ☐ Other: ___________
- ☐ Other: ___________

Calories: ___________

HCGCHICA TIP:

Flavored Stevia Drops...

make everything better and can sometimes be the difference in you getting your water in or not. They can be used in sparkling water to make your own soda, in plain 'ol water, and on your fruits or P2 smoothies.

VLCD 35 (Date): ____________

WEIGHT: ____________

HCG DOSAGE: ____________

HUNGER LEVEL: ____________

BEDTIME/WAKE TIME: ____________

HOURS SLEEP: ____________

TOTAL CALORIES: ____________

SUPPLEMENTS: ____________

☐ Multivitamin ☐ B12 Shot ☐ Lipo Shot

INJECTION LOCATION

TIME: ________

☐ Belly ☐ Deltoid ☐ Thigh ☐ Other: ____________

LIQUIDS:

	LITERS
☐	4 LITERS
☐	3.5 LITERS
☐	3 LITERS
☐	2.5 LITERS
☐	2 LITERS
☐	1.5 LITERS
☐	1 LITER
☐	.5 LITERS

	OUNCES
☐	128 oz = 1 GALLON
☐	120 oz
☐	112 oz
☐	104 oz
☐	96 oz = 3 QUARTS
☐	88 oz
☐	80 oz
☐	72 oz
☐	64 oz = 2 QUARTS
☐	56 oz
☐	48 oz
☐	40 oz
☐	32 oz = 1 QUART
☐	24 oz
☐	16 oz
☐	8 oz = 1 CUP

DROPS / PELLETS DOSE TIMING

1st Dose: ____________ 2nd Dose: ____________

3rd Dose: ____________ 4th Dose: ____________

PERSONAL NOTES

BREAKFAST

Time:

☐ None ☐ Fruit: ____________ ☐ Protein: ____________ Calories: ____________

Serving Size: ____________ Serving Size: ____________

LUNCH Time :

WAS AN ITEM EATEN AS A SNACK? WHICH? Time:

Protein:

- ☐ Chicken breast
- ☐ Beef
- ☐ Veal
- ☐ Shrimp
- ☐ Lobster
- ☐ White fish: ___________
- ☐ Protein Shake
- ☐ Other: ___________

Serving Size:

- ☐ 100 grams/3.5 oz
- ☐ Other: ___________

Calories: ___________

Vegetable:

- ☐ Asparagus
- ☐ Beet Greens
- ☐ Cabbage
- ☐ Celery
- ☐ Chard
- ☐ Cucumber
- ☐ Fennel
- ☐ Lettuce
- ☐ Onions
- ☐ Radishes
- ☐ Spinach
- ☐ Tomatoes
- ☐ Other: ___________
- ☐ Other: ___________
- ☐ Other: ___________

Calories: ___________

Fruit:

- ☐ Strawberries
- ☐ ½ Grapefruit
- ☐ Apple
- ☐ Orange
- ☐ Other: ___________

Starch:

- ☐ Grissini
- ☐ Melba
- ☐ Other: ___________

Calories: ___________

Other:

- ☐ TBS. Milk
- ☐ Juice of 1 Lemon
- ☐ Stevia
- ☐ Shirataki/Miracle Noodles
- ☐ Other: ___________
- ☐ Other: ___________
- ☐ Other: ___________

Calories: ___________

DINNER Time :

WAS AN ITEM EATEN AS A SNACK? WHICH? Time:

Protein:

- ☐ Chicken
- ☐ Beef
- ☐ Veal
- ☐ Shrimp
- ☐ Lobster
- ☐ White fish: ___________
- ☐ Protein Shake
- ☐ Other: ___________

Serving Size:

- ☐ 100 grams
- ☐ Other: ___________

Calories: ___________

Vegetable:

- ☐ Asparagus
- ☐ Beet Greens
- ☐ Cabbage
- ☐ Celery
- ☐ Chard
- ☐ Cucumber
- ☐ Fennel
- ☐ Lettuce
- ☐ Onions
- ☐ Radishes
- ☐ Spinach
- ☐ Tomatoes
- ☐ Other: ___________
- ☐ Other: ___________
- ☐ Other: ___________

Calories: ___________

Fruit:

- ☐ Strawberries
- ☐ ½ Grapefruit
- ☐ Apple
- ☐ Orange
- ☐ Other: ___________

Starch:

- ☐ Grissini
- ☐ Melba
- ☐ Other: ___________

Calories: ___________

Other:

- ☐ TBS. Milk
- ☐ Juice of 1 Lemon
- ☐ Stevia
- ☐ Shirataki/Miracle Noodles
- ☐ Other: ___________
- ☐ Other: ___________
- ☐ Other: ___________

Calories: ___________

Reflections ON WEEK 5

REMEMBER, THIS IS NOT JUST ABOUT LOSING WEIGHT. IT'S ABOUT CHANGING YOUR WHOLE MINDSET ABOUT FOOD AND YOUR BODY.

YOU ARE BREAKING OLD PATTERNS RIGHT NOW. YOU ARE CREATING NEW PATTERNS. TRY NOT TO FOCUS YOUR PROGESS SOLELY ON WEIGHT LOSS.

SO WITH THAT IN MIND, HOW DID THIS WEEK GO?

What are you proud of? Why are you proud of it? What did you struggle with? What would you like to work on changing? What specific logical ways can you think of to make those adjustments? Or maybe you're just burned out at the moment - it's okay to just make it a rant.

Week 6

"I DID THEN WHAT I KNEW
how to do.
Now that I know better,
I do better."

- Maya Angelou

VLCD 36 (Date): ____________

Many people succeed when OTHERS do not believe in them. But rarely does a person succeed when he does NOT BELIEVE IN HIMSELF.

- Herb True

WEIGHT: ____________

HCG DOSAGE: ____________

HUNGER LEVEL: ____________

BEDTIME/WAKE TIME: ____________

HOURS SLEEP: ____________

TOTAL CALORIES: ____________

SUPPLEMENTS: ____________

☐ Multivitamin ☐ B12 Shot ☐ Lipo Shot

INJECTION LOCATION

TIME: ________

☐ Belly ☐ Deltoid ☐ Thigh ☐ Other: ____________

DROPS / PELLETS DOSE TIMING

1st Dose: ____________ 2nd Dose: ____________

3rd Dose: ____________ 4th Dose: ____________

LIQUIDS:

4 LITERS
3.5 LITERS
3 LITERS
2.5 LITERS
2 LITERS
1.5 LITERS
1 LITER
.5 LITERS

128 oz = 1 GALLON
120 oz
112 oz
104 oz
96 oz = 3 QUARTS
88 oz
80 oz
72 oz
64 oz = 2 QUARTS
56 oz
48 oz
40 oz
32 oz = 1 QUART
24 oz
16 oz
8 oz = 1 CUP

PERSONAL NOTES

BREAKFAST

Time:

☐ None ☐ Fruit: ____________ ☐ Protein: ____________ Calories: ____________

Serving Size: ____________ Serving Size: ____________

LUNCH Time :

WAS AN ITEM EATEN AS A SNACK? WHICH? Time:

Protein:

- [ ] Chicken breast
- [ ] Beef
- [ ] Veal
- [ ] Shrimp
- [ ] Lobster
- [ ] White fish: ___________
- [ ] Protein Shake
- [ ] Other: ___________

Serving Size:

- [ ] 100 grams/3.5 oz
- [ ] Other: ___________

Calories: ___________

Vegetable:

- [ ] Asparagus
- [ ] Beet Greens
- [ ] Cabbage
- [ ] Celery
- [ ] Chard
- [ ] Cucumber
- [ ] Fennel
- [ ] Lettuce
- [ ] Onions
- [ ] Radishes
- [ ] Spinach
- [ ] Tomatoes
- [ ] Other: ___________
- [ ] Other: ___________
- [ ] Other: ___________

Calories: ___________

Fruit:

- [ ] Strawberries
- [ ] ½ Grapefruit
- [ ] Apple
- [ ] Orange
- [ ] Other: ___________

Starch:

- [ ] Grissini
- [ ] Melba
- [ ] Other: ___________

Calories: ___________

Other:

- [ ] TBS. Milk
- [ ] Juice of 1 Lemon
- [ ] Stevia
- [ ] Shirataki/Miracle Noodles
- [ ] Other: ___________
- [ ] Other: ___________
- [ ] Other: ___________

Calories: ___________

DINNER Time :

WAS AN ITEM EATEN AS A SNACK? WHICH? Time:

Protein:

- [ ] Chicken
- [ ] Beef
- [ ] Veal
- [ ] Shrimp
- [ ] Lobster
- [ ] White fish: ___________
- [ ] Protein Shake
- [ ] Other: ___________

Serving Size:

- [ ] 100 grams
- [ ] Other: ___________

Calories: ___________

Vegetable:

- [ ] Asparagus
- [ ] Beet Greens
- [ ] Cabbage
- [ ] Celery
- [ ] Chard
- [ ] Cucumber
- [ ] Fennel
- [ ] Lettuce
- [ ] Onions
- [ ] Radishes
- [ ] Spinach
- [ ] Tomatoes
- [ ] Other: ___________
- [ ] Other: ___________
- [ ] Other: ___________

Calories: ___________

Fruit:

- [ ] Strawberries
- [ ] ½ Grapefruit
- [ ] Apple
- [ ] Orange
- [ ] Other: ___________

Starch:

- [ ] Grissini
- [ ] Melba
- [ ] Other: ___________

Calories: ___________

Other:

- [ ] TBS. Milk
- [ ] Juice of 1 Lemon
- [ ] Stevia
- [ ] Shirataki/Miracle Noodles
- [ ] Other: ___________
- [ ] Other: ___________
- [ ] Other: ___________

Calories: ___________

VLCD 37 (Date): ____________

FELLOW HCGER TIP:

Shrimp WITH AN Orange Twist

Saute onion and garlic, add shrimp and cook just until turns pink. Eat with P2 orange slices.

WEIGHT: ____________

HCG DOSAGE: ____________

HUNGER LEVEL: ____________

BEDTIME/WAKE TIME: ____________

HOURS SLEEP: ____________

TOTAL CALORIES: ____________

SUPPLEMENTS: ____________

☐ Multivitamin ☐ B12 Shot ☐ Lipo Shot

INJECTION LOCATION

TIME: ________

☐ Belly ☐ Deltoid ☐ Thigh ☐ Other: ____________

DROPS / PELLETS DOSE TIMING

1st Dose: ____________ 2nd Dose: ____________

3rd Dose: ____________ 4th Dose: ____________

LIQUIDS:

4 LITERS
3.5 LITERS
3 LITERS
2.5 LITERS
2 LITERS
1.5 LITERS
1 LITER
.5 LITERS

128 oz = 1 GALLON
120 oz
112 oz
104 oz
96 oz = 3 QUARTS
88 oz
80 oz
72 oz
64 oz = 2 QUARTS
56 oz
48 oz
40 oz
32 oz = 1 QUART
24 oz
16 oz
8 oz = 1 CUP

PERSONAL NOTES

BREAKFAST

Time:

☐ None ☐ Fruit: ____________ ☐ Protein: ____________ Calories: ____________

Serving Size: ____________ Serving Size: ____________

LUNCH Time:

WAS AN ITEM EATEN AS A SNACK? WHICH? Time:

Protein:

- ☐ Chicken breast
- ☐ Beef
- ☐ Veal
- ☐ Shrimp
- ☐ Lobster
- ☐ White fish: ____________
- ☐ Protein Shake
- ☐ Other: ____________

Serving Size:

- ☐ 100 grams/3.5 oz
- ☐ Other: ____________

Calories: ____________

Vegetable:

- ☐ Asparagus
- ☐ Beet Greens
- ☐ Cabbage
- ☐ Celery
- ☐ Chard
- ☐ Cucumber
- ☐ Fennel
- ☐ Lettuce
- ☐ Onions
- ☐ Radishes
- ☐ Spinach
- ☐ Tomatoes
- ☐ Other: ____________
- ☐ Other: ____________
- ☐ Other: ____________

Calories: ____________

Fruit:

- ☐ Strawberries
- ☐ ½ Grapefruit
- ☐ Apple
- ☐ Orange
- ☐ Other: ____________

Starch:

- ☐ Grissini
- ☐ Melba
- ☐ Other: ____________

Calories: ____________

Other:

- ☐ TBS. Milk
- ☐ Juice of 1 Lemon
- ☐ Stevia
- ☐ Shirataki/Miracle Noodles
- ☐ Other: ____________
- ☐ Other: ____________
- ☐ Other: ____________

Calories: ____________

DINNER Time:

WAS AN ITEM EATEN AS A SNACK? WHICH? Time:

Protein:

- ☐ Chicken
- ☐ Beef
- ☐ Veal
- ☐ Shrimp
- ☐ Lobster
- ☐ White fish: ____________
- ☐ Protein Shake
- ☐ Other: ____________

Serving Size:

- ☐ 100 grams
- ☐ Other: ____________

Calories: ____________

Vegetable:

- ☐ Asparagus
- ☐ Beet Greens
- ☐ Cabbage
- ☐ Celery
- ☐ Chard
- ☐ Cucumber
- ☐ Fennel
- ☐ Lettuce
- ☐ Onions
- ☐ Radishes
- ☐ Spinach
- ☐ Tomatoes
- ☐ Other: ____________
- ☐ Other: ____________
- ☐ Other: ____________

Calories: ____________

Fruit:

- ☐ Strawberries
- ☐ ½ Grapefruit
- ☐ Apple
- ☐ Orange
- ☐ Other: ____________

Starch:

- ☐ Grissini
- ☐ Melba
- ☐ Other: ____________

Calories: ____________

Other:

- ☐ TBS. Milk
- ☐ Juice of 1 Lemon
- ☐ Stevia
- ☐ Shirataki/Miracle Noodles
- ☐ Other: ____________
- ☐ Other: ____________
- ☐ Other: ____________

Calories: ____________

Failure should be our **TEACHER**, not our undertaker. Failure is **DELAY, NOT DEFEAT.** It is a *temporary* detour, **NOT A DEAD END.** Failure is something we can *avoid only by* saying nothing, doing nothing, and being nothing

- Denis Waitley

VLCD 38 (Date): ____________

WEIGHT: ____________

HCG DOSAGE: ____________

HUNGER LEVEL: ____________

BEDTIME/WAKE TIME: ____________

HOURS SLEEP: ____________

TOTAL CALORIES: ____________

SUPPLEMENTS: ____________

☐ Multivitamin ☐ B12 Shot ☐ Lipo Shot

INJECTION LOCATION

TIME: ________

☐ Belly ☐ Deltoid ☐ Thigh ☐ Other: ____________

DROPS / PELLETS DOSE TIMING

1st Dose: ____________ 2nd Dose: ____________

3rd Dose: ____________ 4th Dose: ____________

LIQUIDS:

	4 LITERS
	3.5 LITERS
	3 LITERS
	2.5 LITERS
	2 LITERS
	1.5 LITERS
	1 LITER
	.5 LITERS

	128 oz = 1 GALLON
	120 oz
	112 oz
	104 oz
	96 oz = 3 QUARTS
	88 oz
	80 oz
	72 oz
	64 oz = 2 QUARTS
	56 oz
	48 oz
	40 oz
	32 oz = 1 QUART
	24 oz
	16 oz
	8 oz = 1 CUP

PERSONAL NOTES

BREAKFAST

Time:

☐ None ☐ Fruit: ____________ ☐ Protein: ____________ Calories: ____________

Serving Size: ____________ Serving Size: ____________

LUNCH Time:

WAS AN ITEM EATEN AS A SNACK? WHICH? Time:

Protein:

- ☐ Chicken breast
- ☐ Beef
- ☐ Veal
- ☐ Shrimp
- ☐ Lobster
- ☐ White fish: ___________
- ☐ Protein Shake
- ☐ Other: ___________

Serving Size:

- ☐ 100 grams/3.5 oz
- ☐ Other: ___________

Calories: ___________

Vegetable:

- ☐ Asparagus
- ☐ Beet Greens
- ☐ Cabbage
- ☐ Celery
- ☐ Chard
- ☐ Cucumber
- ☐ Fennel
- ☐ Lettuce
- ☐ Onions
- ☐ Radishes
- ☐ Spinach
- ☐ Tomatoes
- ☐ Other: ___________
- ☐ Other: ___________
- ☐ Other: ___________

Calories: ___________

Fruit:

- ☐ Strawberries
- ☐ ½ Grapefruit
- ☐ Apple
- ☐ Orange
- ☐ Other: ___________

Starch:

- ☐ Grissini
- ☐ Melba
- ☐ Other: ___________

Calories: ___________

Other:

- ☐ TBS. Milk
- ☐ Juice of 1 Lemon
- ☐ Stevia
- ☐ Shirataki/Miracle Noodles
- ☐ Other: ___________
- ☐ Other: ___________
- ☐ Other: ___________

Calories: ___________

DINNER Time:

WAS AN ITEM EATEN AS A SNACK? WHICH? Time:

Protein:

- ☐ Chicken
- ☐ Beef
- ☐ Veal
- ☐ Shrimp
- ☐ Lobster
- ☐ White fish: ___________
- ☐ Protein Shake
- ☐ Other: ___________

Serving Size:

- ☐ 100 grams
- ☐ Other: ___________

Calories: ___________

Vegetable:

- ☐ Asparagus
- ☐ Beet Greens
- ☐ Cabbage
- ☐ Celery
- ☐ Chard
- ☐ Cucumber
- ☐ Fennel
- ☐ Lettuce
- ☐ Onions
- ☐ Radishes
- ☐ Spinach
- ☐ Tomatoes
- ☐ Other: ___________
- ☐ Other: ___________
- ☐ Other: ___________

Calories: ___________

Fruit:

- ☐ Strawberries
- ☐ ½ Grapefruit
- ☐ Apple
- ☐ Orange
- ☐ Other: ___________

Starch:

- ☐ Grissini
- ☐ Melba
- ☐ Other: ___________

Calories: ___________

Other:

- ☐ TBS. Milk
- ☐ Juice of 1 Lemon
- ☐ Stevia
- ☐ Shirataki/Miracle Noodles
- ☐ Other: ___________
- ☐ Other: ___________
- ☐ Other: ___________

Calories: ___________

VLCD 39 (Date): ______________

FELLOW HCGER TIP:

Pre-frozen Lunch Bowls

Vicky says, "I make a huge batch of chicken and veggie soup at the beginning of every round and freeze in bowls. This way on the days I don't have time to fix a meal for work, I grab a bowl and it thaws by lunch time.

WEIGHT: ______________

HCG DOSAGE: ______________

HUNGER LEVEL: ______________

BEDTIME/WAKE TIME: ______________

HOURS SLEEP: ______________

TOTAL CALORIES: ______________

SUPPLEMENTS: ______________

☐ Multivitamin ☐ B12 Shot ☐ Lipo Shot

INJECTION LOCATION

TIME: ________

☐ Belly ☐ Deltoid ☐ Thigh ☐ Other: ____________

DROPS / PELLETS DOSE TIMING

1st Dose: ____________ 2nd Dose: ____________

3rd Dose: ____________ 4th Dose: ____________

LIQUIDS:

	4 LITERS
	3.5 LITERS
	3 LITERS
	2.5 LITERS
	2 LITERS
	1.5 LITERS
	1 LITER
	.5 LITERS

	128 oz = 1 GALLON
	120 oz
	112 oz
	104 oz
	96 oz = 3 QUARTS
	88 oz
	80 oz
	72 oz
	64 oz = 2 QUARTS
	56 oz
	48 oz
	40 oz
	32 oz = 1 QUART
	24 oz
	16 oz
	8 oz = 1 CUP

PERSONAL NOTES

BREAKFAST

Time:

☐ None ☐ Fruit: ____________ ☐ Protein: ____________ Calories: ____________

Serving Size: ____________ Serving Size: ____________

LUNCH Time :

WAS AN ITEM EATEN AS A SNACK? WHICH? Time:

Protein:

- [ ] Chicken breast
- [ ] Beef
- [ ] Veal
- [ ] Shrimp
- [ ] Lobster
- [ ] White fish: ___________
- [ ] Protein Shake
- [ ] Other: ___________

Serving Size:

- [ ] 100 grams/3.5 oz
- [ ] Other: ___________

Calories: ___________

Vegetable:

- [ ] Asparagus
- [ ] Beet Greens
- [ ] Cabbage
- [ ] Celery
- [ ] Chard
- [ ] Cucumber
- [ ] Fennel
- [ ] Lettuce
- [ ] Onions
- [ ] Radishes
- [ ] Spinach
- [ ] Tomatoes
- [ ] Other: ___________
- [ ] Other: ___________
- [ ] Other: ___________

Calories: ___________

Fruit:

- [ ] Strawberries
- [ ] ½ Grapefruit
- [ ] Apple
- [ ] Orange
- [ ] Other: ___________

Starch:

- [ ] Grissini
- [ ] Melba
- [ ] Other: ___________

Calories: ___________

Other:

- [ ] TBS. Milk
- [ ] Juice of 1 Lemon
- [ ] Stevia
- [ ] Shirataki/Miracle Noodles
- [ ] Other: ___________
- [ ] Other: ___________
- [ ] Other: ___________

Calories: ___________

DINNER Time :

WAS AN ITEM EATEN AS A SNACK? WHICH? Time:

Protein:

- [ ] Chicken
- [ ] Beef
- [ ] Veal
- [ ] Shrimp
- [ ] Lobster
- [ ] White fish: ___________
- [ ] Protein Shake
- [ ] Other: ___________

Serving Size:

- [ ] 100 grams
- [ ] Other: ___________

Calories: ___________

Vegetable:

- [ ] Asparagus
- [ ] Beet Greens
- [ ] Cabbage
- [ ] Celery
- [ ] Chard
- [ ] Cucumber
- [ ] Fennel
- [ ] Lettuce
- [ ] Onions
- [ ] Radishes
- [ ] Spinach
- [ ] Tomatoes
- [ ] Other: ___________
- [ ] Other: ___________
- [ ] Other: ___________

Calories: ___________

Fruit:

- [ ] Strawberries
- [ ] ½ Grapefruit
- [ ] Apple
- [ ] Orange
- [ ] Other: ___________

Starch:

- [ ] Grissini
- [ ] Melba
- [ ] Other: ___________

Calories: ___________

Other:

- [ ] TBS. Milk
- [ ] Juice of 1 Lemon
- [ ] Stevia
- [ ] Shirataki/Miracle Noodles
- [ ] Other: ___________
- [ ] Other: ___________
- [ ] Other: ___________

Calories: ___________

VLCD 40 (Date): ____________

WEIGHT: ____________

HCG DOSAGE: ____________

HUNGER LEVEL: ____________

BEDTIME/WAKE TIME: ____________

HOURS SLEEP: ____________

TOTAL CALORIES: ____________

SUPPLEMENTS: ____________

☐ Multivitamin ☐ B12 Shot ☐ Lipo Shot

Whenever you find yourself on the SIDE OF THE MAJORITY, it is time to PAUSE and reflect.

- Mark Twain

INJECTION LOCATION

TIME: ________

☐ Belly ☐ Deltoid ☐ Thigh ☐ Other: ____________

DROPS / PELLETS DOSE TIMING

1st Dose: ____________ 2nd Dose: ____________

3rd Dose: ____________ 4th Dose: ____________

LIQUIDS:

Liters
4 LITERS
3.5 LITERS
3 LITERS
2.5 LITERS
2 LITERS
1.5 LITERS
1 LITER
.5 LITERS

Ounces
128 oz = 1 GALLON
120 oz
112 oz
104 oz
96 oz = 3 QUARTS
88 oz
80 oz
72 oz
64 oz = 2 QUARTS
56 oz
48 oz
40 oz
32 oz = 1 QUART
24 oz
16 oz
8 oz = 1 CUP

PERSONAL NOTES

BREAKFAST

Time:

☐ None ☐ Fruit: ____________ ☐ Protein: ____________ Calories: ____________

Serving Size: ____________ Serving Size: ____________

LUNCH Time :

WAS AN ITEM EATEN AS A SNACK? WHICH? Time:

Protein:

- ☐ Chicken breast
- ☐ Beef
- ☐ Veal
- ☐ Shrimp
- ☐ Lobster
- ☐ White fish: ___________
- ☐ Protein Shake
- ☐ Other: ___________

Serving Size:

- ☐ 100 grams/3.5 oz
- ☐ Other: ___________

Calories: ___________

Vegetable:

- ☐ Asparagus
- ☐ Beet Greens
- ☐ Cabbage
- ☐ Celery
- ☐ Chard
- ☐ Cucumber
- ☐ Fennel
- ☐ Lettuce
- ☐ Onions
- ☐ Radishes
- ☐ Spinach
- ☐ Tomatoes
- ☐ Other: ___________
- ☐ Other: ___________
- ☐ Other: ___________

Calories: ___________

Fruit:

- ☐ Strawberries
- ☐ ½ Grapefruit
- ☐ Apple
- ☐ Orange
- ☐ Other: ___________

Starch:

- ☐ Grissini
- ☐ Melba
- ☐ Other: ___________

Calories: ___________

Other:

- ☐ TBS. Milk
- ☐ Juice of 1 Lemon
- ☐ Stevia
- ☐ Shirataki/Miracle Noodles
- ☐ Other: ___________
- ☐ Other: ___________
- ☐ Other: ___________

Calories: ___________

DINNER Time :

WAS AN ITEM EATEN AS A SNACK? WHICH? Time:

Protein:

- ☐ Chicken
- ☐ Beef
- ☐ Veal
- ☐ Shrimp
- ☐ Lobster
- ☐ White fish: ___________
- ☐ Protein Shake
- ☐ Other: ___________

Serving Size:

- ☐ 100 grams
- ☐ Other: ___________

Calories: ___________

Vegetable:

- ☐ Asparagus
- ☐ Beet Greens
- ☐ Cabbage
- ☐ Celery
- ☐ Chard
- ☐ Cucumber
- ☐ Fennel
- ☐ Lettuce
- ☐ Onions
- ☐ Radishes
- ☐ Spinach
- ☐ Tomatoes
- ☐ Other: ___________
- ☐ Other: ___________
- ☐ Other: ___________

Calories: ___________

Fruit:

- ☐ Strawberries
- ☐ ½ Grapefruit
- ☐ Apple
- ☐ Orange
- ☐ Other: ___________

Starch:

- ☐ Grissini
- ☐ Melba
- ☐ Other: ___________

Calories: ___________

Other:

- ☐ TBS. Milk
- ☐ Juice of 1 Lemon
- ☐ Stevia
- ☐ Shirataki/Miracle Noodles
- ☐ Other: ___________
- ☐ Other: ___________
- ☐ Other: ___________

Calories: ___________

VLCD 41 (Date): ____________

FELLOW HCGER TIP:

"Apple Pie"

Slice an apple into tiny slices and put in a microwaveable dish. Add apple pie spice. Cover with a paper towel and microwave for 3 minutes.

WEIGHT: ____________

HCG DOSAGE: ____________

HUNGER LEVEL: ____________

BEDTIME/WAKE TIME: ____________

HOURS SLEEP: ____________

TOTAL CALORIES: ____________

SUPPLEMENTS: ____________

☐ Multivitamin ☐ B12 Shot ☐ Lipo Shot

INJECTION LOCATION

TIME: ________

☐ Belly ☐ Deltoid ☐ Thigh ☐ Other: ____________

DROPS / PELLETS DOSE TIMING

1st Dose: ____________ 2nd Dose: ____________

3rd Dose: ____________ 4th Dose: ____________

LIQUIDS:

	4 LITERS
	3.5 LITERS
	3 LITERS
	2.5 LITERS
	2 LITERS
	1.5 LITERS
	1 LITER
	.5 LITERS

	128 oz = 1 GALLON
	120 oz
	112 oz
	104 oz
	96 oz = 3 QUARTS
	88 oz
	80 oz
	72 oz
	64 oz = 2 QUARTS
	56 oz
	48 oz
	40 oz
	32 oz = 1 QUART
	24 oz
	16 oz
	8 oz = 1 CUP

PERSONAL NOTES

BREAKFAST

Time:

☐ None ☐ Fruit: ____________ ☐ Protein: ____________ Calories: ____________

Serving Size: ____________ Serving Size: ____________

LUNCH Time:

WAS AN ITEM EATEN AS A SNACK? WHICH? Time:

Protein:

- [ ] Chicken breast
- [ ] Beef
- [ ] Veal
- [ ] Shrimp
- [ ] Lobster
- [ ] White fish: ________
- [ ] Protein Shake
- [ ] Other: ________

Serving Size:

- [ ] 100 grams/3.5 oz
- [ ] Other: ________

Calories: ________

Vegetable:

- [ ] Asparagus
- [ ] Beet Greens
- [ ] Cabbage
- [ ] Celery
- [ ] Chard
- [ ] Cucumber
- [ ] Fennel
- [ ] Lettuce
- [ ] Onions
- [ ] Radishes
- [ ] Spinach
- [ ] Tomatoes
- [ ] Other: ________
- [ ] Other: ________
- [ ] Other: ________

Calories: ________

Fruit:

- [ ] Strawberries
- [ ] ½ Grapefruit
- [ ] Apple
- [ ] Orange
- [ ] Other: ________

Starch:

- [ ] Grissini
- [ ] Melba
- [ ] Other: ________

Calories: ________

Other:

- [ ] TBS. Milk
- [ ] Juice of 1 Lemon
- [ ] Stevia
- [ ] Shirataki/Miracle Noodles
- [ ] Other: ________
- [ ] Other: ________
- [ ] Other: ________

Calories: ________

DINNER Time:

WAS AN ITEM EATEN AS A SNACK? WHICH? Time:

Protein:

- [ ] Chicken
- [ ] Beef
- [ ] Veal
- [ ] Shrimp
- [ ] Lobster
- [ ] White fish: ________
- [ ] Protein Shake
- [ ] Other: ________

Serving Size:

- [ ] 100 grams
- [ ] Other: ________

Calories: ________

Vegetable:

- [ ] Asparagus
- [ ] Beet Greens
- [ ] Cabbage
- [ ] Celery
- [ ] Chard
- [ ] Cucumber
- [ ] Fennel
- [ ] Lettuce
- [ ] Onions
- [ ] Radishes
- [ ] Spinach
- [ ] Tomatoes
- [ ] Other: ________
- [ ] Other: ________
- [ ] Other: ________

Calories: ________

Fruit:

- [ ] Strawberries
- [ ] ½ Grapefruit
- [ ] Apple
- [ ] Orange
- [ ] Other: ________

Starch:

- [ ] Grissini
- [ ] Melba
- [ ] Other: ________

Calories: ________

Other:

- [ ] TBS. Milk
- [ ] Juice of 1 Lemon
- [ ] Stevia
- [ ] Shirataki/Miracle Noodles
- [ ] Other: ________
- [ ] Other: ________
- [ ] Other: ________

Calories: ________

Change
is **HARDEST**
at the beginning,
messiest in the **MIDDLE**
and **BEST AT THE END.**
- Robin S. Sharma

VLCD 42 (Date): ______

WEIGHT: ______

HCG DOSAGE: ______

HUNGER LEVEL: ______

BEDTIME/WAKE TIME: ______

HOURS SLEEP: ______

TOTAL CALORIES: ______

SUPPLEMENTS: ______

☐ Multivitamin ☐ B12 Shot ☐ Lipo Shot

INJECTION LOCATION

TIME: ______

☐ Belly ☐ Deltoid ☐ Thigh ☐ Other: ______

DROPS / PELLETS DOSE TIMING

1st Dose: ______ 2nd Dose: ______

3rd Dose: ______ 4th Dose: ______

LIQUIDS:

4 LITERS
3.5 LITERS
3 LITERS
2.5 LITERS
2 LITERS
1.5 LITERS
1 LITER
.5 LITERS

128 OZ = 1 GALLON
120 OZ
112 OZ
104 OZ
96 OZ = 3 QUARTS
88 OZ
80 OZ
72 OZ
64 OZ = 2 QUARTS
56 OZ
48 OZ
40 OZ
32 OZ = 1 QUART
24 OZ
16 OZ
8 OZ = 1 CUP

PERSONAL NOTES

BREAKFAST

Time:

☐ None ☐ Fruit: ______ ☐ Protein: ______ Calories: ______

Serving Size: ______ Serving Size: ______

LUNCH Time:

WAS AN ITEM EATEN AS A SNACK? WHICH? Time:

Protein:

- [ ] Chicken breast
- [ ] Beef
- [ ] Veal
- [ ] Shrimp
- [ ] Lobster
- [ ] White fish: ___________
- [ ] Protein Shake
- [ ] Other: ___________

Serving Size:

- [ ] 100 grams/3.5 oz
- [ ] Other: ___________

Calories: ___________

Vegetable:

- [ ] Asparagus
- [ ] Beet Greens
- [ ] Cabbage
- [ ] Celery
- [ ] Chard
- [ ] Cucumber
- [ ] Fennel
- [ ] Lettuce
- [ ] Onions
- [ ] Radishes
- [ ] Spinach
- [ ] Tomatoes
- [ ] Other: ___________
- [ ] Other: ___________
- [ ] Other: ___________

Calories: ___________

Fruit:

- [ ] Strawberries
- [ ] ½ Grapefruit
- [ ] Apple
- [ ] Orange
- [ ] Other: ___________

Starch:

- [ ] Grissini
- [ ] Melba
- [ ] Other: ___________

Calories: ___________

Other:

- [ ] TBS. Milk
- [ ] Juice of 1 Lemon
- [ ] Stevia
- [ ] Shirataki/Miracle Noodles
- [ ] Other: ___________
- [ ] Other: ___________
- [ ] Other: ___________

Calories: ___________

DINNER Time:

WAS AN ITEM EATEN AS A SNACK? WHICH? Time:

Protein:

- [ ] Chicken
- [ ] Beef
- [ ] Veal
- [ ] Shrimp
- [ ] Lobster
- [ ] White fish: ___________
- [ ] Protein Shake
- [ ] Other: ___________

Serving Size:

- [ ] 100 grams
- [ ] Other: ___________

Calories: ___________

Vegetable:

- [ ] Asparagus
- [ ] Beet Greens
- [ ] Cabbage
- [ ] Celery
- [ ] Chard
- [ ] Cucumber
- [ ] Fennel
- [ ] Lettuce
- [ ] Onions
- [ ] Radishes
- [ ] Spinach
- [ ] Tomatoes
- [ ] Other: ___________
- [ ] Other: ___________
- [ ] Other: ___________

Calories: ___________

Fruit:

- [ ] Strawberries
- [ ] ½ Grapefruit
- [ ] Apple
- [ ] Orange
- [ ] Other: ___________

Starch:

- [ ] Grissini
- [ ] Melba
- [ ] Other: ___________

Calories: ___________

Other:

- [ ] TBS. Milk
- [ ] Juice of 1 Lemon
- [ ] Stevia
- [ ] Shirataki/Miracle Noodles
- [ ] Other: ___________
- [ ] Other: ___________
- [ ] Other: ___________

Calories: ___________

Reflections ON WEEK 6

REMEMBER, THIS IS NOT JUST ABOUT LOSING WEIGHT. IT'S ABOUT CHANGING YOUR WHOLE MINDSET ABOUT FOOD AND YOUR BODY.

YOU ARE BREAKING OLD PATTERNS RIGHT NOW. YOU ARE CREATING NEW PATTERNS. TRY NOT TO FOCUS YOUR PROGESS SOLELY ON WEIGHT LOSS.

SO WITH THAT IN MIND, HOW DID THIS WEEK GO?

What are you proud of? Why are you proud of it? What did you struggle with? What would you like to work on changing? What specific logical ways can you think of to make those adjustments? Or maybe you're just burned out at the moment - it's okay to just make it a rant.

Reflections ON THIS ROUND

WRITE DOWN 1 MAJOR BREAKTHROUGH YOU HAD.

Breakthrough:

WHAT DID YOU LEARN ABOUT YOURSELF?

Learned:

Reflections ON THIS ROUND

WHAT DO YOU THINK IS THE CAUSE OF ANY STRUGGLES YOU EXPERIENCED? WHAT DO YOU THINK COULD PREVENT THEM NEXT TIME?

Preventing Struggles:

SETTING A GOAL IS NOT THE MAIN THING. IT IS DECIDING HOW YOU WILL GO ABOUT ACHIEVING IT AND STAYING WITH THAT PLAN.

-Tom Landry

It's time for Phase 3 isn't it?
Remember, no need to panic. Gather information so you know what to expect and can form your own personal plan.
Free resource: hcgchica.com/p3
Paid resource: P3 & P4 Workbook at
hcgchica.com/p3workbook

Section 3

CALORIE COUNT CHARTS – Phase 2

Fruits

Quick Glance **MACRO BREAKDOWN**

	SERVING SIZE	INCHES	CALORIES	GRAMS SUGAR	GRAMS FIBER
APPLE	SMALL	2.75	80	16	4
	MEDIUM	3	93	19	4
	LARGE	3.3	120	24	6
ORANGE	SMALL	2.4	45	9	2
	MEDIUM	2.6	62	12	3
	LARGE	3.1	86	17	4
STRAWBERRIES	1/2 CUP		25	3.5	1.5
	1 CUP		49	7	3
	1.5 CUPS		75	10.5	4.5
1/2 GRAPEFRUIT	1/2 MED		41	9	2
	1/2 LARGE		53	11	2
OTHER:					
OTHER:					

Info below based on meat being weighed raw.

Beef

	SERVING SIZE GRAMS	OZ	CALORIES	GRAMS PROTEIN	GRAMS FAT
95% FAT FREE GROUND BEEF	50	1.7	68	11	3
	100	3.5	136	21	5
	150	5.2	204	32	8
LONDON BROIL	50	1.7	61	11	2
	100	3.5	123	21	4
	150	5.2	184	32	5
TOP SIRLOIN STEAK	50	1.7	68	11	2
	100	3.5	136	23	4
	150	5.2	204	34	6
OTHER:					
OTHER:					
OTHER:					
VEAL, GROUND	50	1.7	72	10	3
	100	3.5	144	19	7
	150	5.2	216	29	10
VEAL, LOIN, LEAN	50	1.7	58	10	2
	100	3.5	116	20	3
	150	5.2	174	30	5
VEAL, SIRLOIN, LEAN	50	1.7	55	10	1
	100	3.5	110	20	3
	150	5.2	165	30	4

Chicken & Other

	SERVING SIZE GRAMS	OZ	CALORIES	GRAMS PROTEIN	GRAMS FAT
CHICKEN BREAST	50	1.7	55	12	0.6
	100	3.5	110	23	1
	150	5.2	165	35	2
1 EGG + 3 EGG WHITES			123	17	5
EGG WHITES	50	1.7	26	5	0
	100	3.5	52	11	0
	150	5.2	78	16	0

	SERVING SIZE GRAMS	OZ	CALORIES	GRAMS PROTEIN	GRAMS FAT
COTTAGE CHEESE FAT FREE	50	1.7	36	5	0
	100	3.5	72	10	0
	150	5.2	108	15	0
OTHER:					
OTHER:					
OTHER:					
OTHER:					
OTHER:					

OFF PROTOCOL Proteins

	SERVING SIZE GRAMS	OZ	CALORIES	GRAMS PROTEIN	GRAMS FAT
97% FAT FREE HAM	50	1.7	54	8	2
	100	3.5	107	16	4
	150	5.2	161	24	5
99% FAT FREE GROUND TURKEY	50	1.7	56	12	1
	100	3.5	112	24	2
	150	5.2	168	35	3
WATER PACKED TUNA	50	1.7	64	12	2
	100	3.5	128	24	3
	150	5.2	192	35	4
OTHER:					
OTHER:					
OTHER:					

Seafood

	SERVING SIZE GRAMS	OZ	CALORIES	GRAMS PROTEIN	GRAMS FAT
CATFISH, FARMED	50	1.7	67	8	4
	100	3.5	135	16	8
	150	5.2	202	24	12
CATFISH, WILD	50	1.7	48	8	1
	100	3.5	95	16	3
	150	5.2	143	25	4
COD	50	1.7	41	9	0
	100	3.5	82	18	1
	150	5.2	123	27	1
CRAB, CANNED, DRAINED	50	1.7	42	9	0
	100	3.5	83	18	1
	150	5.2	125	27	1
FLOUNDER	50	1.7	35	6	1
	100	3.5	70	12	2
	150	5.2	105	18	2.5
HALIBUT	50	1.7	55	10	1
	100	3.5	110	21	2
	150	5.2	165	31	3
LOBSTER	50	1.7	45	9	0
	100	3.5	90	19	1
	150	5.2	135	28	1
RED SNAPPER	50	1.7	45	9.5	0
	100	3.5	89	19	1
	150	5.2	134	28	1.6
SEA BASS	50	1.7	49	9	1
	100	3.5	97	18	2
	150	5.2	146	28	3
SHRIMP, WITH SHELL	50	1.7	35	7	0
	100	3.5	70	14	1
	150	5.2	105	21	2
SHRIMP, NO SHELL	50	1.7	53	10	1
	100	3.5	106	20	2
	150	5.2	159	30	3
SOLE	50	1.7	45	9	0
	100	3.5	89	18	1
	150	5.2	137	27	1.5
TILAPIA	50	1.7	48	10	1
	100	3.5	96	20	2
	150	5.2	144	30	3
TROUT, SKINLESS	50	1.7	47	8	1
	100	3.5	94	16	2
	150	5.2	141	24	3

Quick Glance MACRO BREAKDOWN

Veggies

	SERVING SIZE	CALORIES	GRAMS TOTAL CARBS	GRAMS FIBER	NET CARBS
ASPARAGUS	1/2 CUP	14	3	1	1
	1 CUP	27	5	3	2
	1.5 CUPS	41	8	4	4
	2 CUPS	54	10	6	5
BEET GREENS	1/2 CUP	4	1	1	0
	1 CUP	8	2	1	0
	1.5 CUPS	12	2	2	0
	2 CUPS	16	3	3	0
CABBAGE	1/2 CUP	11	3	1	2
	1 CUP	22	5	2	3
	1.5 CUPS	33	8	3	5
	2 CUPS	44	10	4	6
CABBAGE, NAPA	1/2 CUP	6	1	0	1
	1 CUP	12	3	1	2
	1.5 CUPS	18	4	1	2
	2 CUPS	24	5	2	3
CABBAGE, RED	1/2 CUP	14	3	1	2
	1 CUP	28	7	2	5
	1.5 CUPS	42	10	3	7
	2 CUPS	56	13	4	9
CELERY	1/2 CUP	8	2	1	1
	1 CUP	16	3	2	1
	1.5 CUPS	24	5	2	2
	2 CUPS	32	6	3	3
CHARD	1/2 CUP	4	7	0	0
	1 CUP	7	1	1	1
	1.5 CUPS	11	2	1	1
	2 CUPS	14	3	1	1

Quick Glance MACRO BREAKDOWN

Veggies

	SERVING SIZE	CALORIES	GRAMS TOTAL CARBS	GRAMS FIBER	NET CARBS
CUCUMBER, PEELED	1/2 CUP	7	1	0	1
	1 CUP	14	3	2	2
	1.5 CUPS	21	4	1	3
	2 CUPS	28	5	2	3
CUCUMBER, WITH PEEL	1/2 CUP	8	2	0	2
	1 CUP	16	4	0	3
	1.5 CUPS	24	6	1	4
	2 CUPS	32	8	1	6
FENNEL	1/2 CUP	14	3	1	2
	1 CUP	27	6	3	4
	1.5 CUPS	41	9	4	5
	2 CUPS	54	13	5	7
LETTUCE, ROMAINE & ICEBERG	1/2 CUP	4	1	1	0
	1 CUP	8	2	1	1
	1.5 CUPS	12	2	2	1
	2 CUPS	16	3	2	1
LETTUCE, RED & GREEN LEAF	1/2 CUP	3	0	0	0
	1 CUP	5	1	1	1
	1.5 CUPS	8	2	1	1
	2 CUPS	10	2	1	1
ONIONS, CHOPPED	1/2 CUP	34	8	1	7
	1 CUP	67	16	2	14
	1.5 CUPS	100	24	3	21
	2 CUPS	134	32	4	28
RADISHES	1/2 CUP	10	2	1	1
	1 CUP	19	4	2	2
	1.5 CUPS	29	6	3	3
	2 CUPS	38	8	4	4

Quick Glance MACRO BREAKDOWN

Veggies

	SERVING SIZE	CALORIES	GRAMS TOTAL CARBS	GRAMS FIBER	NET CARBS
SPINACH	1/2 CUP	4	6	0	0
	1 CUP	7	1	1	0
	1.5 CUPS	11	7	1	1
	2 CUPS	14	2	1	1
TOMATO	1/2 CUP	16	4	1	2
	1 CUP	32	7	2	5
	1.5 CUPS	48	11	3	7
	2 CUPS	64	14	4	10
TOMATOES, CHERRY	1/2 CUP	14	3	1	2
	1 CUP	27	6	2	4
	1.5 CUPS	41	9	3	6
	2 CUPS	54	12	4	8

OFF PROTOCOL Veggies

	SERVING SIZE	CALORIES	TOTAL CARBS	GRAMS FIBER	NET CARBS
BELL PEPPER	1/2 CUP	23	5	3	3
	1 CUP	46	9	3	6
	1.5 CUPS	69	14	5	9
	2 CUPS	92	18	6	12
BROCCOLI	1/2 CUP	16	3	1	2
	1 CUP	31	6	2	4
	1.5 CUPS	47	9	4	5
	2 CUPS	93	18	7	11
CROOKNECK SQUASH	1/2 CUP	13	3	1	1
	1 CUP	25	5	3	3
	1.5 CUPS	38	8	4	4
	2 CUPS	75	16	8	8

Quick Glance MACRO BREAKDOWN

OFF PROTOCOL Veggies	SERVING SIZE	CALORIES	TOTAL CARBS	GRAMS FIBER	NET CARBS
MUSHROOMS, SLICES	1/2 CUP	8	1	0	1
	1 CUP	15	2	1	2
	1.5 CUPS	23	3	1	3
	2 CUPS	45	7	2	4
ZUCCHINI, CHOPPED	1/2 CUP	10	2	1	1
	1 CUP	20	4	1	3
	1.5 CUPS	30	6	2	4
	2 CUPS	60	12	4	8
OTHER:					
OTHER:					
OTHER:					
OTHER:					

16915467R00077

Made in the USA
Middletown, DE
26 November 2018

THE MODEL RAILROADER'S GUIDE TO

BRIDGES, TRESTLES & TUNNELS

JEFF WILSON

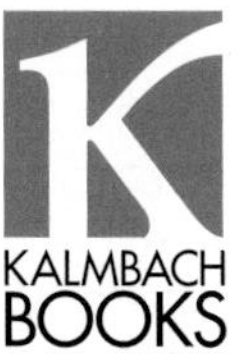

 Published by Kalmbach Publishing Co., 21027 Crossroads Circle, Waukesha, WI 53186.

Printed in the United States of America

05 06 07 08 09 10 11 12 13 14 10 9 8 7 6 5 4 3 2 1

Visit our website at http://kalmbachbooks.com
Secure online ordering available.
Questions or comments? E-mail us at books@kalmbach.com

Publisher's Cataloging-In-Publication Data
(Prepared by The Donohue Group, Inc.)

Wilson, Jeff, 1964-
The model railroader's guide to bridges, trestles & tunnels/Jeff Wilson.

p. : ill. ; cm.
ISBN: 0-89024-596-7

1. Railroads—Models—Design and construction—Handbooks, manuals, etc.
2. Railroad bridges—Models—Design and construction—Handbooks, manuals, etc.
3. Railroad tunnels—Models—Design and construction—Handbooks, manuals, etc.
I. Title.

TF197 .W557 2005
625.19

Senior editor: Lawrence Hansen
Managing art director: Michael Soliday
Art director: Thomas Ford
Book layout: Sabine Beaupré

CONTENTS

INTRODUCTION

A bridge, trestle, or tunnel can be the focal point of the signature scene on almost any model railroad. The key to modeling them realistically is knowing how and why they're used in real life. The goal of this book is to provide you with that background information, along with a range of tips and techniques to help you model these elements. I've tried to keep examples of spectacular, one-of-a-kind structures to a minimum—you'll find plenty of information about those elsewhere—and instead focus on ordinary, commonplace, "working" bridges, trestles, and tunnel portals that will fit in and look realistic on most layouts.

I would like to thank all of the people and companies who helped me by supplying products and information for the many projects shown in this book. Thanks to Mark Ballschmieder of AIM Products, Dale Rush of Blair Line, Jack Parker of Central Valley, Mike O'Connell of Chooch, Rick Rideout of Rix Products, Sermeng Tay-Konkol of Wm. K. Walthers, and Ruean Holt of Woodland Scenics. Their assistance is much appreciated.

Thanks also to the many photographers whose work resides in the David P. Morgan Library at Kalmbach Publishing. I could not have done this project without having access to this priceless resource.

—Jeff Wilson

May 2005

Bridge basics

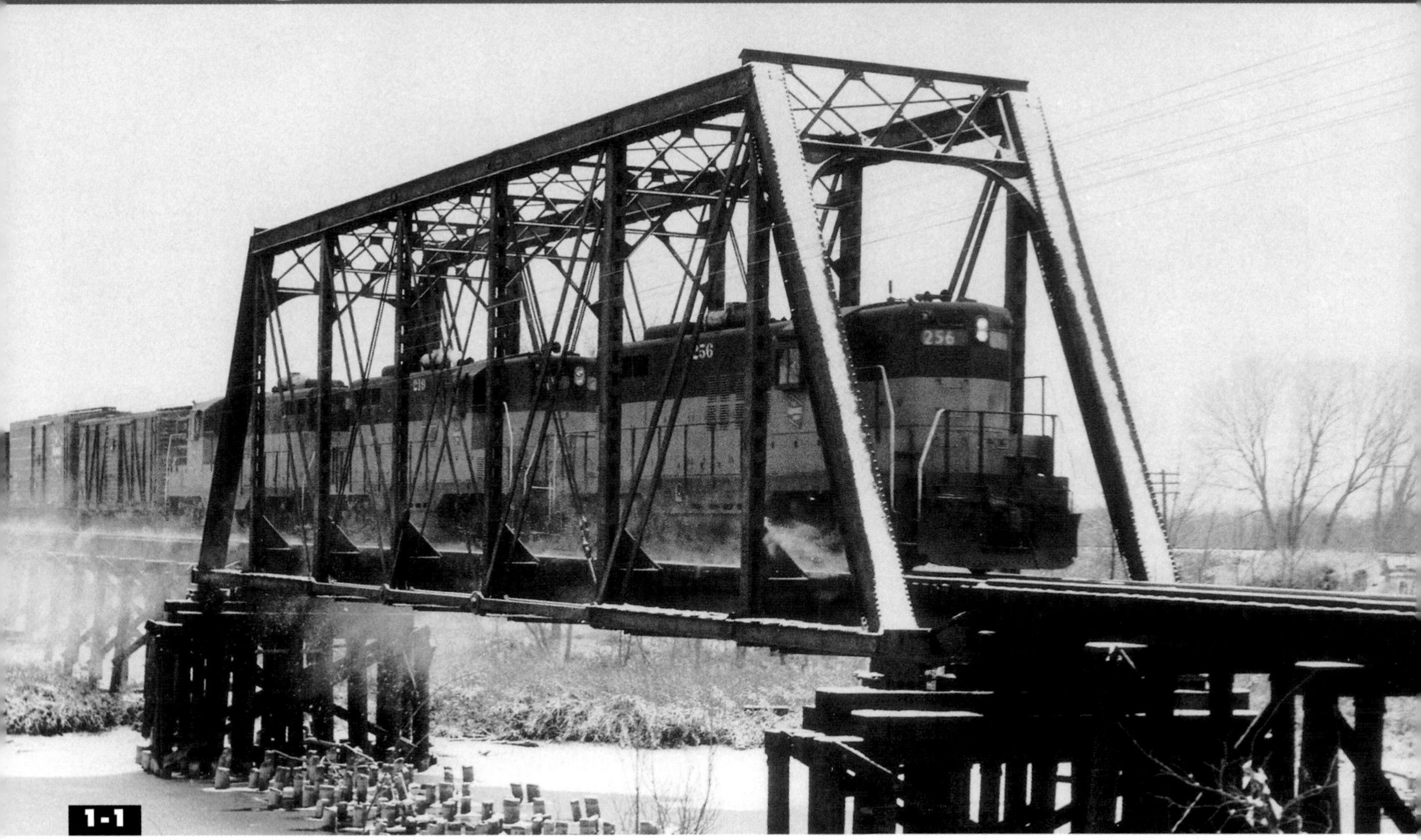

1-1

Railroad photographers tend to gravitate to scenes that include bridges and tunnel portals. After all, bridges and tunnels often accompany dramatic scenery—perhaps a towering mountain, a deep valley, or a wide, rushing river. Modelers naturally want to capture these details on their model railroads, in many cases making a bridge, trestle, or tunnel one of the focal points of a layout.

Bridges and tunnel portals can be signature items for a railroad, either in following a common design throughout a system or as a one-of-a-kind structure that becomes a landmark. They can also serve as simple, common details that lend the final touch of realism to a scene.

A Milwaukee Road freight kicks up a dusting of snow as it crosses a pin-connected Pratt through-truss bridge over the James River in Yankton, South Dakota. The Pratt design was the dominant truss bridge style on railroads between the 1890s and 1920s. Many are still in service today. *Mark Vanderboom*

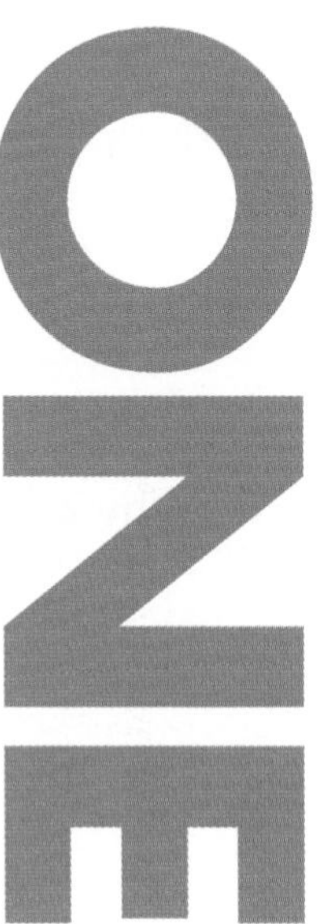

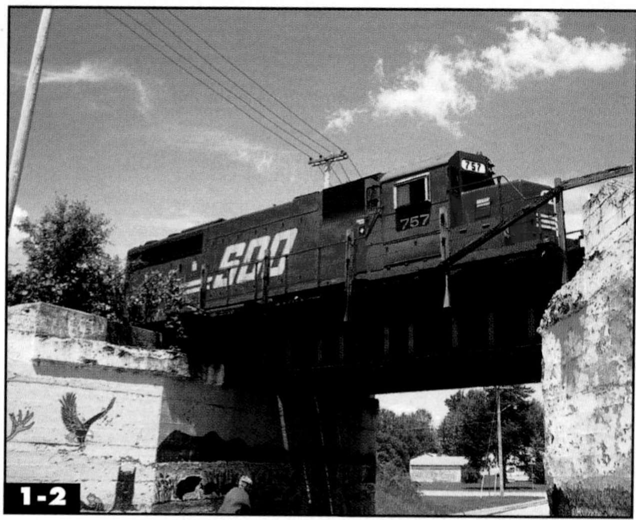

▲ This beam bridge is located on the former Soo Line at Sabula, Iowa. Extensions of the ties provide a base for the walkway. The concrete abutments make a handy canvas for a mural. *Jeff Wilson*

▶ This multiple-span deck plate girder bridge crosses the Fox River in Illinois on the Chicago, Burlington & Quincy. *David P. Morgan Library collection*

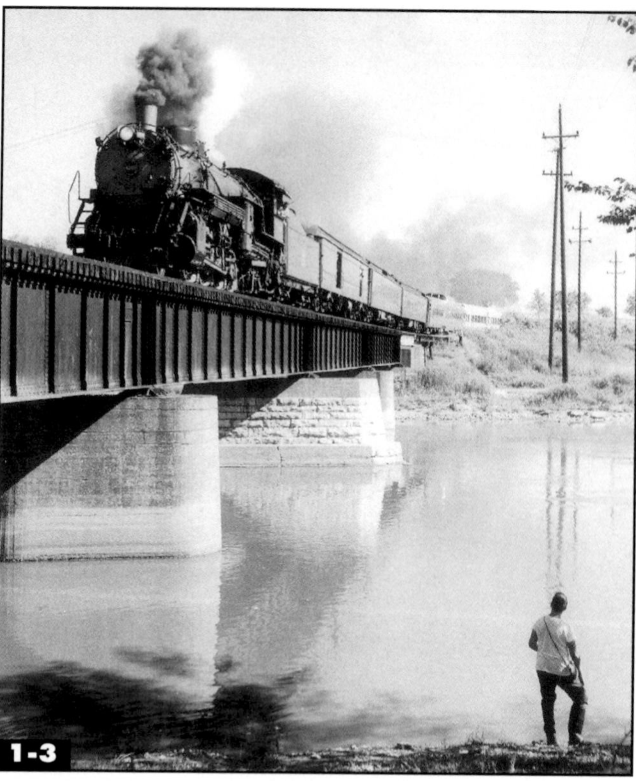

Bridges have been an integral part of railroads since the beginning. Some 211,000 had been built in the U.S. and Canada by 1940, according to the 1942 edition of the *Railway Engineering and Maintenance Cyclopedia*. Railroads employ many types of bridges, and understanding why different bridges are used in different locations will help you make accurate bridge choices for your model railroad. Knowing how bridges are built and how they work will also help you make more realistic models.

Why a bridge?

Some reasons for having a bridge are obvious, such as crossing over a river or highway. Other applications might not be so obvious, such as a culvert or small trestle seemingly in the middle of nowhere with no immediately apparent reason for being there. Look at real-world railroad lines, and you'll notice that they are almost always raised above the surrounding area. However, such structures serve an important purpose: Giving water a clear path under the roadbed is a key to stability.

Railroads consider a number of factors when deciding the type of bridge or trestle to use in a given situation. Questions to consider include: How wide is the span to be crossed? Is it possible to use intermediate piers, or is the gap too deep (or the ground too unstable) for piers? Is below-deck clearance an issue? How much vertical and horizontal clearance is needed for waterway traffic? Will a movable span be needed over a waterway? What will the bridge cost to build and maintain?

Sometimes the answer is a simple single-span bridge; other times the solution is a multiple-span bridge using different bridge types and lengths for each span. Keep your eyes open when railfanning, and you'll notice a wide variety of structures.

When modeling, you must consider these questions as well: What would a full-sized railroad have done? What would it have done in the era that you're modeling? What would your railroad have done when the line was originally built?

If you're modeling a specific railroad, look at prototype photos in books and magazines to see what types of bridges your railroad preferred for various uses.

Bridge types

Bridges are expensive to construct and maintain, so railroads generally try to use the smallest, simplest—that is to say, the least expensive—bridge possible to do the job. Here's a brief look at bridges from the most basic to the most complex.

Pay close attention as you follow a railroad right-of-way, and you'll be astounded at how many culverts you find. You might not think of the lowly culvert as a bridge, but culverts are essential to providing proper drainage.

A culvert is simply a covered opening through the roadbed that allows water, pedestrian traffic, or a narrow road to pass from one side of the right-of-way to the other (see Chapter 2). The culvert is probably the bridge type most overlooked by modelers; many layouts would benefit from having more of them.

Simple beam bridges are next, **1-2**. Wood was originally the most common beam material, with steel and concrete taking over in the 20th century. Modern steel beam bridges are used for spans up to 40′, with concrete used up to 20′ and wood to about 10′.

Plate girder bridges are used for longer spans and are also simple in design, thus relatively inexpensive, **1-3**. Whereas beams are single pieces, plate girders are made from several pieces of steel sheet riveted or welded together. Although average lengths are about 70′ long, some plate girder bridges have spanned lengths 125′ or longer.

Truss bridges are made up of numerous long, slender supports, arranged in triangle patterns for strength (see **1-1**). Truss bridges are used where longer spans are needed and can be 500′ or longer; arch and cantilever bridges (other types of truss bridges) can be more than 1,000′ long. Several different truss designs have been used over the years (see Chapter 5).

Railroads built many stone-arch bridges in the mid-1800s, and although expensive to erect, some were built past the turn of the 20th century. They are extremely strong and durable, and many are still in service, **1-4**. These range from small, simple single-arch bridges to long, tall, multiple-arch structures. Starting around 1900, concrete became the preferred material for masonry bridges, as you'll see in Chapter 6.

Almost an icon of railroads in the 19th century, the wood trestle was the most common bridge type in the early days of railroading, **1-5**. Wood trestles have a series of frame piers (bents) supporting stringers upon which the track is laid, meaning a trestle is basically a series of wood-beam bridges. Although most of the classic tall wooden trestles have long since been replaced, small wood pile trestles are still common across the country. Trestles are also commonly used on approaches to larger steel spans.

Steel viaducts have been common since the early 1900s, **1-6** (page 8). They are often used to cross wide valleys and other depressions, and they usually feature a series of plate-girder spans between steel towers. They can also have longer intermediate spans to accommodate obstructions such as river crossings.

Movable bridges are often used over rivers, bays, and lakes where waterway access is needed. Movable bridges fall into three main types: A swing bridge is on a center pivot that turns horizontally to open a lane on the waterway. On a vertical lift bridge, the bridge span is lifted up on tall towers located on each side of the span. A bascule bridge has one end hinged, and the other end is lifted vertically to clear the waterway. Chapter 7 goes into detail about these types of bridges.

Bridge loading

In looking at bridges, it is apparent that some are built for heavier loads than others, and indeed, the load a bridge can carry is of prime importance to railroads. In general, the later a bridge was built, the heavier load it is designed to carry. Heavier bridges are usually built on main lines, with lighter bridges found on branch and secondary lines. Light bridge loading was a key factor in many branchline abandonments with the coming of heavier locomotives and 100- and 110-ton capacity cars in the mid- and late 1900s.

Bridges are usually classified by carrying capacity using loading formulae developed by Theodore Cooper, a 19th century engineer and pioneer in calculating strain on bridge members. His system is based on axle loading, so that, for example, a bridge with an E-60 loading can carry 60,000 pounds on each axle.

In the early 1900s, loadings of E-40 were common, moving to E-50, E-55, E-60, and E-72 by the end of the steam era to E-80 and even E-90 ratings today. To railway

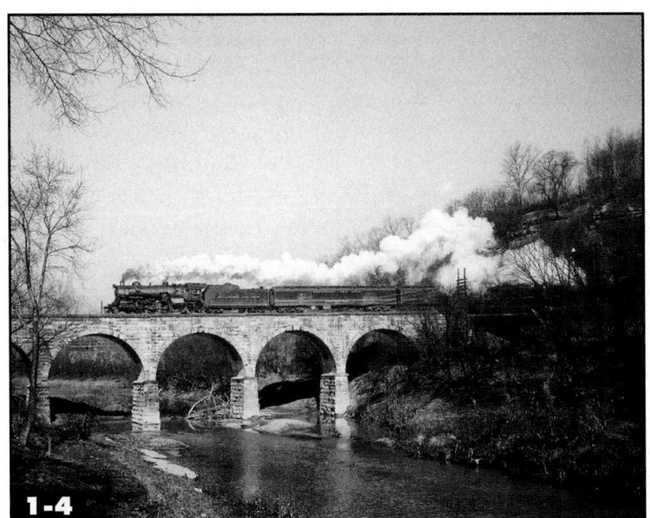

1-4

Many stone viaducts and bridges built in the 1800s were still in use well into the 20th century—some still serve even today. This Baltimore & Ohio viaduct is at Wheeling, West Virginia. *J.J. Young, Jr.*

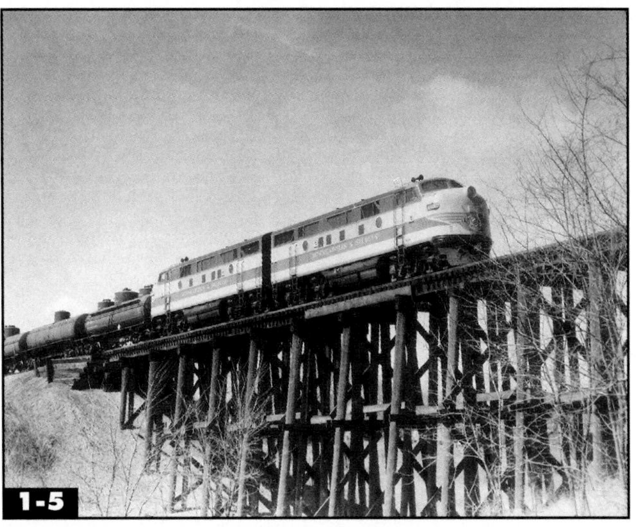

1-5

This wood pile trestle is on the Minneapolis & St. Louis near Oskaloosa, Iowa, in 1948. Trestles will be discussed in depth in Chapter 3. *Robert H. Milner*

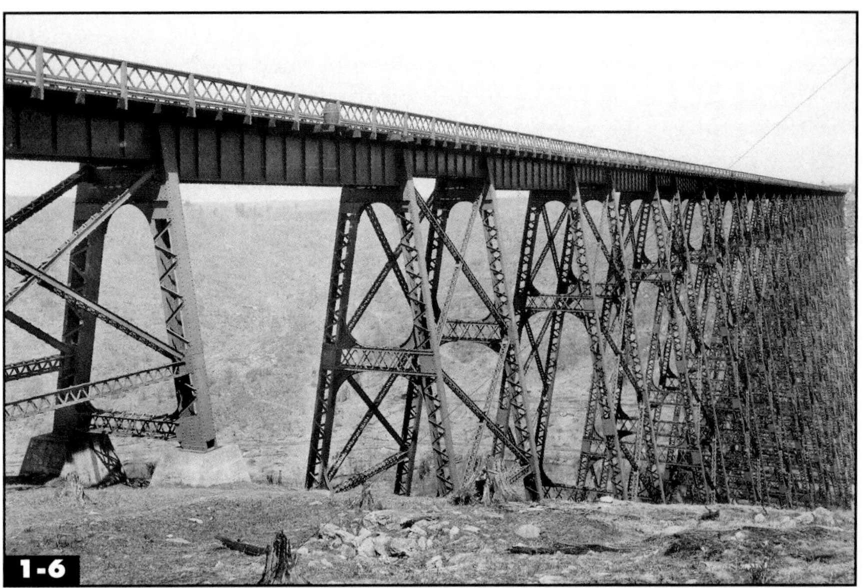

Since 1900, the steel viaduct has been the preferred way to cross wide valleys. Plate girder spans like this one are supported by steel piers. *David P. Morgan Library collection*

engineers, following Cooper's formulae means using heavier materials for a given. Railroads maintain a list of ratings for their bridges, and motive-power assignments can be made based on loading. If you read through employee timetables and special instructions, you'll often find lists of certain locomotives that aren't allowed on specific track or routes, especially on branch and secondary lines.

Space doesn't permit detailing the specifics of each rating in Cooper's system, but for modelers, the key is that the heavier the locomotives and cars you use, the more substantial your bridge models should be. For example, a pair of AC4400CWs pulling a coal train on a main line simply won't look right on a lightweight, pin-connected Pratt truss bridge or tall four-post frame trestle, but they'll look at home on a heavy plate girder span.

Putting it all together

The following chapters will look in depth at each type of bridge, outlining the history and typical usage of each bridge type. We'll look at the basics of bridge modeling, along with many hints, guidelines, and modeling projects. We'll also cover ancillary details such as piers and abutments (Chapter 9) and take a look at highway bridges (Chapter 8) and tunnel portals (Chapter 10). A list of available bridge models is provided on pages 86-88.

Throughout the book, the emphasis is on modeling bridges and trestles in a realistic manner. You won't find coverage of toy-train style trestle "riser" sets, piers with slots cut into them, or similar models. The goal of this book is to take you beyond the toy level to realistic modeling.

Even in a specialized book the size of this one, it's impossible to cover everything. If you still have questions, try looking at what real railroads do. It's hard to go wrong by copying the real thing.

Now, turn the page and we'll start our bridge explorations by looking at culverts and simple beam bridges.

Engineering Cyclopedia

One of the handiest sources of prototype information on bridges and trestles is the *Railway Engineering and Maintenance Cyclopedia*, which has been published periodically since the early 1900s by Simmons-Boardman. The *Engineering Cyc* follows the same style as the better-known *Car Builders' Cyclopedia* and *Locomotive Cyclopedia*.

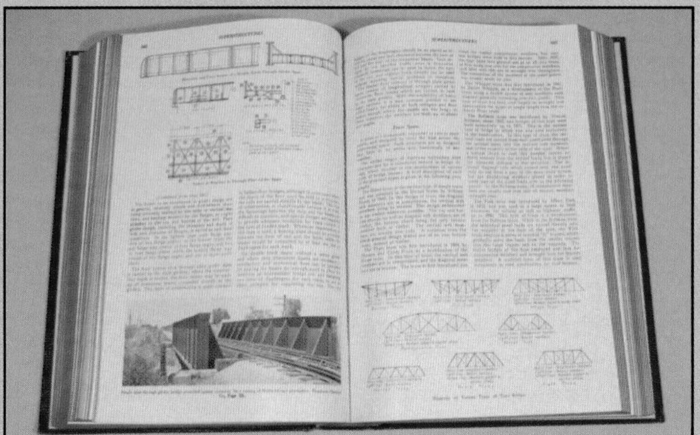

The *Engineering Cyc* covers many aspects of railroad rights-of-way, including bridges, trestles, tunnels, and retaining walls, as well as trackwork, ballast, signaling, turntables, locomotive terminals, and other subjects. Features include extensive prototype drawings and specifications, as well as history and usage. These are large books; each edition runs more than 1,000 pages.

You can track down old issues of the *Cyc* through dealers specializing in railroad books and documents. Copies also turn up often on eBay and other online auction sites.

Culverts and beam bridges

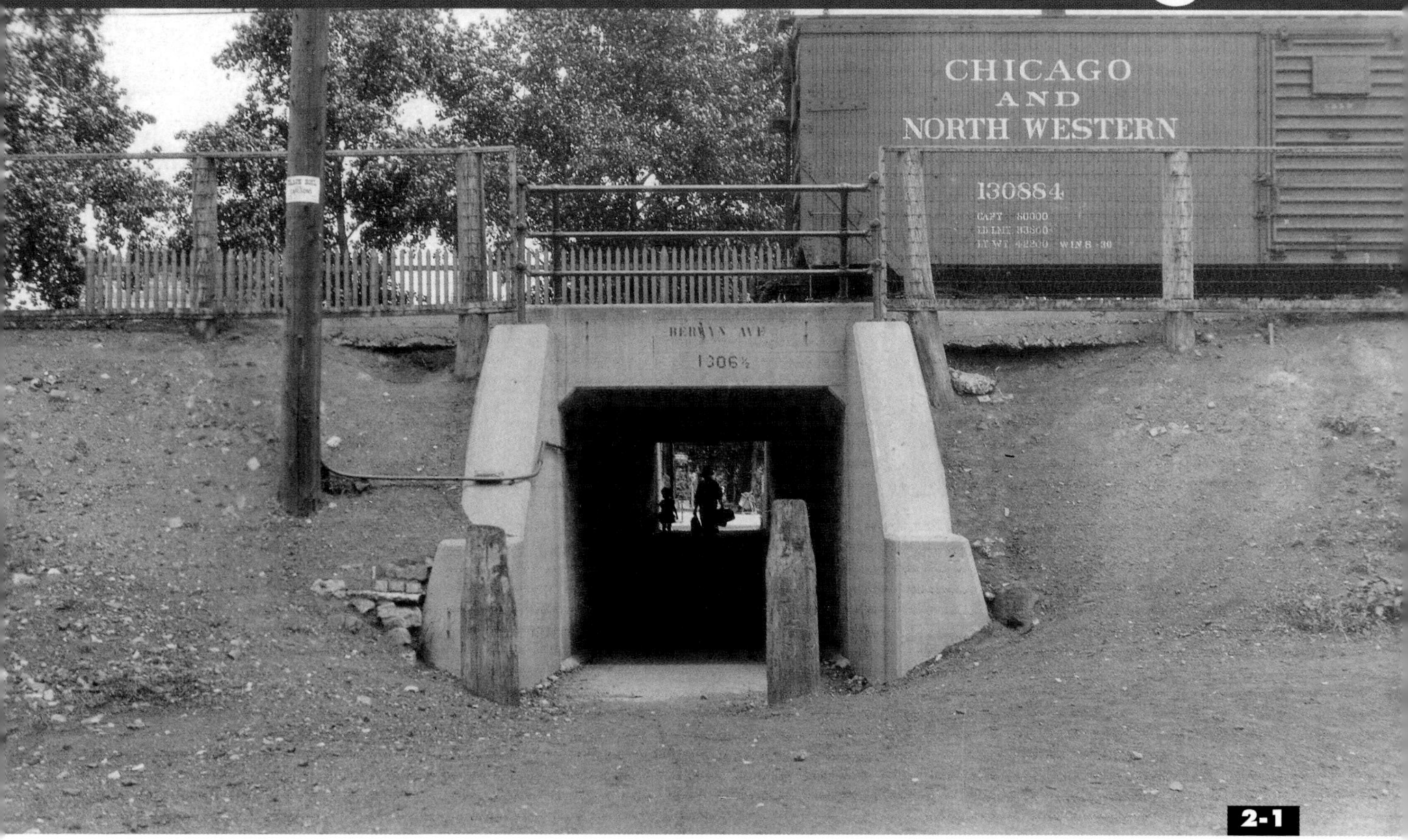

2-1

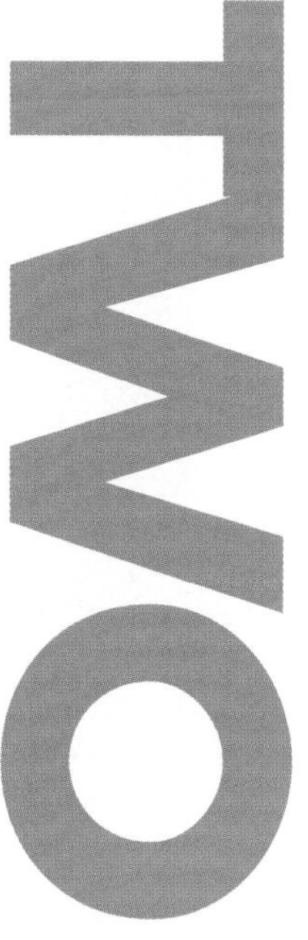

Many modelers don't even consider the most basic type of bridge a true bridge, but technically it is. The lowly but extremely important culvert is simply a covered opening under the roadbed that allows water, a walkway, or a narrow road to pass from one side of the right-of-way to the other, **2-1**. Culverts can be pipes of various types, or can be small masonry (stone or concrete) structures. Some modern metal culverts are large enough for a track to pass through.

Also vital to ensuring proper drainage, beam bridges—made from wood, concrete, or steel—are the other type of basic railroad bridge. These structures often ignored by model railroaders because they are not very exciting; most layouts would benefit from having more culverts and beam bridges.

Essentially small tunnels under the roadbed, culverts are the most basic type of bridge. They can be made of wood, stone, or concrete, like this one used for pedestrian traffic, or they can be simple pipes. *David P. Morgan Library collection*

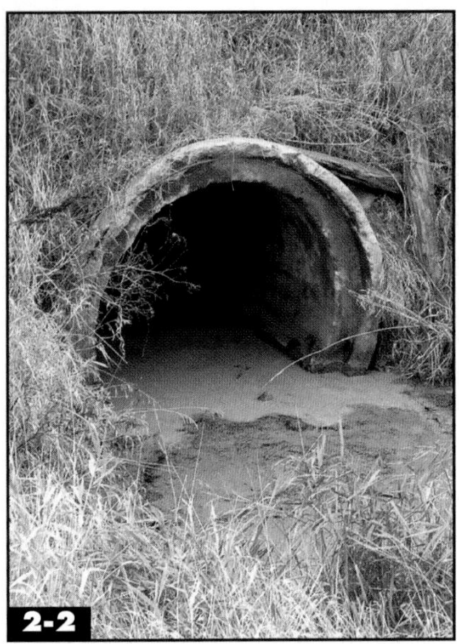

2-2

This concrete pipe is typical of the simplest culverts along railroad rights-of-way. Culverts are also made from corrugated metal, iron, and clay pipes. *Jeff Wilson*

Culverts

Railroads decide what type of culvert or small bridge to use based on the conditions of surrounding ground: whether it is normally dry, wet, or swampy, and whether the runoff characteristics of the surrounding land are good or poor. Another factor is typical weather conditions, such as whether the area is subject to heavy rainfall or experiences frequent flash floods. In general, the higher the likelihood of heavy water, the larger the openings.

In wet areas, culverts are generally not placed at the lowest surrounding ground level. Instead, the bottom of the culvert is a few feet above the bed of the neighboring surrounding stream or pond. This cuts down on sediment collecting in the culvert. Culverts also often have a slight slope to aid drainage and prevent sediment buildup.

Culverts fall into three basic categories: pipe, box, and arch. The most basic type of culvert is a pipe, **2-2**. These come in many sizes and are made from a variety of materials, including clay, cast iron, and corrugated metal. Clay was popular through the early 1900s, and saw occasional use later, especially in areas with alkaline soils or other conditions that could be corrosive to other materials. Clay pipe culverts could be found in various sizes up to 36″ in diameter.

Cast iron was also a popular culvert material through the late steam era. These pipes had thinner, stronger walls than clay. Cast iron pipes ranged from 24″ to 48″ in diameter, with even larger sizes used in some applications.

Galvanized corrugated metal became very popular for new and replacement installations in the 1930s. The material's strength, durability, and flexibility (corrugated culverts are much less prone to breakage compared to clay or iron) made this type ideal for use under railroad roadbeds. They range in size from a foot or two to six feet and more in diameter.

Concrete pipe (see **2-2**) became popular in the early 1900s. It resists corrosion and can be made to almost any size and strength (by making the walls thicker). Sizes range from 24″ to 7′ in diameter.

Box and arch culverts

As the name implies, box culverts have a structure including side walls, roof, and floor. This allows for a larger opening than a simple pipe. Concrete became popular for box culverts in the early 1900s (see **2-1**), but wood and steel have also been used. Concrete box culverts can span up to 12′, with walls up to 10′. If a larger opening is required, a double-box design is used, or an arched structure or bridge is used.

Stone arch culverts were popular for medium to large openings from the 1800s through the early 1900s, **2-3**. These can be found with openings from a few feet across up to bridge-sized spans—in fact, it can be difficult to tell when an arch culvert becomes a bridge. Masonry culverts can be eye-catching, and their design is often fancier than their use would seem to require. See Chapter 6 for other examples of small and large concrete and stone structures.

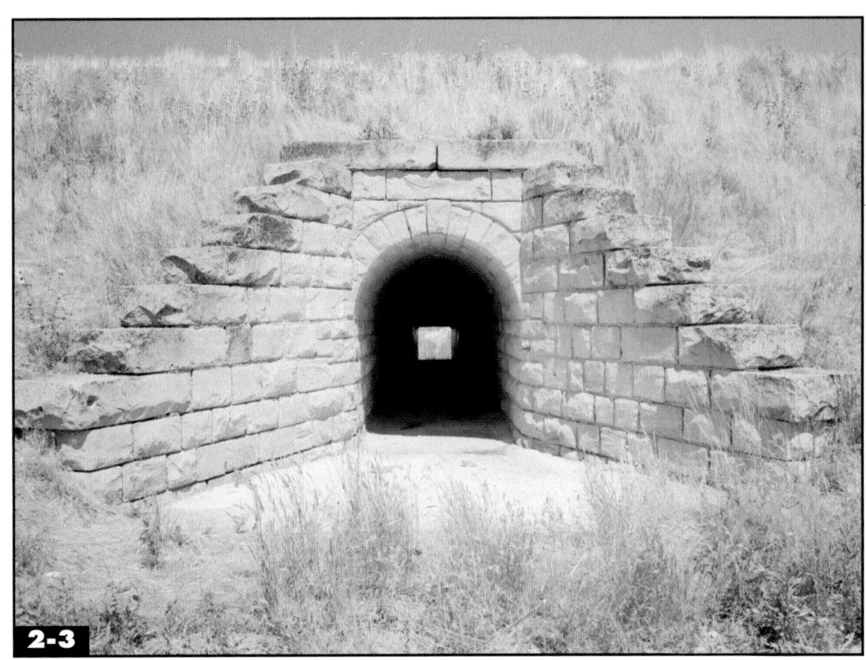

2-3

Stone culverts were built from the 1800s into the early 1900s. This culvert with wing walls is on the old Chicago & North Western line in Wyoming. *Historic American Engineering Record; Jack Collier*

Beam bridges

Beam bridges are the most basic railroad spans. They are easy and inexpensive to build, and can be found using wood, steel, or concrete members. These bridges are always deck style, and they sup-

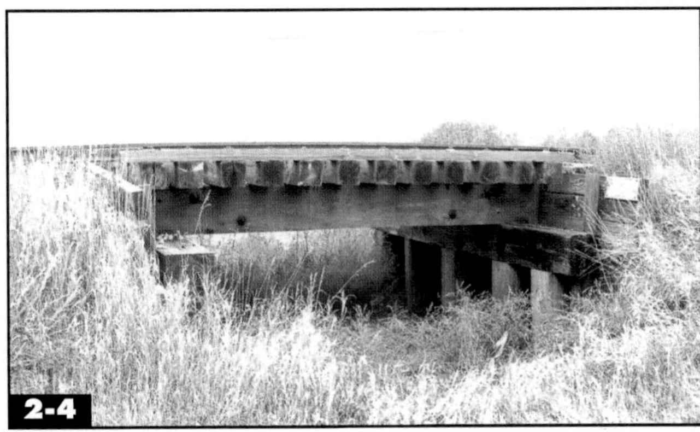
2-4

Used for short spans, wood beam bridges are basically trestles without bents. *Jeff Wilson*

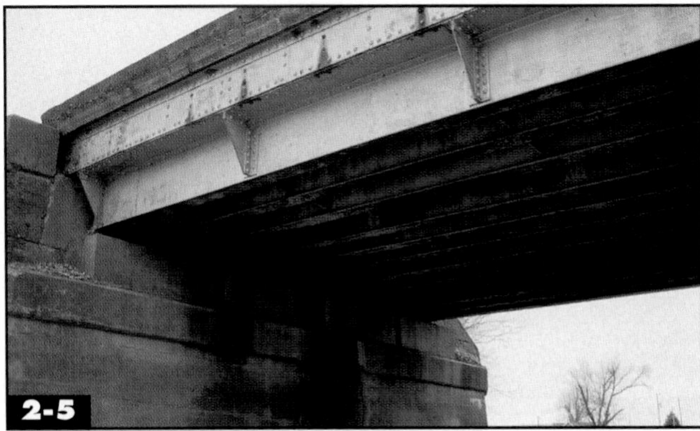
2-5

This double-track beam bridge has six steel I-beams under each track. Note the steel pieces that connect the I-beams, providing stability. *Jeff Wilson*

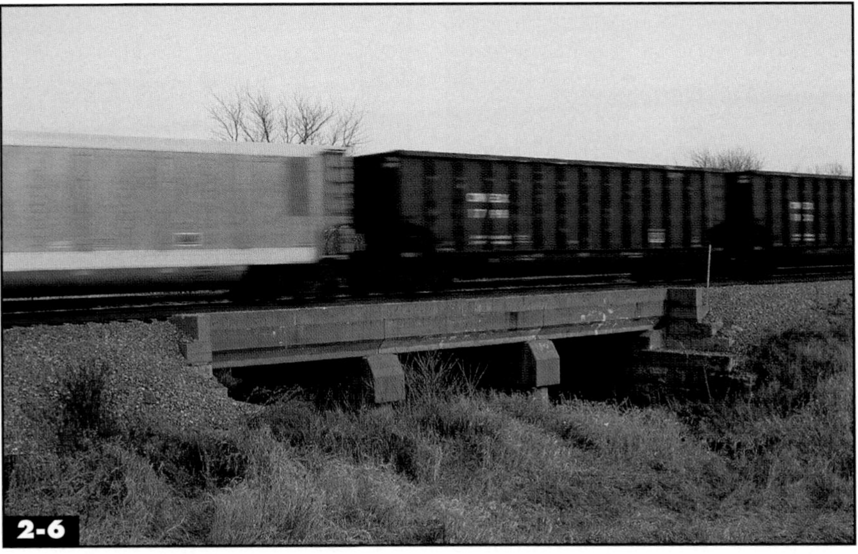
2-6

Concrete beam bridges are usually topped by a trough for a ballasted deck. This one is on the Union Pacific main line in Iowa. *Jeff Wilson*

port the track on beams that are single pieces—as opposed to a plate girder, which is made from five or more pieces.

You can think of a wood beam bridge as a trestle without intermediate bents. Photo **2-4** shows an example, which uses wood beams resting on bulkheads consisting of a timber wall with wood pilings and cap (more on those in Chapter 3).

Steel I-beams are often used for beam bridges, as photo **2-5** shows. As with plate girder bridges (more on those in chapter 4), beam bridges can have ballasted decks (as does the bridge in the photo), or the bridge ties can rest directly on the beams. Steel beams are used for spans to around 25′. Note that several beams are used to support the tracks (six under each track in the bridge in **2-5**), with plates connecting them.

Concrete has also been used for beam bridges, **2-6**. These are usually used to support a concrete trough for ballasted track. Concrete beam spans are kept fairly short, about 15′ or less, although you'll find longer spans that use steel I-beams encased in concrete.

Modeling culverts

Several companies offer culvert models. Woodland Scenics has several simple cast-plaster N and HO scale kits for concrete and stone culverts, **2-7** (page 12). Photo **2-8** (page 12) shows an HO stone culvert from Woodland Scenics and a corrugated pipe culvert from Pre-Size Model Specialties.

Assembling one of these kits is fairly simple. Simply glue the cast pieces together with white glue, being careful to not get glue on the visible surface (doing so will seal the plaster, making it difficult to color). If some glue does get on the surface, sand the area lightly (after the glue has dried) with fine sandpaper.

Occasionally plaster kits—especially those with thin cross-sections—will break. Broken pieces usually can be fixed by applying white glue along the break, **2-9** (page 12), then pressing the pieces firmly together. It's not a problem if a slight crack or chip is visible, as that can give the piece a realistic aged appearance.

Plaster pieces often have stray material from the molding process. Remove this material and smooth it with a hobby knife, **2-10** (page 12).

For a simulated concrete culvert, paint the culvert a shade of gray or tan, **2-11** (page 12). You can use Woodland Scenics' earth coloring set (No. 1215), which includes concrete, white, and various shades of gray, or you can use almost any type of water-based model paint.

Real concrete varies in color from nearly white (new concrete) to light and medium gray to tan, depending upon its age and weathering. I've found that many model paints labeled "concrete"

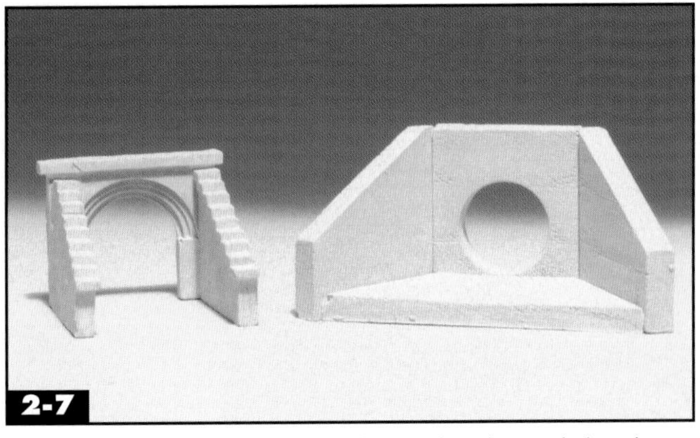

2-7 Woodland Scenics has many cast-plaster culvert kits, including these HO masonry arch (No. 1263), left, and concrete (No. 1262), right, models. *Jeff Wilson*

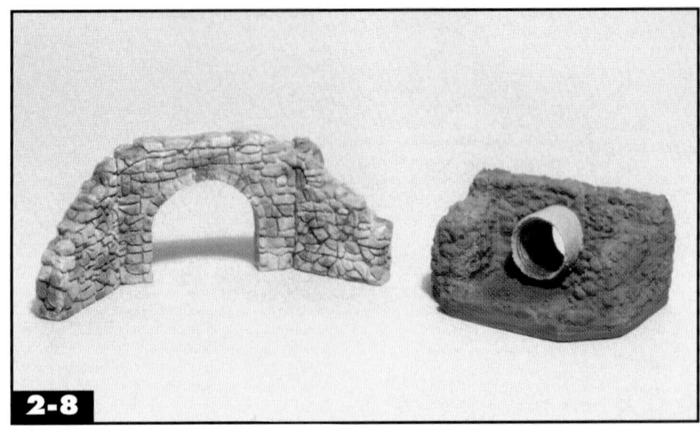

2-8 Stone culverts include these HO models: Woodland Scenics random stone (No. 1264) and Pre-Size Model Specialties random stone with corrugated pipe (No. 122). *Jeff Wilson*

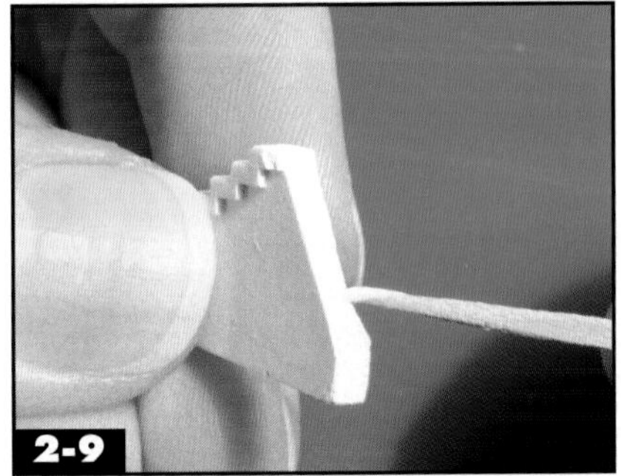

2-9 To fix a broken piece, apply a thin coat of white glue to one of the broken edges, then press the halves together firmly. *Jeff Wilson*

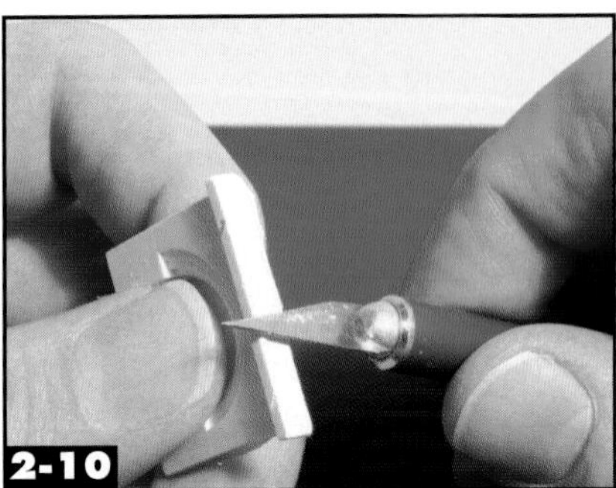

2-10 Use a hobby knife to remove flash and other stray material from plaster and plastic parts. *Jeff Wilson*

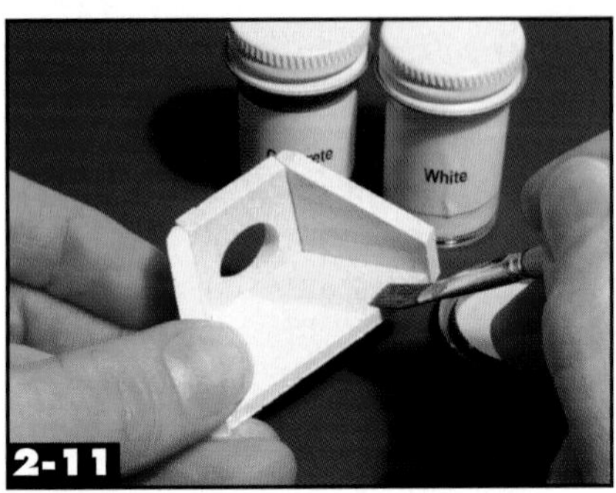

2-11 To give this culvert a concrete color, the author mixed white and concrete from the Woodland Scenics earth coloring set. *Jeff Wilson*

are too dark for my tastes, so I mix them with white or light gray to lighten them. Photo **2-12** shows a chart I made to use as a starting point for mixing Polly Scale paints, including concrete, aged concrete, white, and SP lettering gray. Make up your own mixes to match the effects you're looking for.

You can use a brush to apply the color, **2-11**. You can also use an airbrush or spray can for a more even finish.

Photo **2-8** shows a stone arch culvert from Woodland Scenics. Chapter 10 includes some tips for painting and weathering cast-plaster models of stone structures. Photo **2-8** also shows a cast-resin HO culvert, featuring a corrugated pipe, from Pre-Size Model

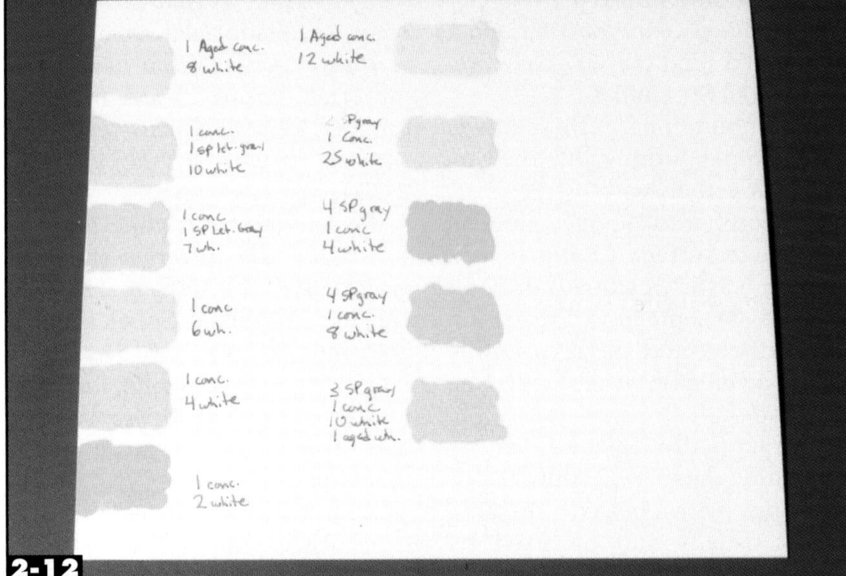

2-12 A color mixing chart is a handy reference when blending paint to create different effects or to match specific prototypes. *Jeff Wilson*

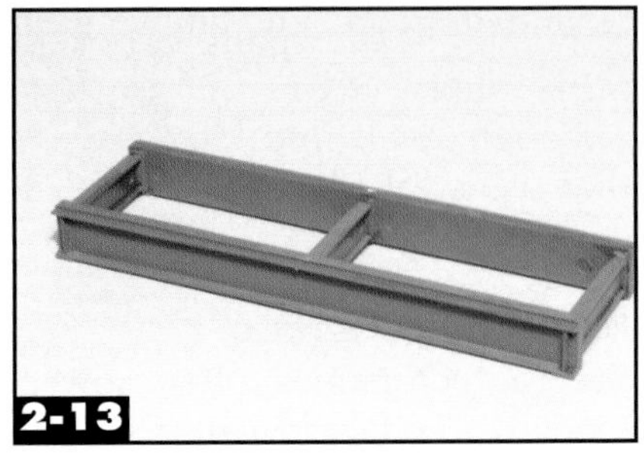

2-13 Walthers offers a simple HO steel beam bridge as part of a trestle and bridge kit. *Jeff Wilson*

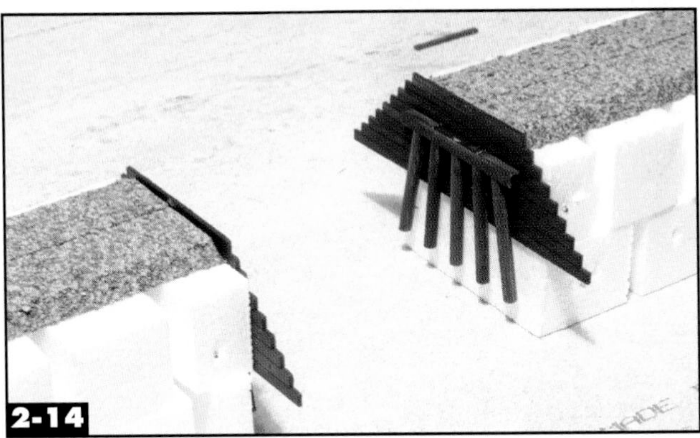

2-14

Position the kit's bulkheads at each end of the gap. Make sure the gap is the proper distance to match the bridge. *Jeff Wilson*

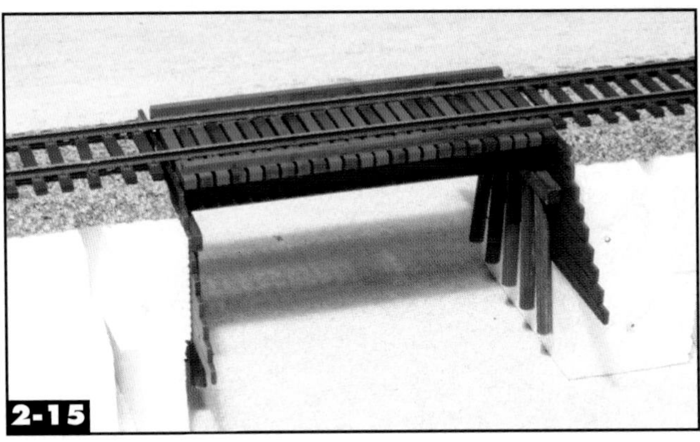

2-15

Here's the completed beam bridge, with Central Valley bridge track laid on top. You can substitute concrete or stone abutments for a different look. *Jeff Wilson*

Specialties. Paint items such as this to match your scenery, then add them to your layout and blend them into your layout's scenery.

You can also make your own simple pipe culverts using brass or styrene tubing painted appropriate colors to match cast iron, clay, or concrete pipes. Keep your eyes open for photos and prototype examples.

Modeling beam bridges

Whether you use a commercial kit or try your hand at scratchbuilding, installation of a beam bridge follows the same steps. A good starting point in HO is the Walthers injection-molded styrene trestle and bridge kit (No. 933-3147). It includes several trestle bents, bulkheads, pile piers, and a short beam bridge. It's a great source of raw materials for trestle building as well.

Photo **2-13** shows the assembled bridge from the Walthers kit, which is simply a pair of beams with cross members. You can use it with the trestle approaches included in the kit, but you can use just the bridge itself.

I used a trestle bent and wood wall from the kit for the bulkhead, gluing the bent to the abutment wall. You can also use a commercial concrete or stone abutment or make your own as demonstrated in Chapter 9.

Position a bulkhead at each end of the bridge gap, so the level of the bridge track will match the level of the approach track on your roadbed, **2-14**. When the bulkheads are aligned, they can be glued in place. Chapters 3 and 4 will go into greater detail on aligning abutments and bulkheads, as well as installing bridge track.

The easiest approach is to complete the surrounding scenery before adding the bridge deck and track, but photo **2-15** shows the completed bridge in place with the bridge track installed before the scenery is added. It's nothing spectacular, but it looks good simply because it is so typical of the small spans found in thousands of locations across the country.

The beauty of small bridges like these is that, because of their small size, it's very easy to work them into tight areas. You can also blend them into existing layouts and scenes by cutting away just a minimal amount of track and surrounding scenery.

The simplest type of beam bridge in real life—wood—is also probably the simplest to model. Follow the guidelines for trestles in Chapter 3, without the intermediate bents. You can use wood stringers from a commercial trestle kit or plastic molded (simulated wood) stringers from the Walthers kit, but the easiest way is to just use appropriate sizes of scale stripwood. Chapter 3 includes dimensions for these pieces, as well as tips on staining and working with wood.

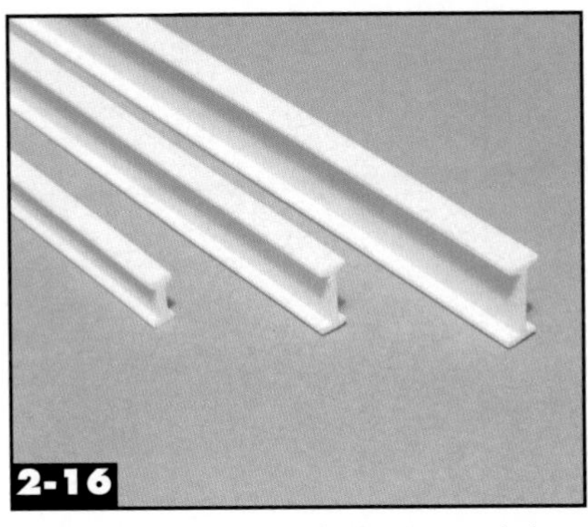

2-16

Styrene beams suitable for bridges include (left to right) Plastruct $^{3}/_{16}''$ and Evergreen $^{1}/_{4}''$ and $^{5}/_{16}''$ strips. *Jeff Wilson*

You can also construct your own steel-beam bridges using styrene I-beams available from Evergreen or Plastruct, **2-16**. Follow the same guidelines described for the Walthers bridge shown earlier by placing the beams across the gap and gluing commercial bridge track across the beams.

Be sure to paint the beams an appropriate color—usually black, dark gray, or brown. Use prototype photos and observation as your guide; these bridges vary in style from one railroad and one installation to the next.

Next, we're going to take a look at modeling wood trestles.

Trestles

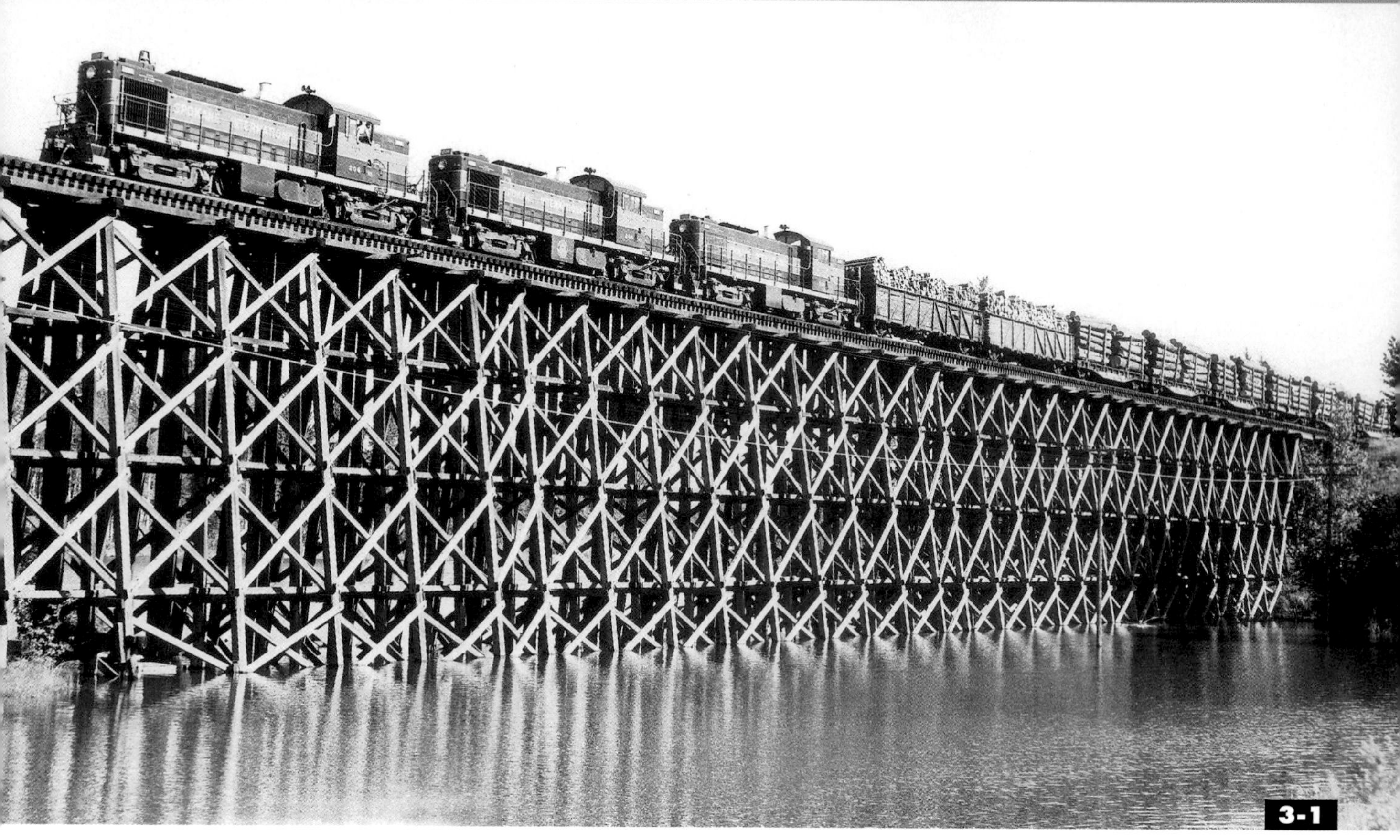

3-1

THREE

This tall frame trestle on the Spokane International is typical of many found all over the U.S. into the early 1900s. Located in lumber country, this wood trestle was still receiving heavy use in 1955. *L.E. Shawver*

When most model railroaders hear the word "trestle," they think of the classic tall wood structure that dominated early years of railroading, especially in the Midwest and West, **3-1**. Although most of the large, towering structures have been replaced, many small wood trestles still exist. They remain an economical way of bridging small gaps where drainage is required and where below-deck clearance isn't an issue.

A trestle is essentially a series of short spans over multiple supports—in the case of a wood trestle, a series of short wood-beam bridges on wood bents. And, regardless of size, wood trestles just look impressive, which is why they find their way onto so many model railroads.

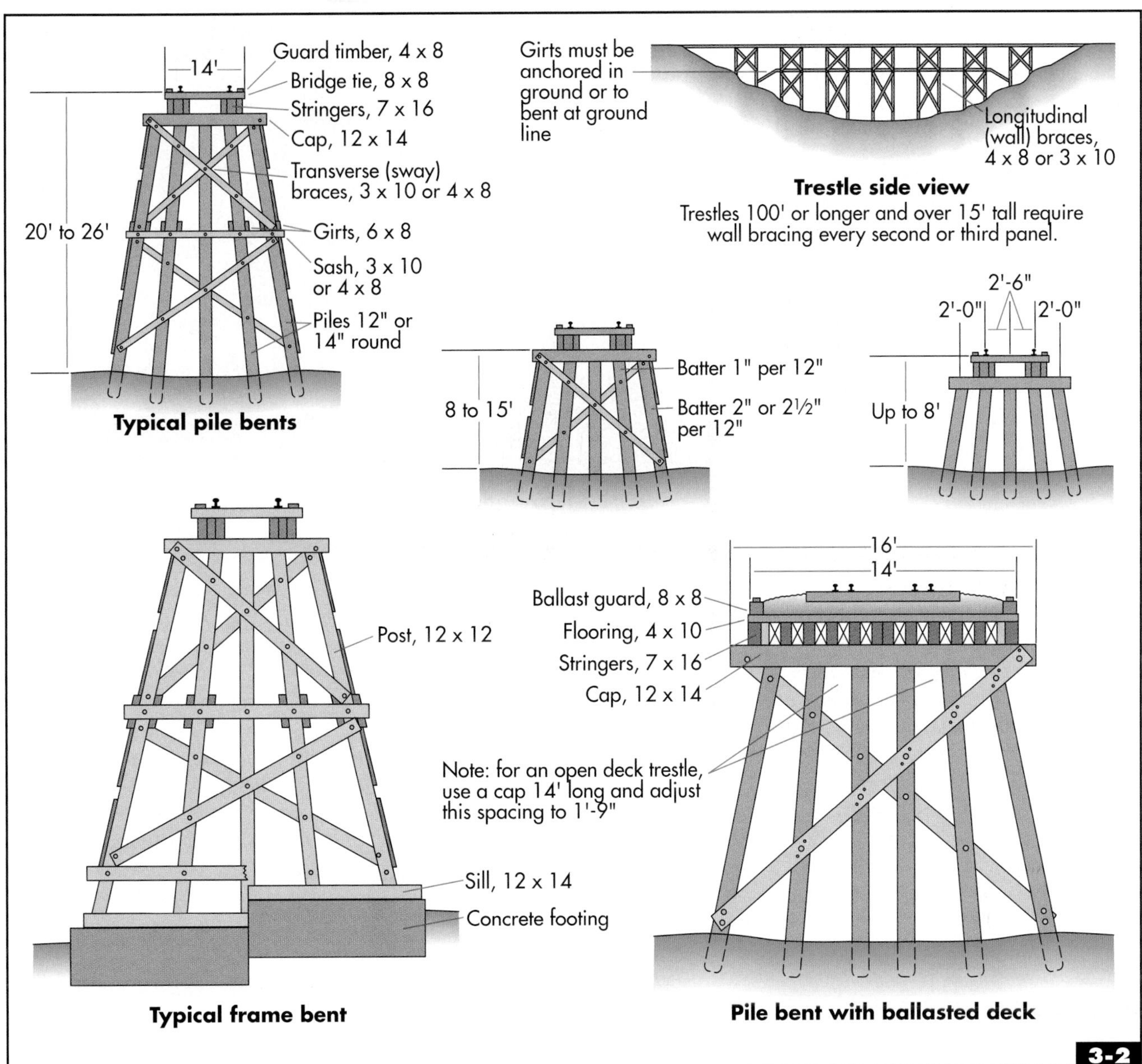

3-2

Wood trestles

Wood trestles were popular in the early days of railroading because of their ease and speed of construction, particularly in areas that had a plentiful local supply of timber. Most trestles have a common look, **3-2**, with vertical supports called "bents" made of five or six vertical posts. Some early light-duty trestles have four-post bents, **3-3** (page 16). The outermost posts of the bents angle outward, with cross- and X-bracing for rigidity.

The bents are spaced about 12′ to 15′ apart, with wood stringers placed across the tops. Wood ties—spaced much more closely than on conventional track—are laid across the stringers, as you can see in the prototype photos throughout this chapter.

Wood trestles fall into two categories: frame and pile. Frame trestles have bents with posts that aren't driven into the ground, but are framed and rest on a solid foundation, **3-4** (page 16). Square timbers were typically used for the posts on frame trestles, although round posts were not unheard of.

Pile trestles have round posts that are driven into the ground by a pile driver. Most trestles still in service, including those being built today, are pile trestles, **3-5** (page 16).

Bracing on trestles includes X-braces, called sway or transverse braces, on the bents. The straight horizontal pieces between stories are called sash braces. X-braces that connect adjacent bents are called wall or longitudinal braces. If a trestle is more than one story tall, the bents are connected by straight horizontal members called girts.

Most trestles have open decks, with the ties laid on the stringers, **3-6** (page 16). Guard timbers at the outside of the ties keep the ties aligned. Many trestles have guardrails inside the running rails, although these are omitted on some short spans.

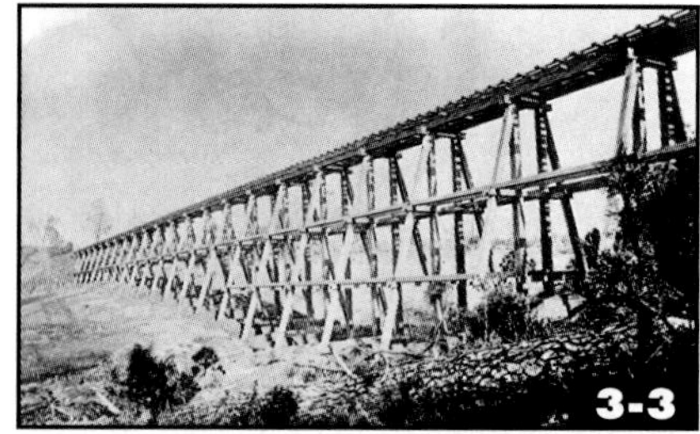

▲ Lightweight four-post trestles, like this 1860s structure on the Central Pacific, were common before the turn of the 20th century. *D.L. Joslyn collection*

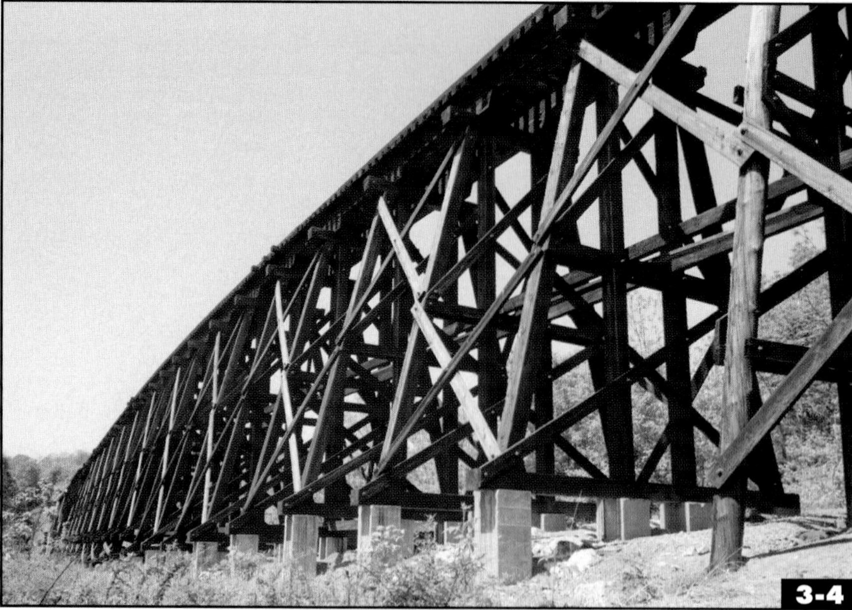

► The sills at the base of frame trestle bents rest on solid stone or concrete footings. The footings sometimes run the length of the sill, or may just be under the vertical posts. *Historic American Engineering Survey; E.Q. Johnson*

Trestles with ballasted decks have floors, with the track (laid on standard ties) resting on top of the ballast on the deck, **3-7** (see illustration **3-2** for a cross-section of a ballasted-deck trestle). Ballasted deck trestles are often used for heavy mainline applications and are therefore built stronger to support the weight of the ballast and flooring. They have bents with wider caps and more posts, and they have additional (sometimes heavier) stringers compared to standard trestles.

Tall frame trestles have dwindled in number, and are now very rare on main lines. Many were filled in by simply dumping dirt through the tracks (often after having a culvert or culverts added between bents); others were replaced by concrete trestles or bridges of various types. Trestles still in service are mainly low pile trestles, **3-7**.

Trestles are also often used as approaches to other bridges (see photo **1-1** in Chapter 1). Longer trestles sometimes have bridges of various types (often steel beam or plate girder, sometimes wood truss) in the middle. These give multi-span bridges an asymmetrical look that is interesting to model.

The drawings in **3-2** show trestles in the E-60 range; for more modern trestles with E-72 loading, use six-pile bents with 12′ spacing, and use four stringers per side instead of three. Heavier trestles can be modeled with seven-post bents (24″ spacing between all posts, with the middle three posts vertical) and heavier stringers (9 x 16 or 10 x 16).

Steel and concrete

Around 1900, railroads started turning to steel for the tall, dramatic valley crossings once accomplished with wood trestles. With their tall steel towers connected by girder bridges, these

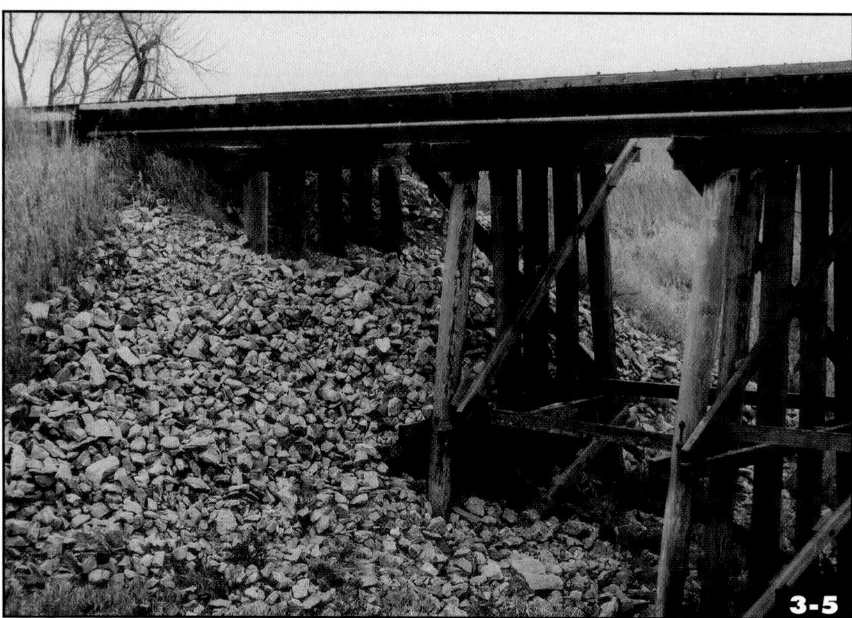

The posts on a pile trestle are driven directly into the ground, and therefore don't require footings like frame trestles. *Jeff Wilson*

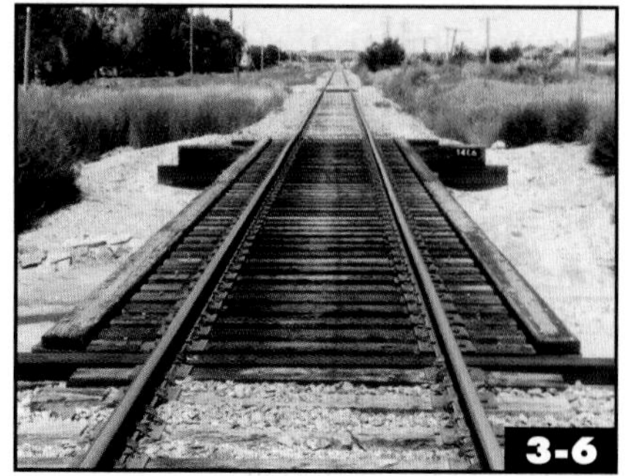

Note how the rails pass over the timber bulkheads at each end of this open-deck trestle. *Jeff Wilson collection*

large steel trestles—often called viaducts—became common in the 20th century. (For a more in-depth discussion of steel viaducts, see pages 29-30 in Chapter 4.)

Concrete came into common use for trestles in the 1930s, **3-8**. Although not as common as wood, they can be found in many areas in configurations resembling wood trestles. They are often used to span short crossings as replacements for old wood trestles.

Modeling wood trestles

The intricate structures of wood trestles make for eye-catching models on a layout. Although trestles look complex, their construction is basic, and if you divide models into simple subassemblies, you'll find they are easy to build. Several companies also make kits for timber trestles in HO and N scales (see the list of available kits starting on page 86). Most of these feature stripwood construction, but a few (Walthers among others) use plastic. (See page 24 for some tips on making plastic bents look like wood.)

Plastic models go together quickly and easily, and usually have nice details including nut-bolt-washer details molded in place. However, many modelers will tell you that nothing replicates the look of wood like real wood. You can start with a wood kit for a trestle, or you can buy your own dimensional stripwood to make a trestle of almost any size or design.

Basswood works well for this application because it is strong but easy to cut and shape, and it accepts stain and glue well. Use the proper-size scale lumber for your project (see **3-2** for the typical sizes of prototype components). Scale lumber is available from Kappler, Midwest, Mt. Albert, Northeastern, and others. Most of these companies sell lumber in scale dimensions, but the chart in **3-9** (page 19) will help you convert measurements from fractions or decimals to scale sizes.

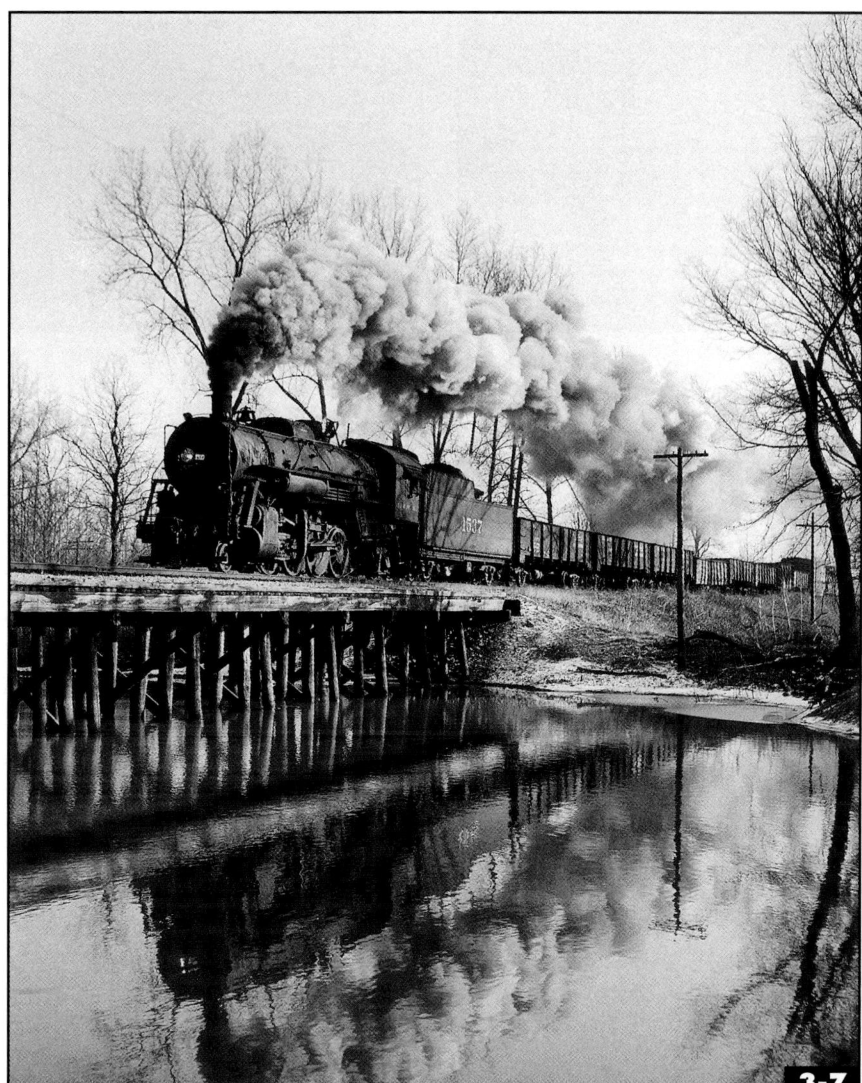

Look above the stringers and you'll see the ends of the planks that make up the deck of this ballasted-deck trestle. The rail and standard ties are visible on top of the ballast. *J. Parker Lamb, Jr.*

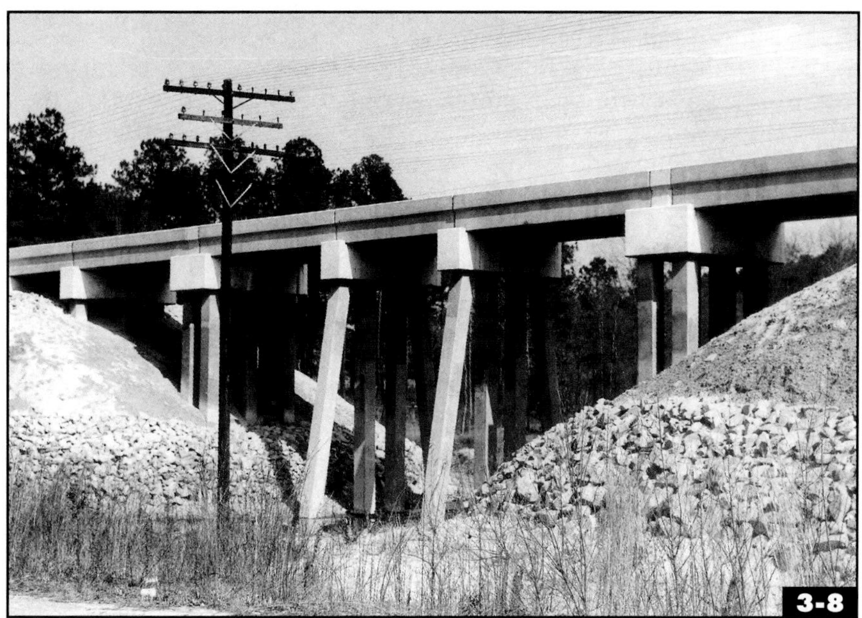

Concrete trestles replaced timber in many locations starting in the 1930s. *G.E. Roshley*

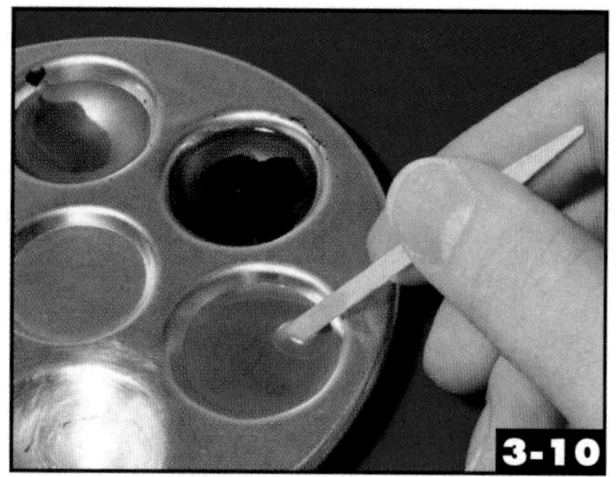

Various colors of artist's acrylic paint, thinned with water, make great stains for scale lumber. *Jeff Wilson*

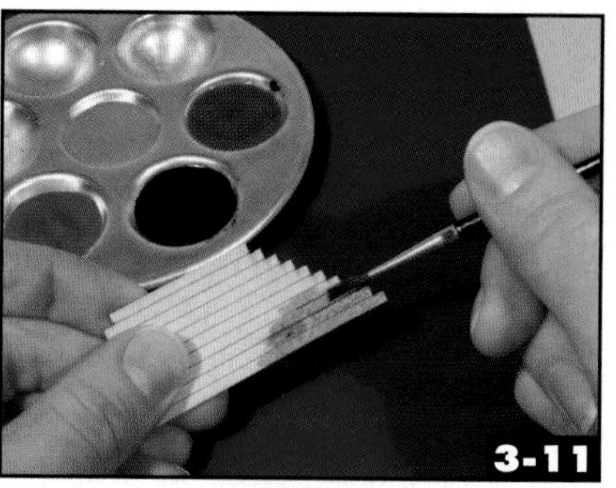

Brush the thinned acrylic paint onto the wood. You can mix and blend the colors with your brush as you go. *Jeff Wilson*

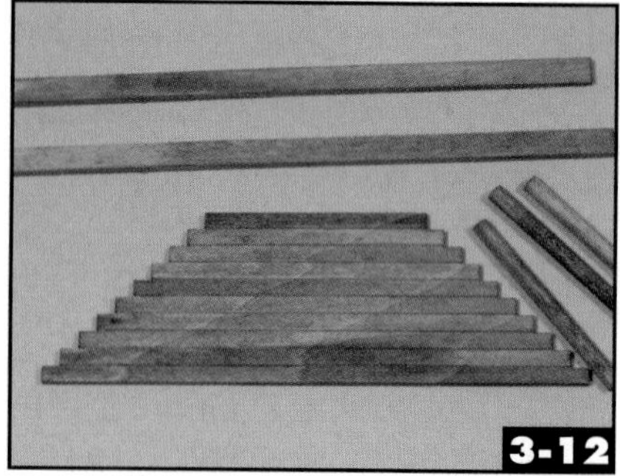

Vary the appearance of individual boards. This is especially important when coloring scribed sheet material. *Jeff Wilson*

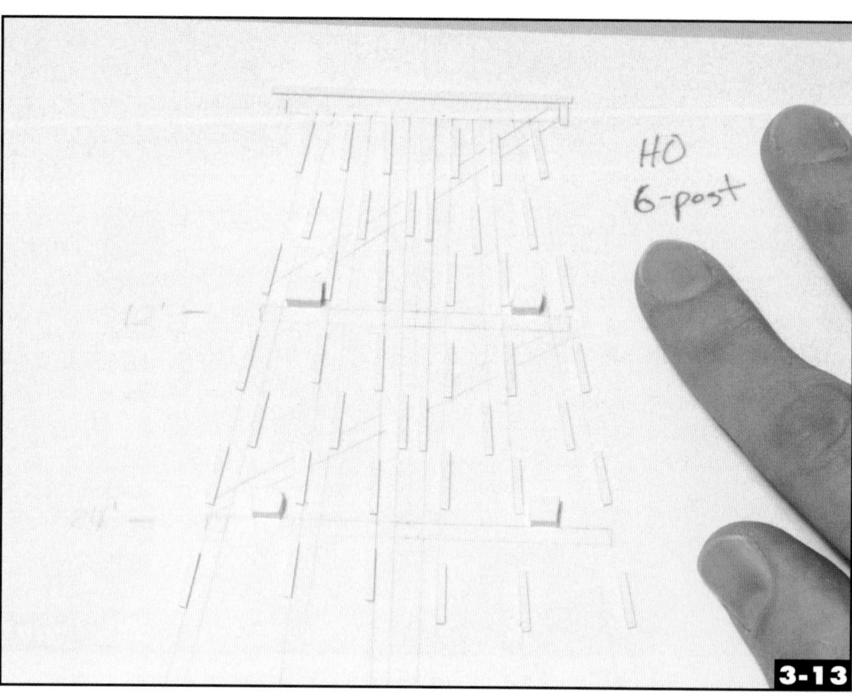

◀ Glue small strips of styrene next to the post locations. The thicker pieces of styrene will keep the sashes aligned. *Jeff Wilson*

▼ A NorthWest Short Line Chopper is a useful tool for cutting multiple pieces of stripwood and styrene to the uniform lengths. *Jeff Wilson*

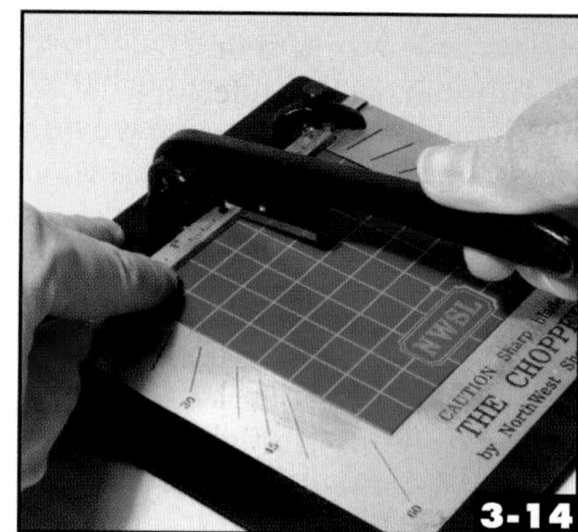

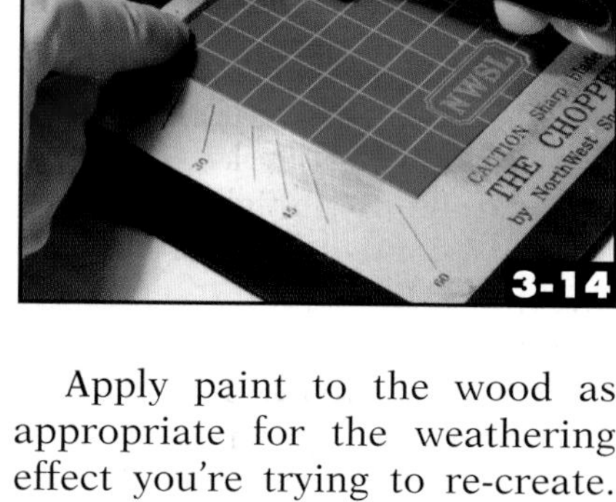

Staining wood

The look of weathered wood is vital to the appearance of the finished trestle. Lumber used in full-scale trestles is treated with creosote or other preservatives to protect it from the elements and termites. Colors range from almost black to many shades of brown and gray, depending upon the type of treatment, type of wood, age, and weather conditions.

The initial staining and coloring of stripwood is best done before beginning assembly. Otherwise, any glue that seeps out of a joint during construction will seal the wood, keeping the stain from penetrating. The result will be unrealistic patches of unweathered wood.

You can use many methods to color the wood, including commercial wood stains like Minwax. These are easy to use and come in a wide variety of colors.

I've had good good results mixing my own "stains" using artist's acrylic paint. Good weathered-wood colors include black, burnt sienna, burnt umber, raw umber, and raw sienna. Squeeze a small amount of paint into a small aluminum palette (available at art-supply or craft stores), then add some water, **3-10**.

Use a large toothpick to stir the paint into the water, but don't mix the paint thoroughly. The goal is to have a thin wash of the color on top, but thicker paint at the bottom. This lets you just touch the tip of your brush into the mix for a light wash, or dip it way down for a heavy dose of color, **3-11**.

Apply paint to the wood as appropriate for the weathering effect you're trying to re-create. Follow initial light coats of color with heavier doses to get different effects, **3-12**. Make sure the stain is completely dry (let it sit at least overnight) before beginning construction.

Bents

The first step in constructing a trestle is to build the bents. As you'll find throughout this book, I'm a big fan of jigs. Jigs speed construction and improve the quality of the finished model by working as a third hand to hold pieces in place during assembly, guaranteeing uniform results. A jig is particularly handy when you have to assemble a lot of bents or

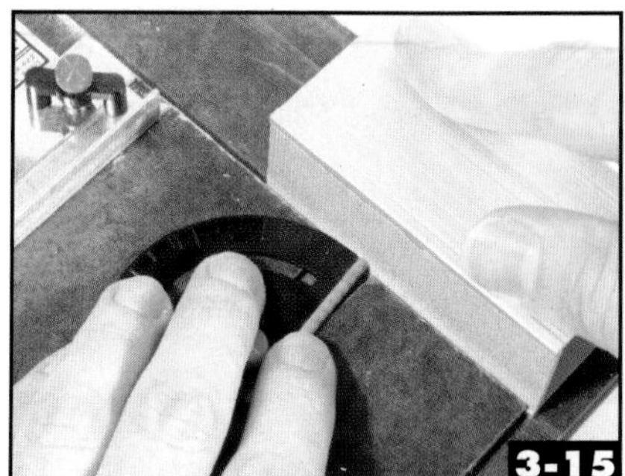

The NorthWest Short Line True Sander keeps parts aligned when truing the edges of strip and sheet material. *Jeff Wilson*

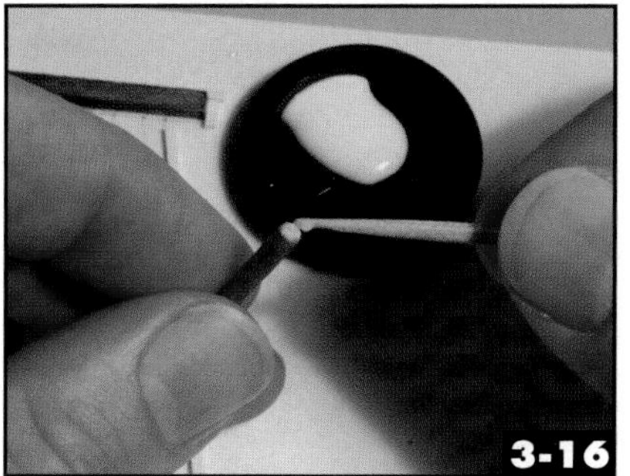

A toothpick is useful for applying small, precise quantities of glue to post ends and other tight areas. *Jeff Wilson*

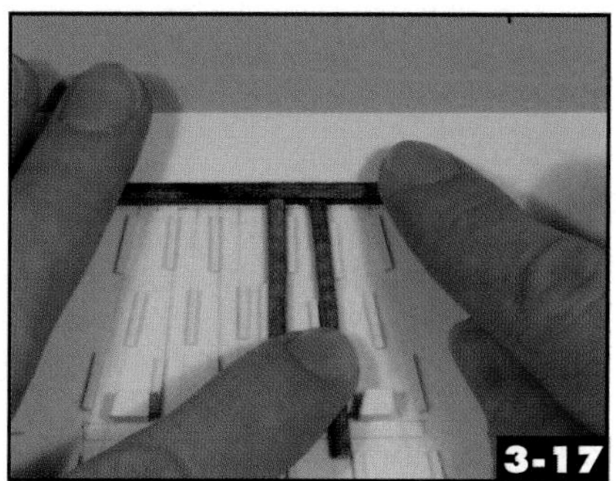

The jig holds the posts in line as the glued end is pushed against the cap. *Jeff Wilson*

are building especially tall ones.

To build a bent-assembly jig, get a piece of plain sheet styrene at least .040″ thick. Styrene works well because the white glue used in construction won't stick to it. Trace the outlines of the bent onto the plastic with a pencil; include the span and cross-bracing. Use the drawings in **3-2** or other published plans as a guide.

The jig I built for the project shown here is based on the six-post bent of the ballasted-deck trestle shown in **3-2**. Glue strips of plastic along both sides of each post location, **3-13**. The fit should be snug enough to hold the pieces in line, but not too tight.

A NorthWest Short Line Chopper makes quick work of cutting the posts and other trestle components, **3-14**. I used the adjustable sliding guide with a NorthWest Short Line True Sander to sand the tops of the posts at the proper angles, **3-15**.

Place the cap of the bent in the jig. Put a dab of white glue on top of each post, **3-16**, then press it into place, **3-17**. I like using white glue; yellow carpenter's glue or thick super glue (cyanoacrylate adhesive) will also work. If you're using super glue, be especially careful that no glue seeps onto the jig or the bent will be glued in place. In any case, use glue sparingly and avoid getting it on (or allowing it to seep onto) visible surfaces of the wood.

If your bents are taller than 10 scale feet or so, you'll need to add sway bracing and sashes as **3-2** shows. Drawing the diagonal braces on the jig will aid in placing glue before installing the braces, **3-18**.

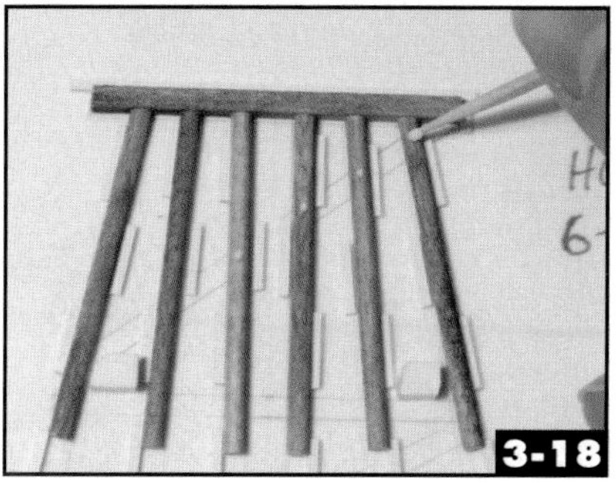

The sash drawing on the jig is a handy reference for adding glue before adding the sash. *Jeff Wilson*

You can detail trestles with nut-bolt-washer castings, **3-19** (page 20). These are available in different sizes and styles from Detail Associates, Grandt Line, and other companies. Drill holes in the wood where you want to install them. Cut a casting from its sprue, dip the end of the stem into a drop of super glue, then care-

DIMENSION CONVERSIONS

	N scale		HO scale		O scale	
Board size	**Decimal**	**Fractional**	**Decimal**	**Fractional**	**Decimal**	**Fractional**
2 x 4	.010″ x .020″	1/64″ x 1/32″	.020″ x .040″	1/32″ x 1/16″	.040″ x .080″	1/32″ x 3/32″
3 x 10	.020″ x .060″	1/32″ x 1/16″	.030″ x .120″	1/32″ x 1/8″	.060″ x .200″	1/16″ x 7/32″
4 x 4	.020″-sq.	1/32″-sq.	.040″-sq.	1/16″-sq.	.080″-sq.	3/32″-sq.
4 x 8	.020″ x .040″	1/32″ x 1/16″	.040″ x .080″	1/16″ x 3/32″	.080″ x .160″	3/32″x 5/32″
4 x 10	.020″ x .060″	1/32″ x 1/16″	.040″ x .100″	1/16″ x 1/8″	.080″ x .200″	3/32″ x 7/32″
6 x 8	.030″ x .040″	1/32″ x 1/16″	.060″ x .080″	1/16″ x 3/32″	.125″ x .160″	1/8″ x 5/32″
7 x 16	.040″ x .100″	1/32″ x 3/32″	.080″ x .180″	3/32″ x 3/16″	.140″ x .320″	5/32″ x 5/16″
8 x 8	.040″-sq.	1/16″-sq.	.080″-sq.	3/32″-sq.	.160″-sq.	5/32″-sq.
12 x 12	.080″-sq.	1/16″-sq.	.140″-sq.	1/8″-sq.	.250″-sq.	1/4″-sq.
12 x 14	.080″ x .100″	1/16″ x 3/32″	.140″ x .160″	1/8″ x 5/32″	.250″ x .300″	1/4″ x 9/32″

Note: The dimensions above are approximations. To calculate the exact size for a given scale, multiply the size by .00625 for N scale, .01148 for HO, and .2083 for O scale. For example, 4″ in HO scale is 4 x .01148, or .04592″.

3-9

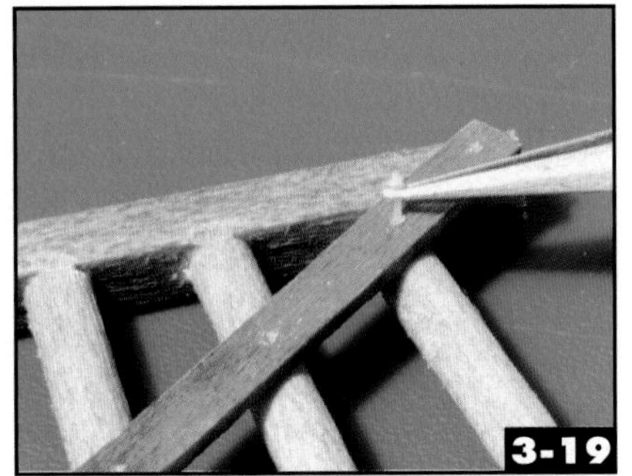

Use tweezers to place nut-bolt-washer castings in their mounting holes. *Jeff Wilson*

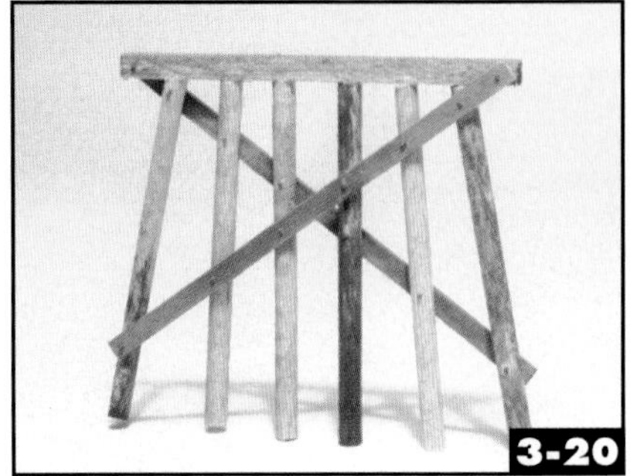

The finished bent, with weathered wood and cast details, looks realistic. *Jeff Wilson*

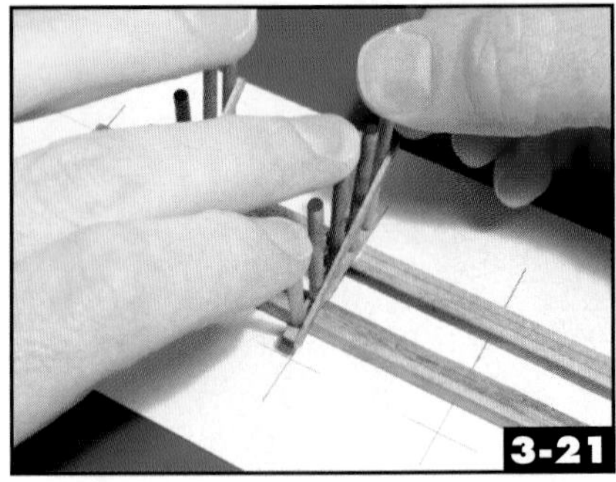

Mark the bent location on the bottoms of the stringers, apply a drop of white glue, and press the bent in place. *Jeff Wilson*

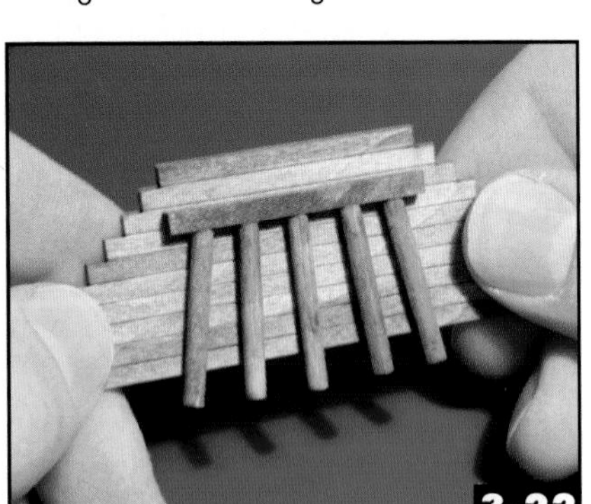

Glue the pile/cap assembly to the wood wall, making sure the distance from the top of the cap to the top of the wall is correct. *Jeff Wilson*

fully place it in the hole. The process goes quickly, and the extra detail looks great. Paint these dark brown or grimy black to finish them, **3-20**.

When modeling a pile trestle, leave the posts at the bottom of the trestle unfinished and "plant" them in the scenery when installing the trestle on your layout. If you're modeling a frame trestle, you'll need to end the bottom of the bent in a sill (see **3-2**) that will rest on a foundation when installed.

Ties, stringers, and bracing

You have two choices with ties: Use wood ties or use bridge track. Commercial kits are available both ways; if you're building from scratch, you can pick the method you want.

Bridge ties are available precut in HO scale from Campbell and Kappler; you can also cut your own from scale stripwood. Bridge track, which includes ties and—depending upon the brand—may include

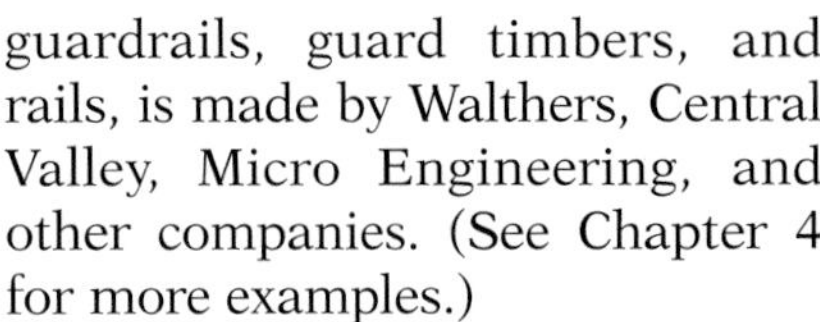

guardrails, guard timbers, and rails, is made by Walthers, Central Valley, Micro Engineering, and other companies. (See Chapter 4 for more examples.)

If you're using commercial bridge track, proceed by gluing the bents to the stringers. Glue the stringers together, then use double-sided tape to hold them in alignment on a piece of cardboard, **3-21**.

Mark the bent location lightly across the stringers with a pencil or scriber. Use a toothpick to place dots of white glue on the stringers, then position the bent in place. Make sure it is centered side-to-side on the stringers. Hold it firmly until the glue begins to set. When the glue is set, remove the assembly from the tape.

Assemble the bulkhead separately; the one shown in photo **3-22** is from Blair Line, but the process is similar if you're building one from scratch. (A plastic bulkhead from Walthers is shown in photos **2-14** and **2-15** in Chapter 2.) Glue the end bent to the bulkhead, making sure the resulting space from the tops of the stringers to the top of the bulkhead is slightly less than the thickness of one tie. Glue the bulkhead assemblies to the trestle, **3-23**.

Add the remaining bracing, if any, to your trestle. The wall bracing is the most prominent. One- to two-story trestles typically have wall bracing between every other bent; trestles taller than two stories should have wall bracing for two consecutive gaps. Frame trestles often have wall bracing on every gap. In general, the taller and longer the trestle, the more wall bracing it has.

The sample trestle I built here is a short one, but as **3-2** shows, tall trestles have girts. These

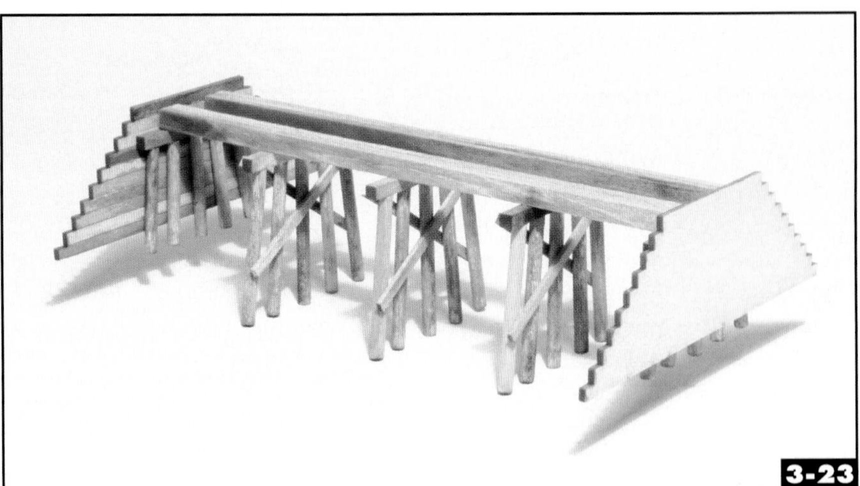

Glue the bulkhead assemblies to the trestle prior to installing the trestle (this one's a Blair Line HO kit) on the layout. *Jeff Wilson*

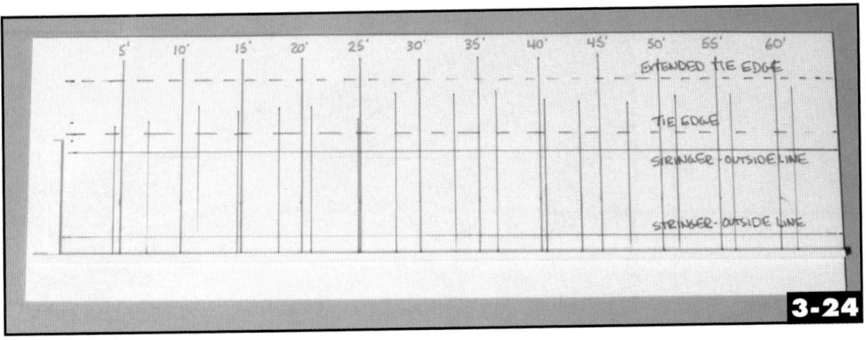

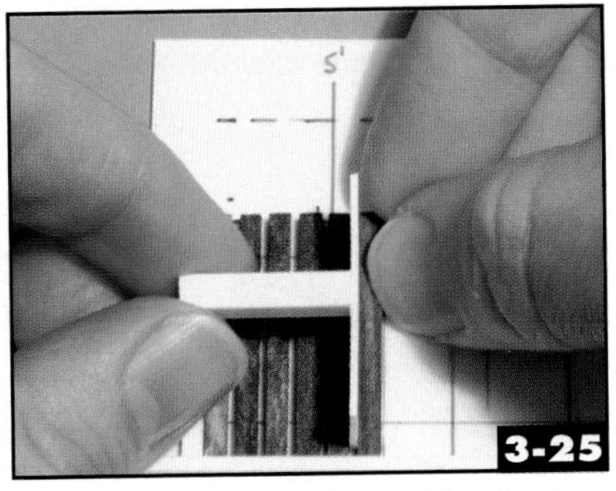

Above left: This jig can be used for aligning ties for trestles or deck girder or beam bridges. The strip at the bottom keeps the ends of the ties aligned; other markings are for reference. *Jeff Wilson*

▲ A piece of .040″ styrene (with a styrene strip handle) keeps ties spaced properly. Double-sided tape holds the ties in place. *Jeff Wilson*

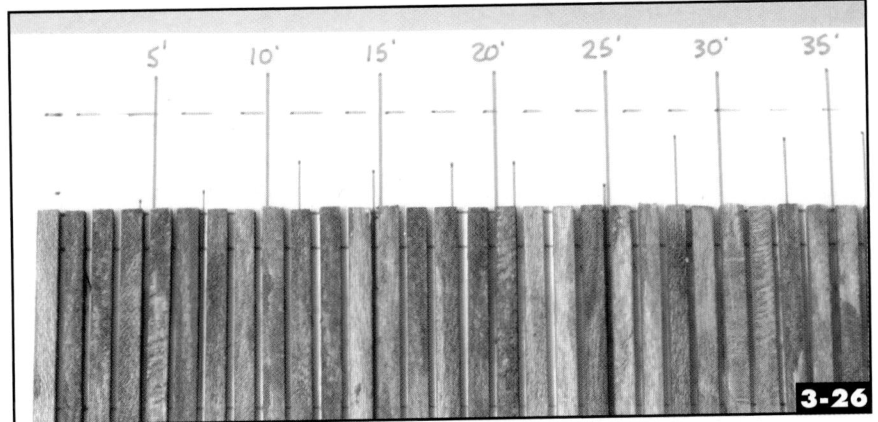

◄ The finished strip of ties is ready for installing on a trestle or bridge. *Jeff Wilson*

continue into the ground or to a bent at ground level on each end of the trestle.

If you're using commercial bridge track, add it after installing the trestle. More on that in a bit.

Individual ties

If you're using individual wood ties, you'll need to alter the construction order a bit. Make another jig to hold the ties in alignment. I like to use a sheet of styrene with a straight strip of styrene along its length to keep the ends of the ties even and another strip at a right angle to the first strip at one end, **3-24**. Mark the jig as shown with lines to help keep the ties perpendicular to the guide strip. Marks at intervals of five scale feet provide a length guideline, and additional lines mark the outside locations of the stringers.

Ties on trestles are typically 8″ square and 10′ long. Ties on trestles are spaced much more closely than normal track—on 12″ centers, meaning there's a gap of just 4″ between ties.

Place a strip of double-sided cellophane tape on the jig down the center of the ties the length of the deck. Fresh tape may pull the finish off of weathered wood, so press the tape with your fingers a few times to make it less sticky.

Press the first tie in place at the end guide. Continue pressing ties in place, using a piece of .040″ styrene (for HO; use .020″ for N and .080″ for O scale) as a spacer. Glue a small handle to the spacer to make it easier to use, **3-25**.

Once all the ties are in place, **3-26**, glue on the stringers following the guidelines on the jig, then add the bents.

Installation

The technique for installing a trestle will depend on the type of subroadbed, roadbed, and track you're using, along with the type of scenery you're planning. The key is to make sure the trestle is level and follows the line of the roadbed. It must also match the level of the adjoining trackwork.

I tacked my Blair Line trestle in place in a gap left in Woodland Scenics foam riser subroadbed and cork roadbed, **3-27** (page 22). The bulkhead wall should be slightly above the level of the top of the roadbed, but not so tall that the rails will touch it.

Depending on your scenery plans, you might want to add surrounding scenery before installing the trestle. Once you're ready to install it permanently, set it in place and position the bridge track on the trestle, making sure it lines up with the adjoining track, **3-28** (page 22). If you plan to paint the bridge track (see Chapter 4), do so before installing it on the trestle.

After gluing the bridge track in place, glue the trestle onto the layout. If necessary, you can shim the approach tracks slightly with thin styrene sheet to raise the height. When the glue sets, the scene will be ready for scenery.

If you've built a trestle with separate bridge ties, add the rails prior to installing the trestle as discussed in the section on girder bridges in Chapter 4 (pages 30-31).

Guardrails

Short trestles often don't have guardrails, but you'll find them on longer trestles and most other types of bridges. Commercial bridge track from Walthers has them; with other brands of bridge

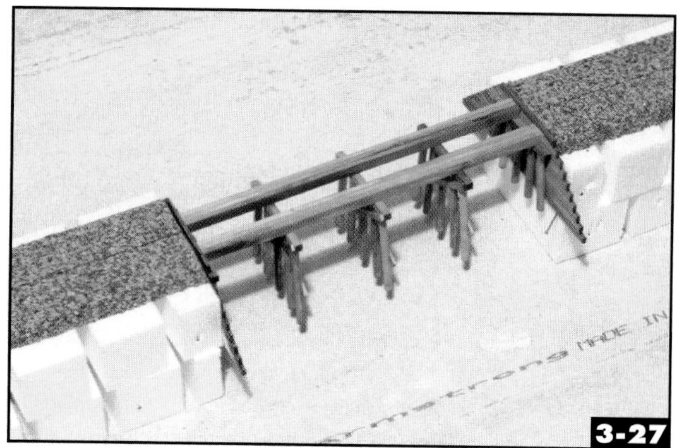
Test-fit the trestle. The top of the bulkhead wall should be less than a tie-thickness above the top of the roadbed. *Jeff Wilson*

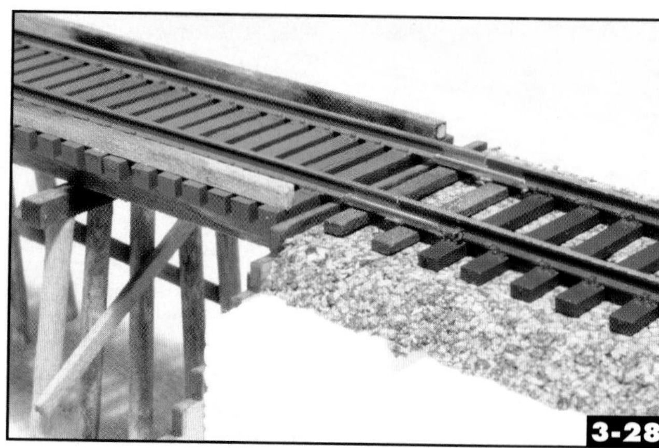
The rails of the bridge track just clear the bulkhead. A couple of ties glued in place under the rail joint improve the appearance of the track. *Jeff Wilson*

track (or if you're using separate ties) you're on your own. Here's how to make guardrails.

Guardrails usually start at a frog (yes, just like at a turnout) 30′ to 50′ from the end of the trestle or bridge, **3-29**. Guardrails are usually smaller in size than the running rails (and are never taller). Full-size railroads use scrap or used rail for this, and you can too. Watch as I make guardrails from a cut-off piece of Atlas N scale code 55 track that I had on hand (the running rails are code 83).

Use a large flat file to bevel the end of a piece of rail to form the frog, **3-30**. Positioning the rail at the end of a board helps brace it while filing. Bevel a second piece of rail on the opposite side, **3-31**.

Soldering will provide the strongest joint. I made a jig by cutting a V shape in a piece of thin basswood, then gluing it to a scrap board, **3-32**. The angle isn't critical—it just needs to hold the rail ends in position. Slide the rails into place, then secure them with tape or a clamp.

Apply heat to the end of both rails using a soldering iron as shown in photo **3-32**. When they're hot, touch solder to the joint, and the solder will flow into it. When the area cools, use a large flat file to shape the frog end, removing any sharp points or burrs. Set the frog and rails in place on the track and mark locations for the spikes that will hold it in place, **3-33**.

It's a good idea to insulate one side of the guardrail; otherwise, if a metal wheel happens to bump spikes or rail on both sides (especially in a derailment), you'll have a short circuit. To do this, simply cut one of the guardrails near the frog and file both ends flat. When laying the guardrails, super glue a small bit of styrene or gray ABS plastic (Plastruct) in the gap to keep the rails apart, **3-34**.

Use super glue or spikes to secure the guardrail in position, **3-35**. Needle-nose pliers work well for pushing the spikes in place. Do the same at the other end of the trestle or bridge. You can simply butt the two ends together, or use rail joiners.

Ballasted decks

You can model a ballasted deck trestle using methods similar to those described above. The drawing in **3-2** shows the cross-section of one of these trestles, and a prototype example can be seen in photo **3-7**. Ballasted deck trestles have wider bent caps (usually 16′ for a single track) to support the 14′-wide deck.

To model one of these, start with the deck. On real trestles, the deck boards are usually 4″-thick planks (see the prototype in photo **3-7**), but since only the ends of the individual boards can be seen once the ballast is in place, I use ¹⁄₁₆″-thick sheet basswood oriented side-to-side so the end grain shows at the sides of the deck. Stain this end grain using the technique described in "Staining wood" on page 18.

Prototype ballasted deck trestles have many stringers spaced across the underside of the deck. Since they can't be seen when the model is installed on a layout, I used only four on the example

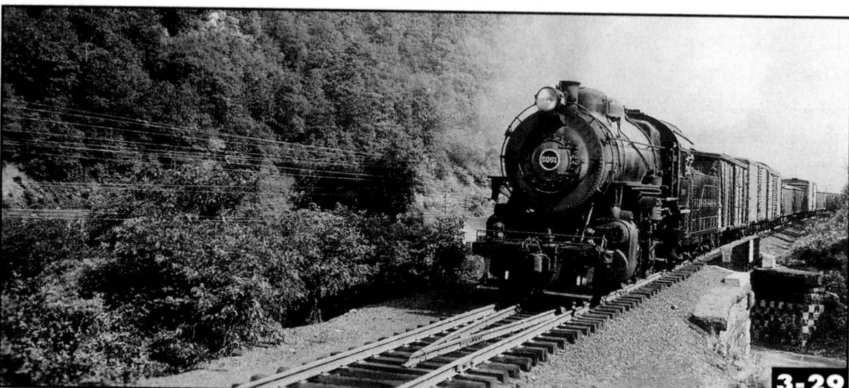
Guardrails typically extend 30′ to 50′ from the end of a bridge or trestle and usually come together at a frog. *Norman Cooper*

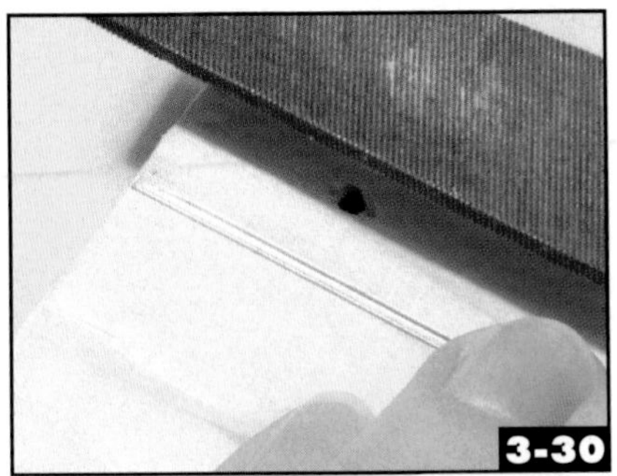
3-30

Bevel one end of a rail using a large flat file. A board holds the rail in place while filing. *Jeff Wilson*

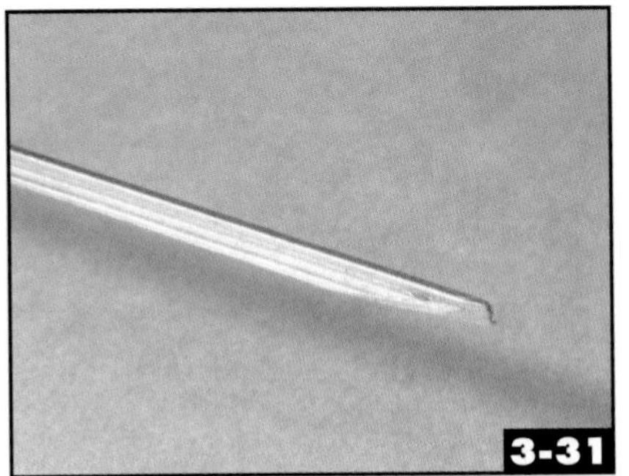
3-31

For the other side of the guardrail frog, bevel the end of another length of scrap rail to a mirror image of the first. *Jeff Wilson*

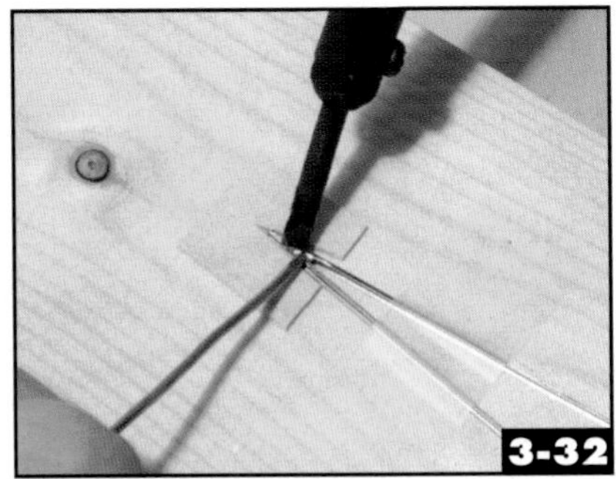
3-32

A V-groove cut into a thin wood piece, glued to a larger board, holds the rails in place for soldering. *Jeff Wilson*

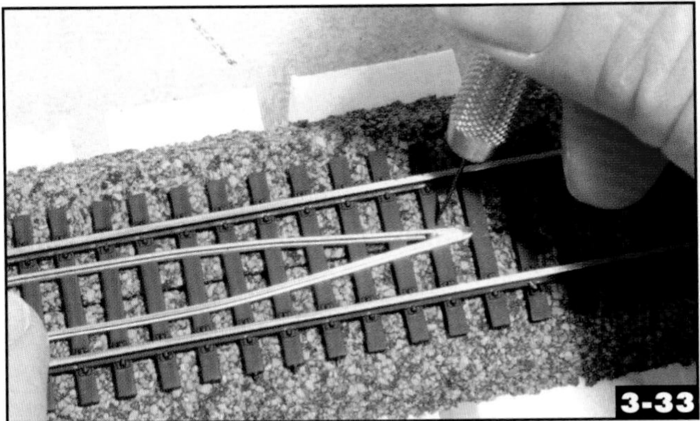
3-33

Position the frog and drill holes for the spikes that will hold it in place. *Jeff Wilson*

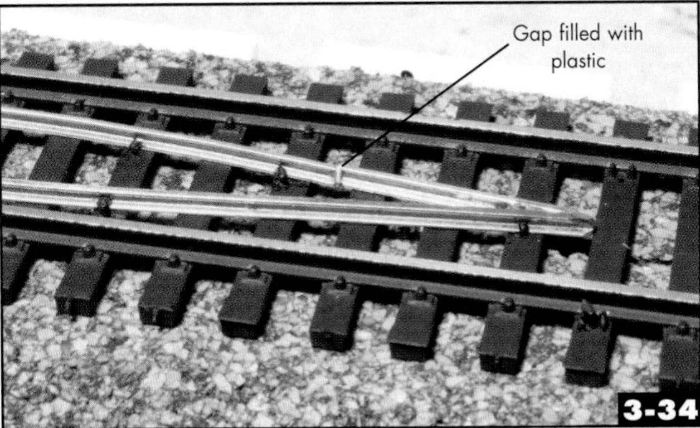

3-34

A small piece of styrene or ABS in the guardrail gap will prevent short-circuits. Painting the rails will hide the styrene. *Jeff Wilson*

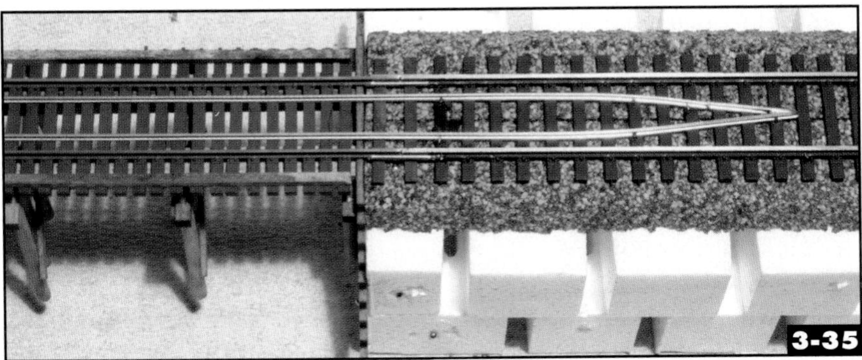
3-35

The finished guardrail is spiked in place on the trestle. *Jeff Wilson*

shown here, **3-36** (page 24). You certainly may use more stringers if you like.

Once the stringers are in place, mark the location of the bents (see **3-36**). I use a scriber to mark one edge of each bent across all the stringers. Add a bit of white glue at each stringer, then press the bent in place.

When the bents are in place and the glue is dry, flip the trestle upright. The next step is to add the ballast guards along the outside edges of the deck. These are 8 × 8 boards on real trestles, so I used white glue to secure scale stripwood in place.

The track should be elevated slightly above the deck, but most HO roadbed is too thick. Instead, I use N scale cork that is not split apart to elevate the track the correct amount. Photo **3-37** (page 24) shows the deck with the cork, track, and ballast in place.

The ballasted deck trestle can be installed using the same techniques shown earlier in this chapter (see "Installation" on page 21). You can add the cork to the bridge deck beforehand, making sure that it aligns with the roadbed on the layout when the trestle is installed. When laying track, simply continue it across the trestle.

Be sparing in the amounts of water and diluted glue you use when ballasting the deck because the wood is thin and will warp easily if it gets too wet. It's not a bad idea to give both sides of the deck a coat of paint before gluing it in place to seal it from water.

Curved trestles

Decks for curved trestles can be made in a similar fashion to straight trestles. The only thing that's different is the design of the stringers, which must be cut to fit between the bents. On a curved trestle, the stringers themselves aren't curved—they are a series of straight sections between bents.

Draw the outline of the stringer locations in a curve on a piece of cardstock. (I use an old yardstick with holes drilled in it as a compass to get the proper radii.) Next, add extended lines showing the

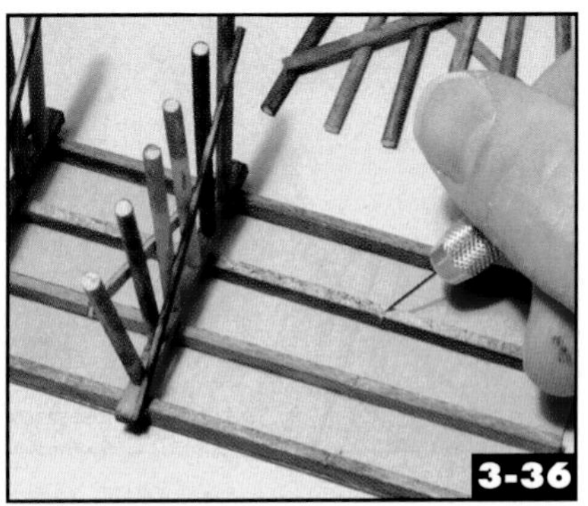

Mark the bent location on the stringers with a pin or fine scriber, then glue the bents in place. *Jeff Wilson*

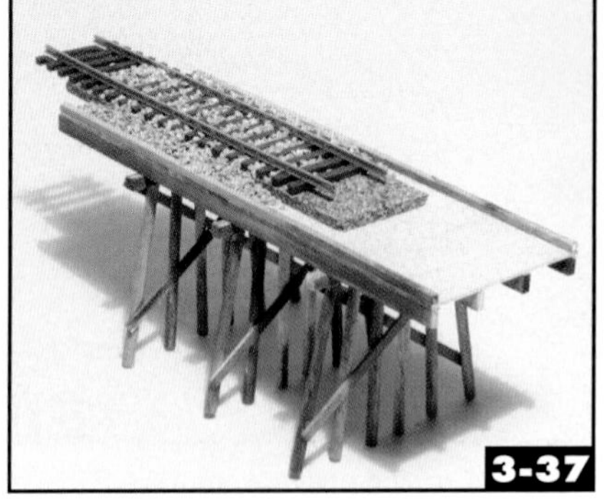

This view shows how N scale cork elevates the track. The cork will be hidden by the ballast. *Jeff Wilson*

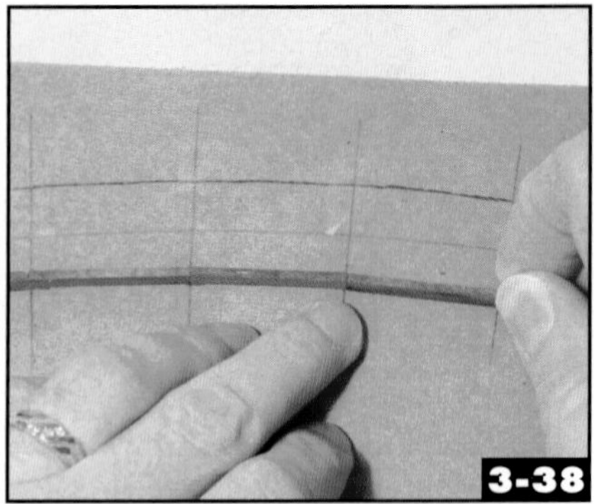

Cut stringers to fit, using the bent-center-line marks as a guide. *Jeff Wilson*

bent locations, **3-38**. Place strips of double-sided tape along the stringer positions.

Lay a stringer in place, mark it, and cut it so it runs from center to center of the caps. Repeat the process until the stringers are all in place, and glue adjoining stringers to each other.

When the stringers are done, glue the bents in place just as you would on a straight trestle. For the track, you can use a flexible bridge track (such as Micro Engineering), or you can place individual bridge ties by hand.

Most curves are superelevated—the outer rail is raised. This is done by installing wedge-shaped shims under the ties or by beveling thicker-than-normal ties. Model this with shims of 1⁄16" or less, or by sanding the ties.

Conclusion

Building larger trestles is simply a matter of using the techniques described in this chapter on a larger scale. Each railroad has its own standards regarding bracing, size of members, bent spacing, number of piles, and other details. The standards have been adjusted many times over the years to accommodate increased train weights. If you're modeling a specific trestle or railroad, check prototype photos and engineering drawings (if you can find them).

Now it's time to look at one of the simplest and sturdiest bridge types: the plate girder bridge.

Painting plastic trestles

You can improve the appearance of plastic trestle components that come in kits. Start by roughing up the plastic to make it look more like rough-cut wood. The photo at the far left shows how to use coarse (80-grit) sandpaper to enhance the effect of wood grain. Rub the sandpaper hard along all the surfaces of the bent. While you're doing that, make sure you remove mold parting lines along the edges of the poles.

Use a brush to paint the parts with medium to dark gray paint. Placing a few drops of several colors (black, grays, and browns) on a palette and mixing them with your brush as you apply them will result in a nice varied look. Apply brown or black washes (one part acrylic paint to eight or nine parts water) to some areas to further vary the appearance of the surface.

The photo at the far right shows a completed bent next to a raw plastic one. The texture and weathering make the plastic parts much more realistic.

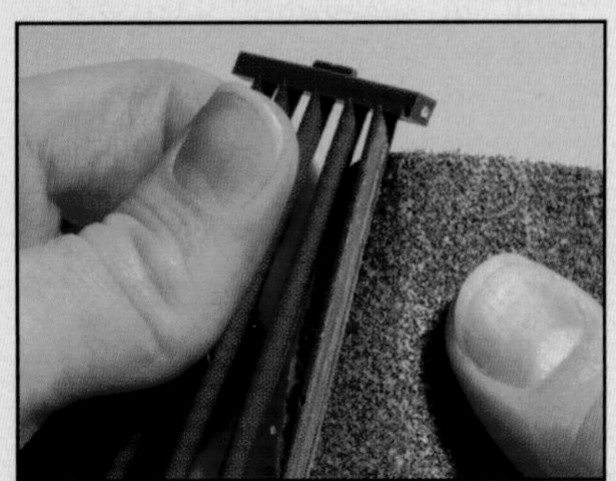

Rub coarse sandpaper along the bents and caps to enhance the effect of rough wood grain. *All photos: Jeff Wilson*

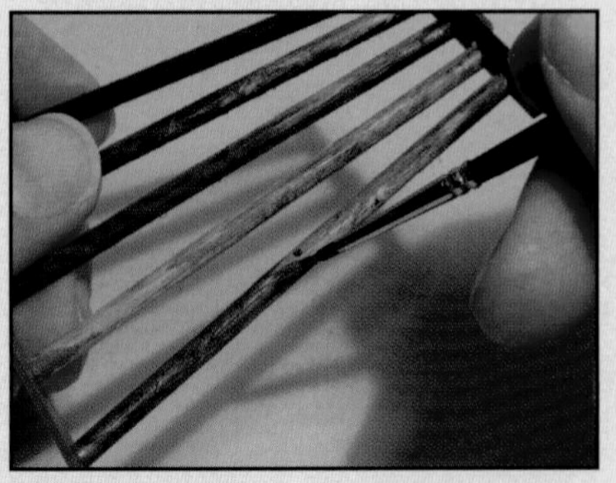

Paint the members with black and various shades of brown and gray to represent weathered, treated wood.

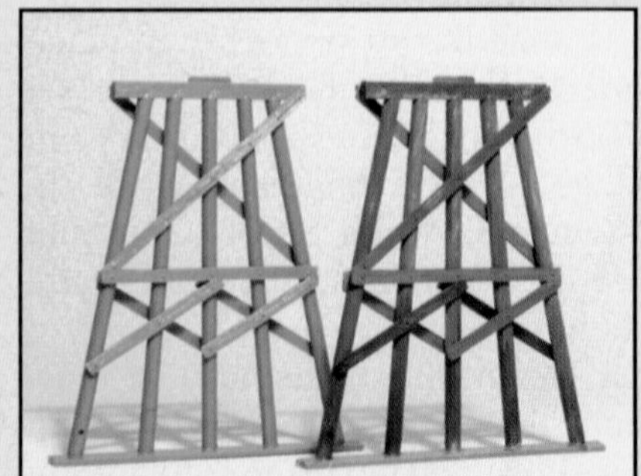

Compare the appearance of the roughed-up, weathered bent at right to the raw plastic, fresh-from-the-kit-box bent at left.

FOUR

Plate-girder bridges

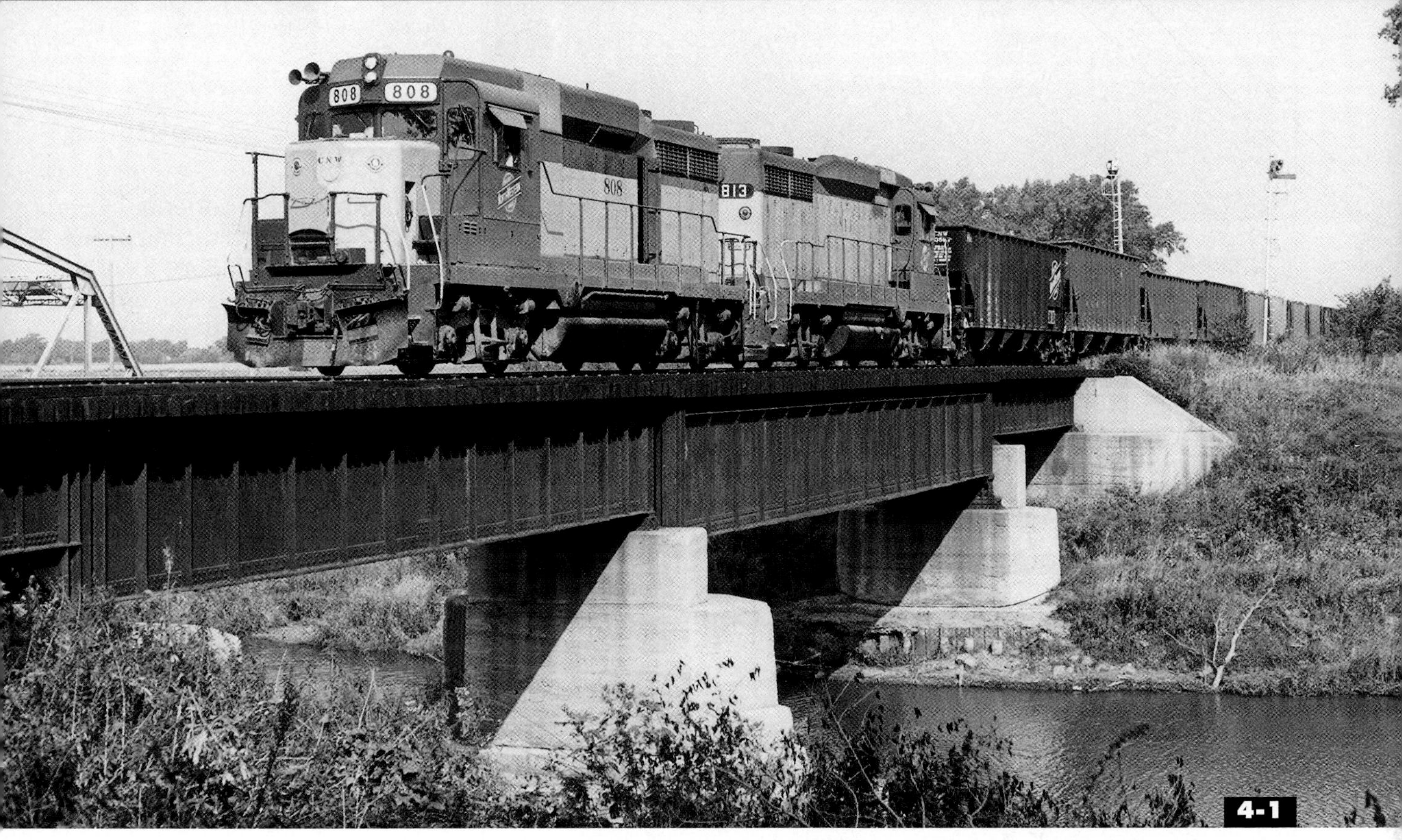

Plate-girder bridges are among the most common bridge types on full-scale railroads. Here, a Chicago & North Western freight rolls across a four-span deck plate-girder bridge in Sioux City, Iowa, in 1980. *Mike Schafer*

The steel plate-girder bridge is one of the most common bridge types used by railroads, **4-1**. A plate-girder bridge differs from a beam bridge in that the carrying girders are fabricated from several pieces of flat steel joined together.

Plate-girder bridges became popular early in the 1900s because they are simple, sturdy, easy to construct, and easy to transport to the job site. They are common for spans from about 40′ to 125′, though some are longer. They are generally not the most dramatic or picturesque of bridge types, but because they are the most common, most model railroad layouts should have at least several.

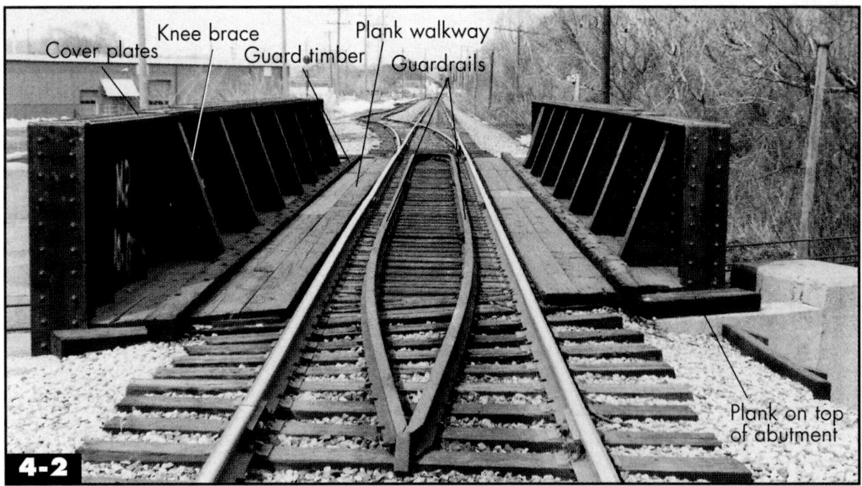

◀ Note how the ties on this skewed bridge are angled where the bridge meets the abutment. *Sy Dykhouse*

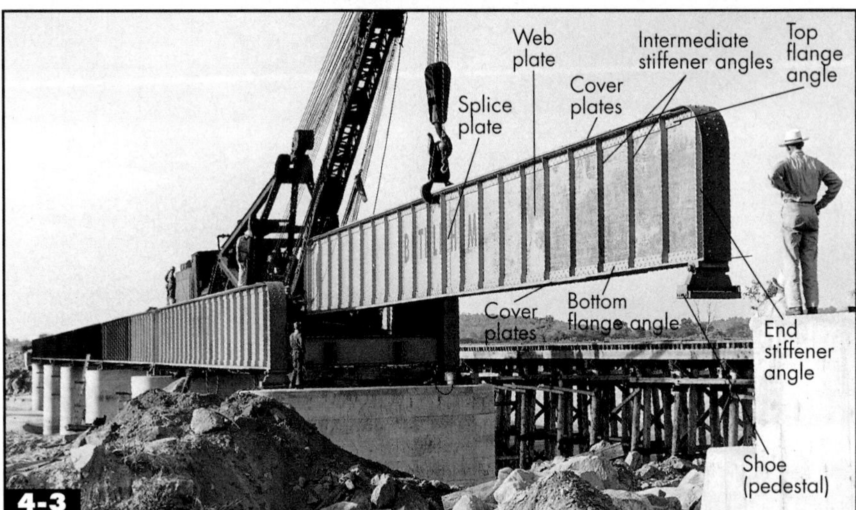

The components of this plate girder are in plain view as it is lowered into place. *Missouri-Kansas-Texas Railroad*

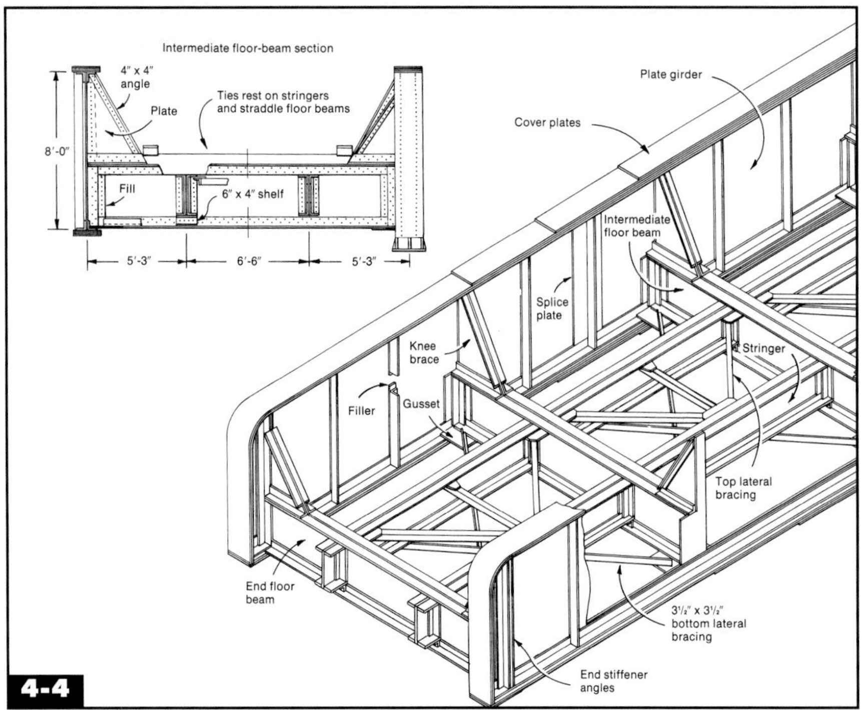

Plate-girder bridge construction is simple and straightforward.

Plate-girder components

Photo **4-2** shows the components of a plate-girder bridge (looking through the bridge); **4-3** shows a girder being installed on a bridge. Both photos help show how the bridge components come together.

The keys of a plate-girder bridge are the two side girders. The steel sheet itself is called the "web plate." It is reinforced with flange angles and cover plates around the edges. The vertical angles along the length of the girder are called "stiffener angles."

If more than one web plate is used to build a longer bridge, splice plates are used to join the web plates. These are riveted flat panels. Splice plates are generally located about a third of the way in from the ends, but they aren't placed in the center of the span.

Floor beams connect the girders from side to side, with stringers running between the floor beams, **4-4**. Knee braces solidify the connection between floor beams and girders, and lateral (cross) bracing also contributes to stability.

Plate-girder bridges come in two types: deck and through. The simpler design, the deck girder bridge, is used where below-bridge clearance is not an issue (see **4-1**). Through bridges are used where additional clearance is required below the bridge, typically for crossing highways and railroad tracks but also sometimes for navigable waterways.

As with trestles, plate-girder bridges can have either open-deck or ballasted-deck construction. On an open-deck through bridge, the ties—spaced more closely than conventional track—rest on the stringers and straddle the floor beams, **4-5**.

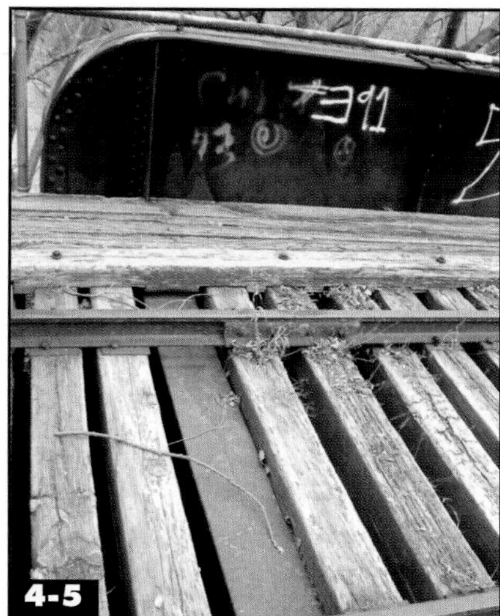

Note how the wood ties straddle the steel floor beam, which is taller than the stringers that the ties rest upon. This through-girder bridge has rounded corners. *Jeff Wilson*

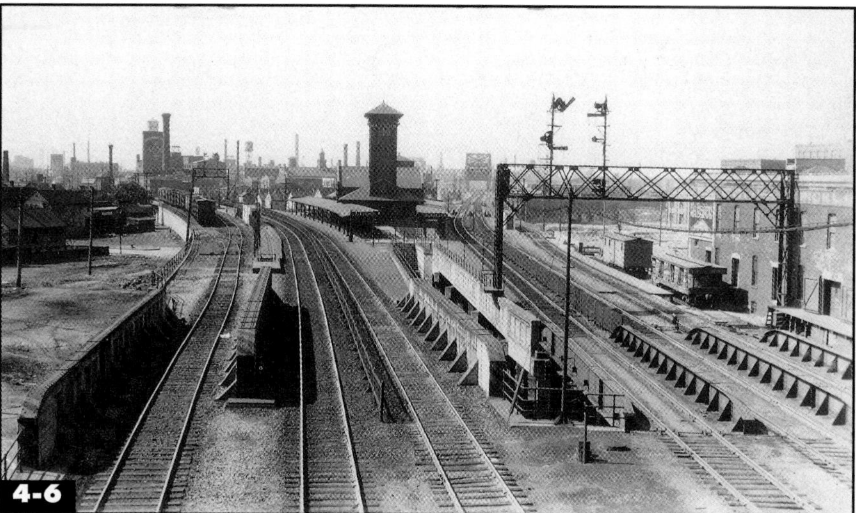

The three-track plate-girder bridge at left has a ballasted deck, while the three-track bridge at right is an open-deck that's been covered by metal plates. *David P. Morgan Library collection*

Through bridges have plate girders with either squared-off ends (see **4-2**) or rounded top corners (see **4-5**). Girders on deck bridges always have squared-off ends.

Ballasted-deck through bridges have a concrete trough that holds ballast, with standard track running atop the ballast, **4-6**. Decks are also often covered by metal plates or wood planks. This is usually done where a bridge spans a road or railroad, to keep debris from falling onto vehicles or trains below. It also makes it easier to adjust the height of track for optimum alignment and to superelevate curves without tapered or shimmed ties.

Deck bridges may also have ballasted decks, **4-7**. The concrete trough holding the ballast is quite apparent on this type of bridge.

Support for any bridge, including plate girders, is vital. Each end of each girder must be firmly supported on a pier or abutment by a bridge pedestal or shoe, **4-8**. Since metal bridges (plate-girder or truss) are subject to expansion and contraction due to temperature changes, the bridge must be allowed to move slightly on its length. One end of the bridge is anchored, with the other end on a pedestal that is allowed to move.

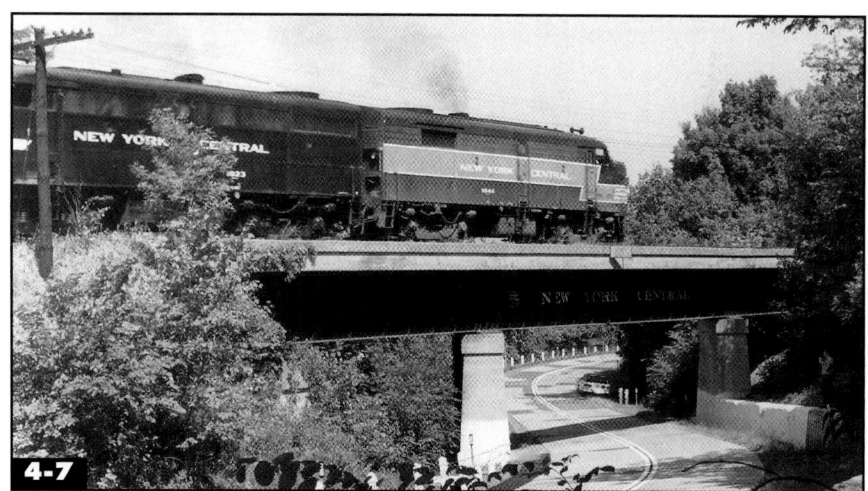

Ballasted deck girder bridges have a concrete trough atop the girders to hold the ballast and track. *Jim Shaughnessy*

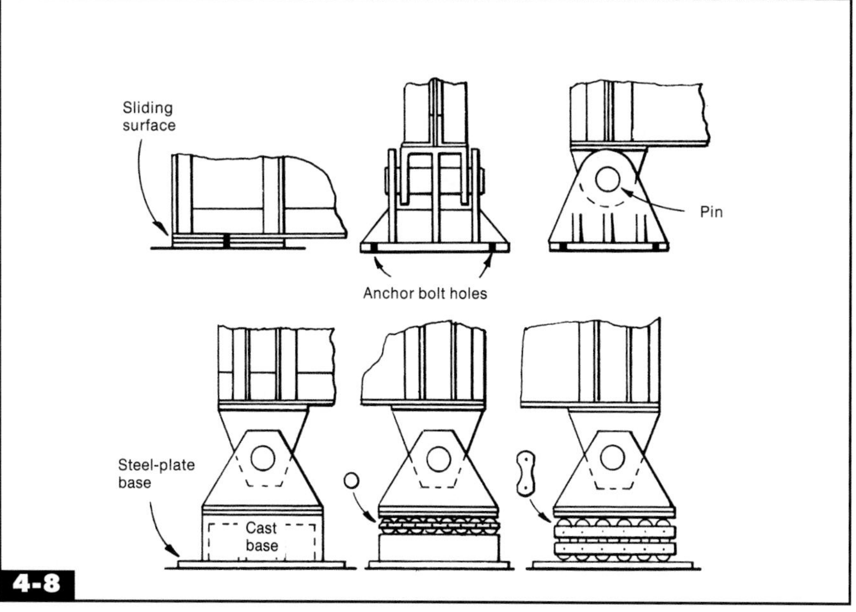

The girders on plate-girder bridges are connected to abutments or piers by bridge pedestals (also called shoes). Pedestal configuration depends on the type of bridge and the application.

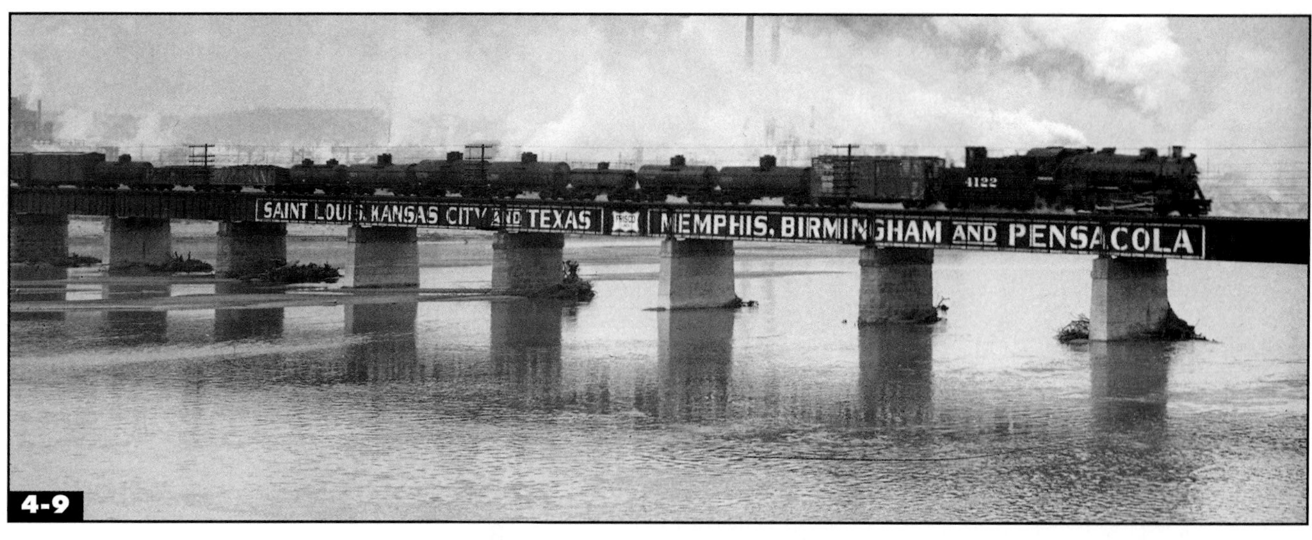

4-9

BRIDGE RATINGS

Span length:	30′	50′	70′	90′	110′
Girder height, E-50 loading:	4′-1 1/2″	5′-8 1/2″	7′-3 1/2″	8′-5 1/2″	9′-6 1/2″
Girder height, E-72 loading:	5′-9″	6′-0 1/2″	8′-0″	9′-4″	10′-0″

4-10

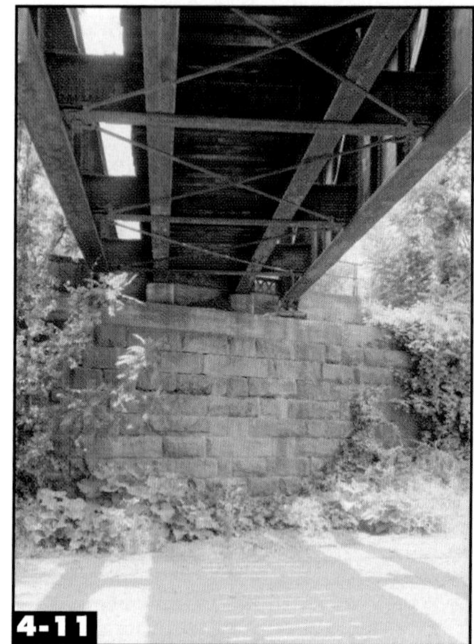

4-11

▲ (top) The St. Louis-San Francisco used this long multi-span deck plate-girder bridge as a billboard. *St. Louis-San Francisco Ry.*

► Note the angle of the abutment on this skewed through bridge. The extensions of the stringers beyond the last floor beam rest on their own concrete footings atop the abutment; other components remain the same. *Historic American Engineering Record*

On short spans, the pedestals can be simple flat sliding bearings, as on the bridge in **4-7** (page 27). Long bridges often have a rocker shoe beneath one end (see the girder in **4-3**, page 26), with a rolling shoe at the other, **4-8** (page 27). Check prototype photos throughout this chapter and Chapter 5 to see the variety of bridge pedestals in use.

Multiple spans of plate-girder bridges are common, **4-9**. Sometimes, the spans are the same length and style; other multiple spans have bridges of differing lengths and styles (through and deck, sometimes mixing truss and girder styles as well).

Regardless of the length or style, the end of each bridge girder must rest on top of an abutment or pier. Every joint between spans must rest on a pier, or the bridge would not support its own weight—much less that of a train. Chapter 9 goes into more detail on the use and placement of piers and abutments.

Plate-girder bridges, like other bridges, are rated for strength by Cooper's system (explained in Chapter 1). To modelers, this simply means that the longer the bridge and the heavier the trains, the heavier (deeper) the girders should be. Table **4-10** has guidelines for E-50 and E-72 spans; look at prototype photos (and engineering drawings if you can get them) for additional guidance. A length-to-width ratio of 7:1 is typical for railroad bridges.

Skewed bridges

Railroads often use skewed bridges where a bridge crosses a road, river, or other railroad at an angle other than 90 degrees. On these spans, the ends of the girders are not parallel. The through bridge in **4-2** (page 26) is a skewed span.

When modeling skewed spans, remember that each girder end must still be supported by a pier or abutment. Piers are angled to match the direction of flow in rivers, and to fit between other obstructions such as highways and railroads.

On a skewed bridge, the floor beams are still at a 90-degree angle to the girders, the beams still meet the girders at a stiffener angle, and other bracing remains the same. However, on the ends the stringers are extended to rest on the pier or abutment, as the under-bridge view in **4-11** shows.

Multi-track and curved bridges

Multiple through plate girders are sometimes used for parallel tracks (see **4-6**, page 27). They come in two varieties. Some, like the one in **4-6**, have an additional girder

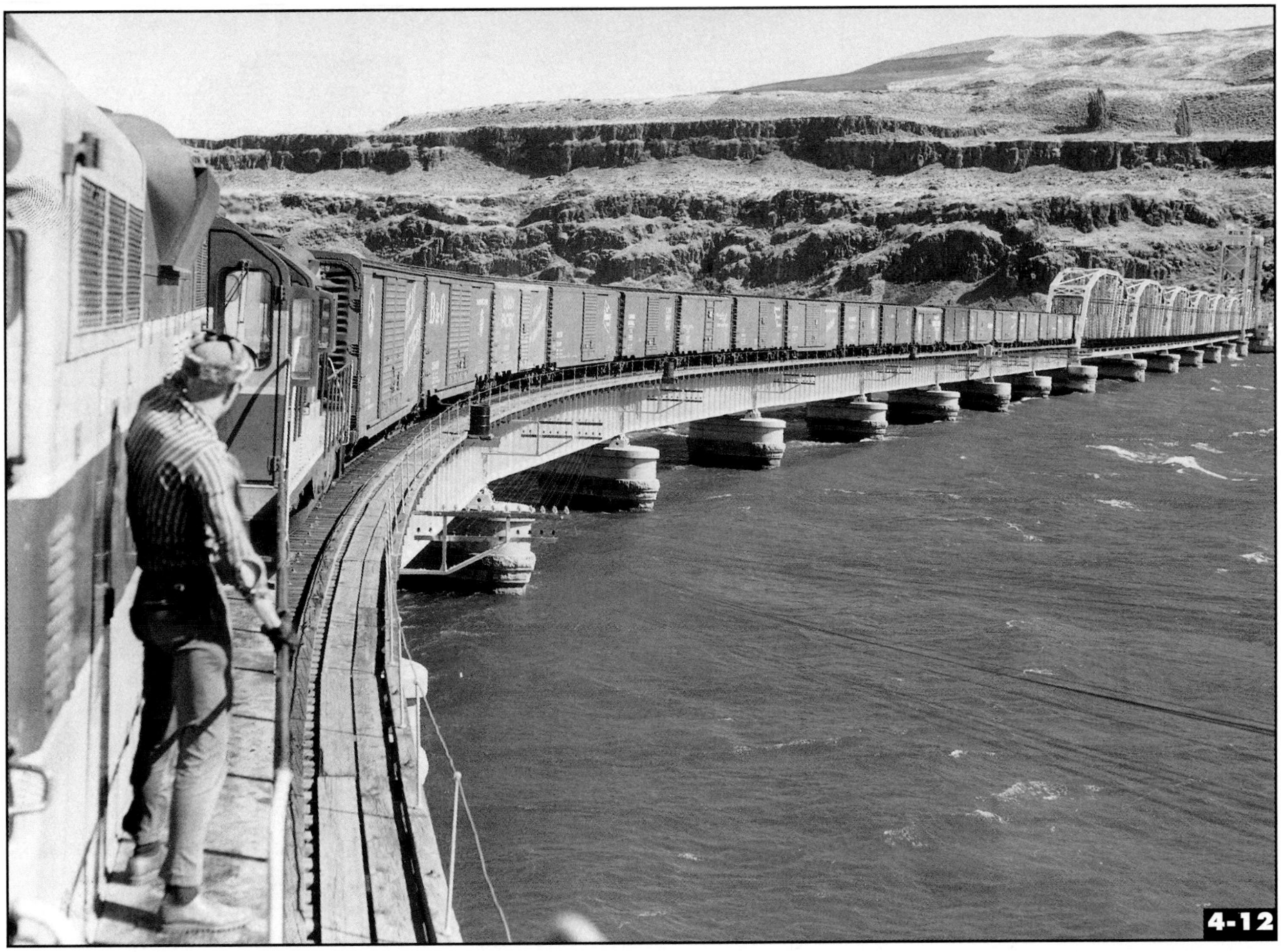

4-12

▲ Curved plate-girder bridges are actually a series of straight spans, each joined at a slight angle to the next. *Donald Sims*

between the tracks. This girder is a foot deeper than the outside girders. Other double-track bridges omit the center girder; however, on these, the outside girders will be deeper than those of an equivalent single-track span to support the extra load.

Double-track deck bridges are sometimes built, but they aren't as common as double-track through bridges. Instead, railroads often use parallel single-track deck bridges.

Plate-girder bridges are often used on curves, but the model railroader must keep in mind that the individual girders comprising a bridge are straight. Curved steel girders are now used sometimes in highway construction, but they are extremely rare on railroads because of the stresses involved. Instead, curves are made by connecting several straight spans, each of which is at a slight angle to the next span, **4-12**.

Steel viaducts

Around 1900, tall viaducts comprised of steel towers connecting multiple plate-girder bridge sections became the preferred method of crossing wide valleys and other broad depressions, **4-13**. Steel viaducts, the successors to tall wood-frame trestles, are among the most impressive bridges in modern railroading. They feature a

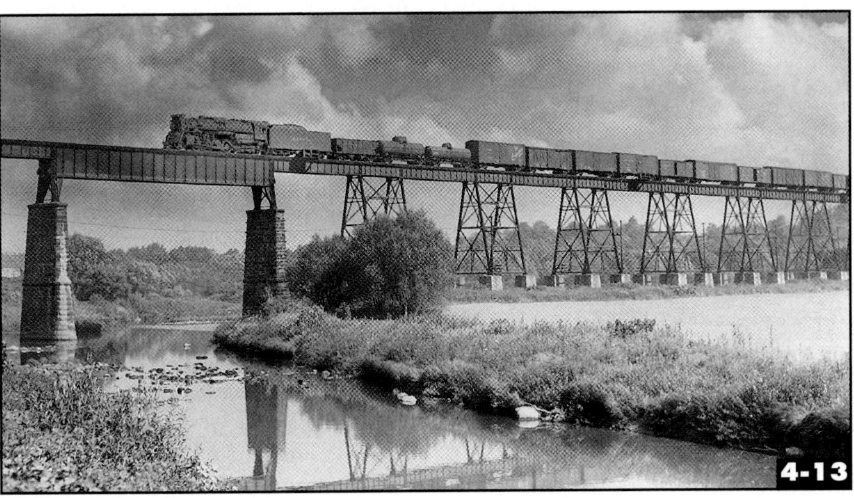

▼ This Nickel Plate Road viaduct at Conneaut, Ohio, includes a couple of longer plate-girder spans in the middle to bridge the river and another railroad. The structure is 1,320 feet long and 54 feet tall. *Richard J. Cook*

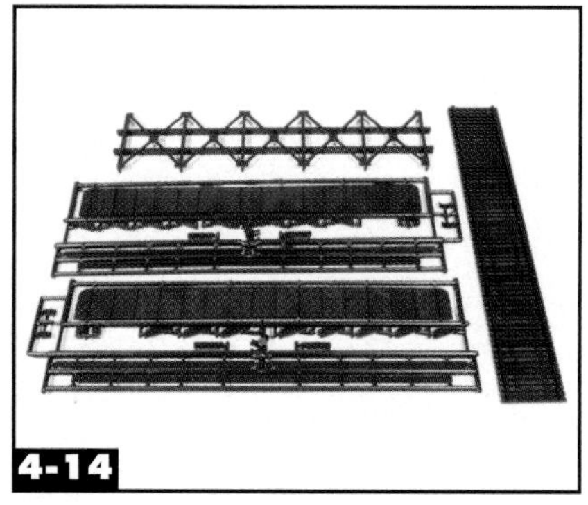

4-14

The easy-to-assemble Central Valley through truss bridge kit is made of injection-molded styrene plastic. *Jeff Wilson*

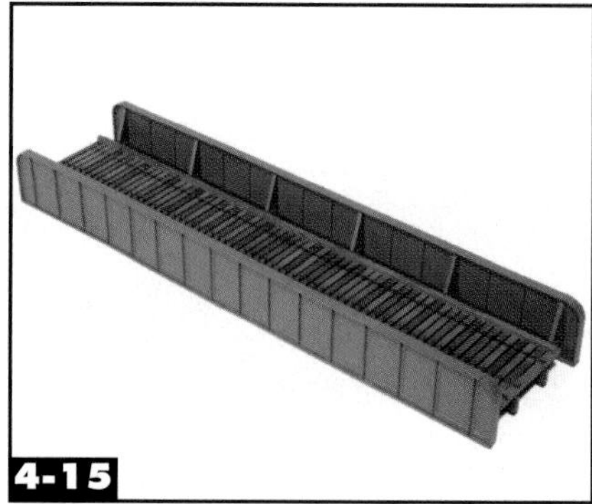

4-15

The Central Valley kit builds into an attractive model. *Jeff Wilson*

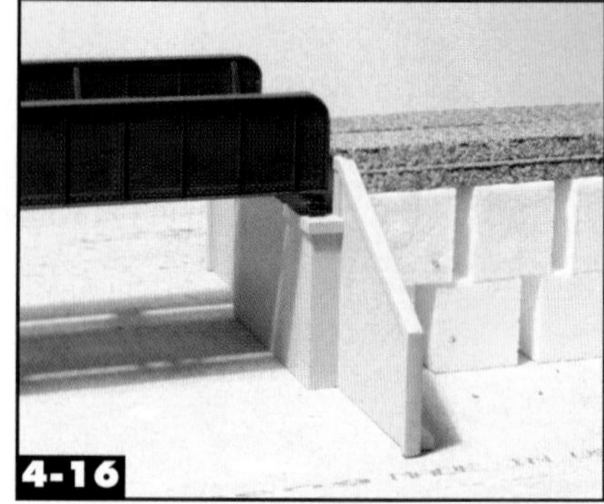

4-16

Make sure the bridge track aligns properly with your roadbed, and that the bridge feet rest firmly on the abutment. *Jeff Wilson*

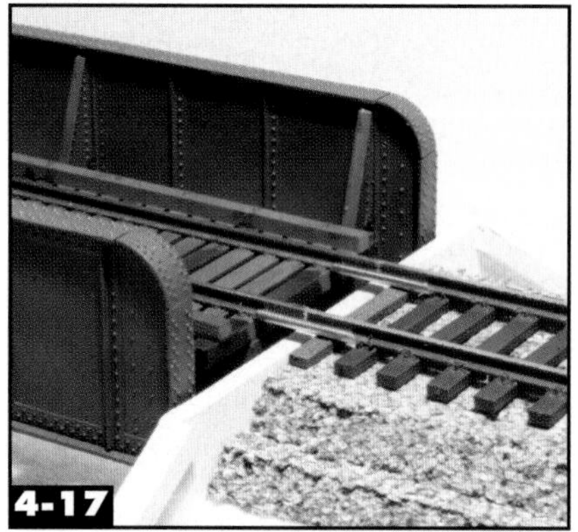

4-17

The rails just clear the top of the abutment. Add a filler tie if needed next to the abutment. *Jeff Wilson*

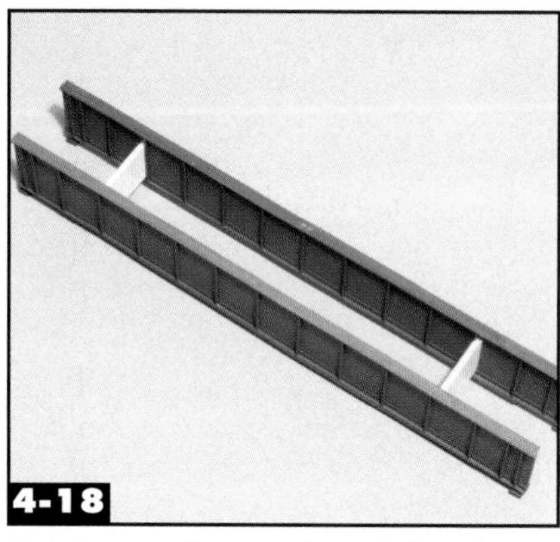

4-18

You can use a kit to model a deck girder bridge, or you can simply use styrene spacers to join two girders. *Jeff Wilson*

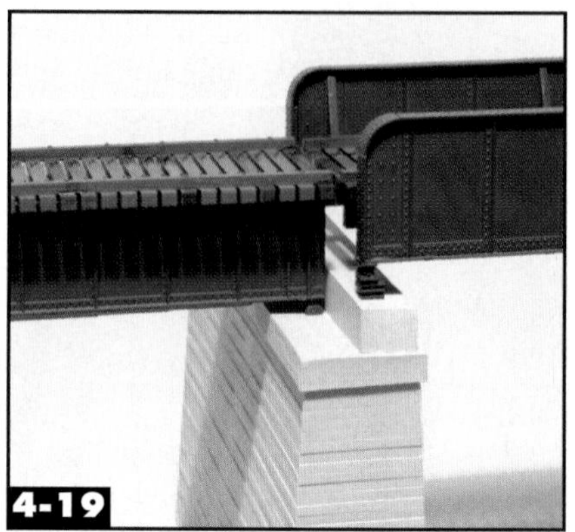

4-19

The deck bridge (left), made with Central Valley bridge track and Micro Engineering girders, meets the Central Valley through bridge atop a Walthers abutment. *Jeff Wilson*

common appearance, and they are found on railroads across the country. They can range from a couple hundred to several thousand feet in length.

A viaduct is built with several towers, each of which is made up of two steel trestle bents joined by bracing. The towers rest on concrete or stone abutments at each corner. Photo **4-13** (page 29) shows the tower-and-abutment structure, as does **1-6** in Chapter 1.

The bridges between towers are the intermediate spans, and the bridge across the top of each tower is called the tower span. The spans are generally spaced so that the distance between adjacent towers is double the distance across the top of each tower.

Although similar in appearance, viaducts vary in their details. On some viaducts, the girders used for the tower and intermediate spans are the same depth, **4-13**. On others, because of their shorter length, the girders for the tower spans aren't as deep (see photo **1-6** in Chapter 1). The towers also vary in design.

If a viaduct crosses an intermediate obstacle, such as a river, a longer span might be used over the longer gap. This long span can be another plate-girder bridge (see **4-13**), or it can be a truss bridge.

Viaducts sometimes follow curves. As with other bridges, each segment is straight, placed at a slight angle to its neighbor.

Modeling plate-girder bridges

When it comes to replicating plate-girder bridges, modelers have a wide variety of products to choose from. (A list of available models begins on page 86.) Commercial models in several sizes are available, and you can also kitbash your own bridge using a kit as a starting point.

Central Valley offers a well-detailed injection-molded styrene model of a 72′ through plate-girder bridge in HO scale, **4-14**. Kits such as this one are not difficult to build, **4-15**.

Once your bridge is built, the next step is to install it on your layout. It's important to keep the bridge track at the same level as the approach track. The bridge feet must also rest firmly on their abutments or piers.

Make sure the abutment you've chosen fits the bridge you're using. Abutments are relatively easy to make and can be custom built to the bridge you are using. I built an abutment from styrene to fit the Central Valley through bridge, **4-16**, following techniques demonstrated in Chapters 6 and 9.

You can make bridges fit available abutments by using larger or smaller pedestals. You can also trim the top of the abutment back

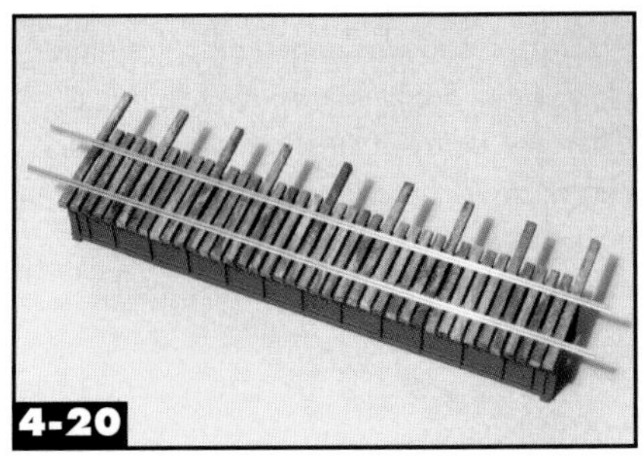

The long ties will support a walkway at the side of the bridge. The rails are glued in place with super glue. *Jeff Wilson*

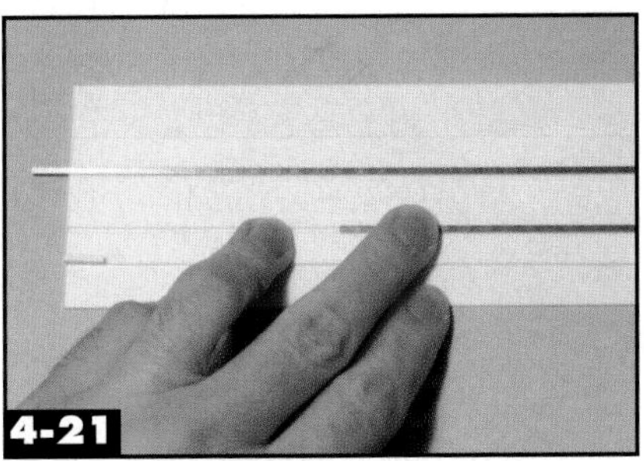

This styrene jig holds the rails in gauge upside down. The larger pieces of plastic at lower left and lower right align the edges of the ties. *Jeff Wilson*

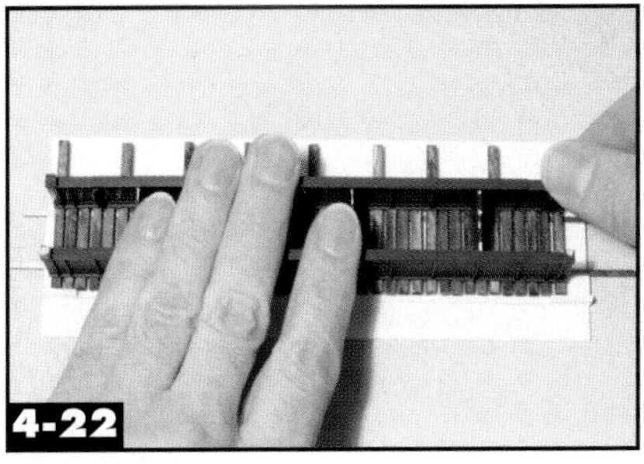

Run a bead of super glue along the bottom of each rail, then press the bridge in place. Hold it firmly for a few seconds until the glue takes hold. *Jeff Wilson*

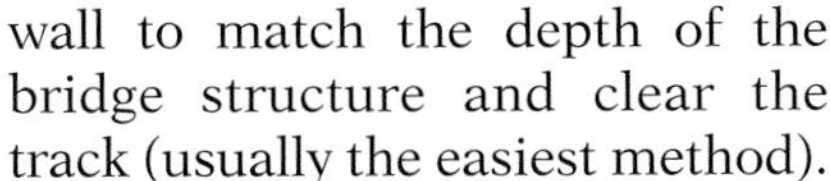

wall to match the depth of the bridge structure and clear the track (usually the easiest method).

On many bridges, the bottoms of the rails just clear the top of the abutment, **4-17**. On others, the rails rest on a tie placed directly on top of the abutment (see photo **4-2**, page 26). I like to model the rails clearing the wall because it provides a bit more leeway when making final adjustments.

The bottoms of the ties on my model bridge are just below the top of the abutment, **4-17**. I added rail to the Central Valley bridge track, then joined it to the flextrack on the layout. Make sure this joint is level. If necessary, add some thin styrene shims under the flextrack to bring the track to the same level.

Both bridge pedestals should be firmly in contact with the abutment (see photo **4-16**). A bit of super glue under the pedestals will help keep them that way in case the bridge is bumped while track is being cleaned or scenery is added to the layout.

If possible, install and align bridges before the surrounding scenery is in place, but wait to secure bridges permanently until after the scenery is complete.

Deck bridges

Deck girder bridges are easy to model. The only visible elements are the girders themselves with the ties and rail on top. Except in rare cases where the model can be viewed from underneath, there's no need to model the interior bracing. Several companies make kits for deck bridges, but any pair of square-ended girders can be used (rounded-end girders are only used for through bridges).

I modeled a deck bridge with a spare pair of HO scale Micro Engineering girders, **4-18**. (The company also offers a kit for a deck bridge, but I already had the girders on hand and wanted to use them.) Cut a few pieces of .080"-thick styrene to a scale 6'-6" width and fit them between the girders, making sure the ends are square. (I used a True Sander to clean up the styrene spacers in the photo.) Glue them to the inside of one of the girders at a flange angle, making sure the bottom of the styrene is down against the rivet plate for proper alignment.

Once that's dry, glue the second girder to the styrene spacers. Paint the spacers grimy black to make them less visible.

You can use any commercial bridge track atop the girders (see sidebar on page 36 for more on bridge track). For my sample bridge, I chose to use the Central Valley bridge track because I like the appearance of the realistic guard timbers molded in place. Another benefit of this bridge track is that it can be glued with styrene cement.

Cut the bridge track to length, then glue it in place atop the girders, making sure the track is centered side-to-side on the girders. Photo **4-19** shows this bridge meeting the Central Valley through bridge. More on that in a bit.

You can also model a deck girder bridge using real wood ties. Use a jig for aligning the bridge ties as demonstrated in Chapter 3. Once your bridge is built, run a thin bead of super glue on the inside edge of the top of each girder, then press the girders firmly down onto the strip of ties, **4-20**.

If you're modeling a single-span bridge, you can lay rail on it at this point. If you're using multiple spans with natural ties, it's often easier to wait until the bridges are in place on the layout and lay the rails in a continuous strip across the span.

For single spans using wood ties, I glue the rails in place with the aid of another jig, **4-21**. It's a piece of sheet styrene, with strips of .060" styrene glued on top to form guides for holding parallel pieces of upside down code 83 rail. Use a piece of sectional track to place the styrene guides the proper distance apart. Two additional small pieces of plastic rest against the bridge ties, keeping things aligned when the bridge is set in place.

Place two pieces of rail in the jig and run a light bead of medium-viscosity super glue along each rail. Place the bridge ties-down atop the rails and press firmly until the super glue sets, **4-22**.

If you use Central Valley's plastic ties, the best way to attach rail is to coat the bottom of the rail with Barge cement (used by shoe repair shops) thinned with methyl ethyl ketone (MEK). Let it dry,

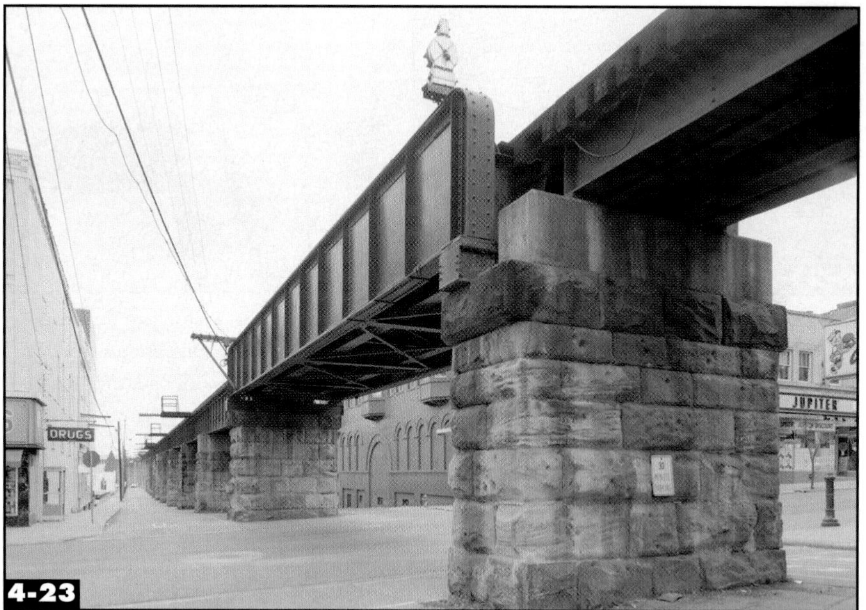

4-23

A concrete pad was added atop this stone abutment to accommodate the height difference between these plate-girder (left) and beam (right) bridges, which replaced earlier truss bridges. *Historic American Engineering Survey, Wm. E. Barrett*

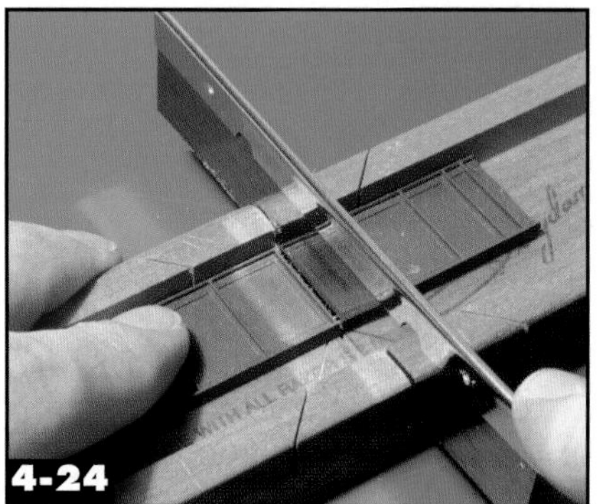
4-24

Use a razor saw and miter box to cut the girder next to a stiffener angle. *Jeff Wilson*

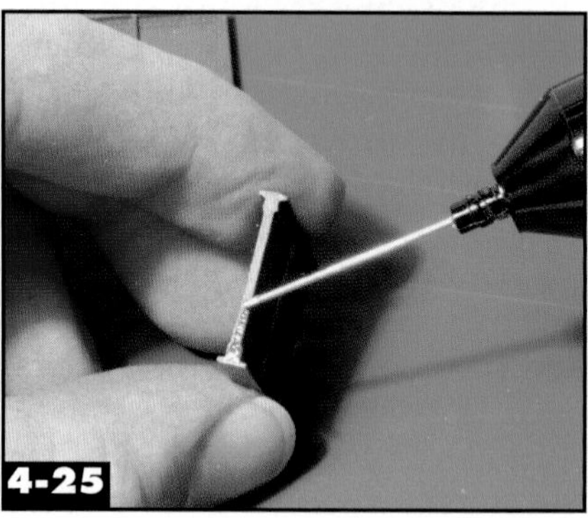
4-25

Spread liquid plastic cement on one of the mating surfaces. *Jeff Wilson*

position the rail, and re-wet the Barge cement and tie strip with MEK. It locks in place right away but can be adjusted by re-wetting the joint with MEK.

To lay the rails from above, use a fine-point scriber (or a straight pin in a pin vise) to lightly mark the outside location of one rail along the ties. Lay the first rail in place by running a thin bead of super glue along the underside of the rail and pressing it in place, carefully following the marks on the ties.

Position the second rail on the ties, using several track gauges to keep the rail in alignment. Use the scriber to lightly mark one edge of the rail on the ties.

Lay the second rail the same way as the first, following the scribed mark, and immediately check the track for proper gauge.

Installing a deck bridge

You can install a deck bridge in the same way as a through bridge, but the depth will be different compared to the through bridge shown earlier. On multiple spans, you'll often have to join a deck bridge end-to-end with a through plate-girder bridge, a truss bridge, or another deck bridge with girders of different heights.

Full-scale bridges either have a pier with two levels or a concrete pad atop an existing pier, **4-23**. You can do the same thing on your model.

Place the adjoining bridges on a flat surface, butting them together end-to-end. Measure the height difference from tie top to tie top. That's the distance you'll need to make up.

The easiest way to do this is to build a small box from styrene and then glue it to the pier. This replicates the concrete extension found on many prototype piers. In photo **4-19** (page 30), an extension box is installed on a Walthers pier and painted concrete color. (Chapters 6 and 9 discuss working with styrene in greater depth.)

Another way to do it is to make a custom stepped pier for your bridge, like the prototype piers shown in photo **4-1** (page 25) and **9-9** in Chapter 9.

Modifying girders

Bridges and bridge kits are available with girders in several lengths, but it's also possible to shorten a girder to provide a better fit for a specific space on a layout. Bridges can be lengthened using the same technique, but be careful: It's easy to wind up with a bridge that wouldn't realistically carry a heavy load. Remember the 7:1 ratio.

I shortened a Micro Engineering HO scale 50′ girder by one panel length (about 4′). Keep splices on panel lines, and be sure to keep the intermediate stiffener angles and rivet plates intact. Start by cutting the girder at a panel edge, **4-24**. Use a razor saw and miter box to keep the cut square. Make the next cut the same way.

On my sample project, I used a True Sander on both pieces to ensure that the joint would be square. Spread a little plastic cement on one of the mating surfaces, **4-25**, and press the pieces firmly together. Work on a flat surface, holding the parts against a steel rule or other straightedge to keep the girder aligned. If you work carefully, the splice line on the shortened (or lengthened) girder will be almost invisible, **4-26**.

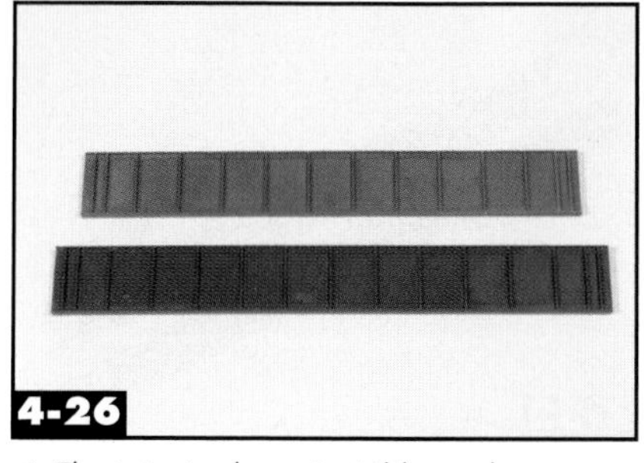

▲ The joint is almost invisible on the top girder; an unaltered girder is at bottom. *Jeff Wilson*

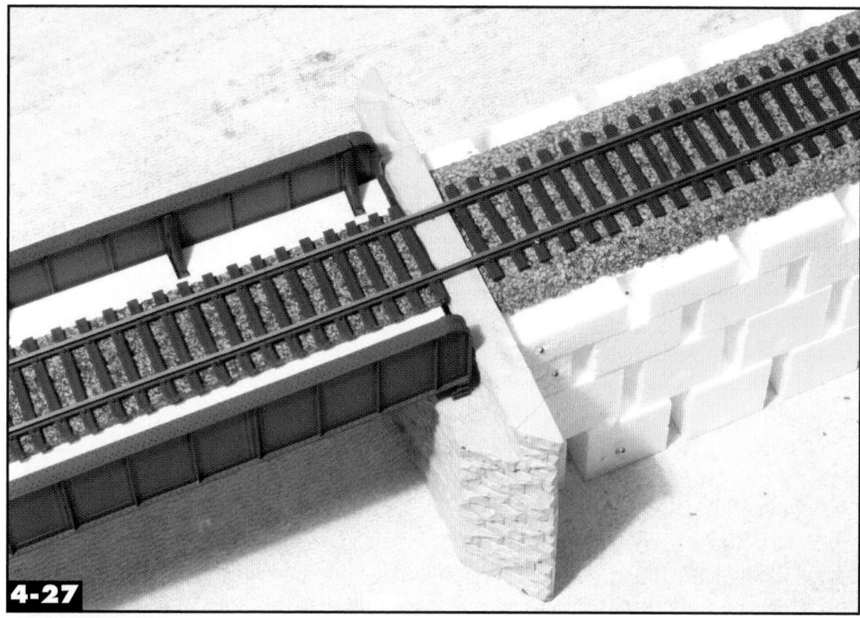

► Add a piece of plastic to the bridge as a deck, then add roadbed. The track is a continuation of flextrack, with a gap in the ties over the abutment. *Jeff Wilson*

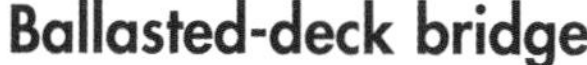

Ballasted-deck bridge

Ballasted-deck bridges are fairly common on real railroads, and they're relatively easy to model. Several companies offer them as kits, including Micro Engineering.

Converting a through open-deck bridge to a ballasted-deck bridge is fairly simple. For my sample project, I started with an HO Central Valley through bridge, adding a sheet of .020" styrene cut to fit between the girders and atop the stringers and floor beams. Glue the plastic deck in place, **4-27**. I used a bridge I already had on hand; it would have been easier to add the styrene floor before gluing the knee braces in place. Seal any gaps around the edges of the styrene with thick super glue or other filler to keep ballast from dropping through.

To provide a bed for the track I used N scale cork roadbed (HO roadbed elevates the track too much). Don't separate the cork strip—simply glue it in place with super glue as shown. If you're modeling a bridge in N scale, go ahead and use N scale cork.

Install the bridge the same way the through bridge was installed earlier in this chapter. Build the subroadbed and roadbed up to the abutment (I used a stone abutment from Chooch) as before, making sure the rails will clear the top of the abutment. You can use thin strips of styrene to shim up the track if necessary.

Glue the bridge in place, making sure it is properly aligned at both ends with the abutments and the track leading up to it. If you're using flextrack, cut away a tie at each end of the bridge where the track will pass over the top of the abutment wall.

Ballast the track the same way you would ballast regular track, **4-28**. Painting the styrene deck concrete gray beforehand will help hide it from view once the ballast is in place. When gluing the ballast on the bridge, have some paper towels ready in case glue seeps through the bridge deck.

As with other bridges, you may want to complete the surrounding scenery before gluing the bridge in place.

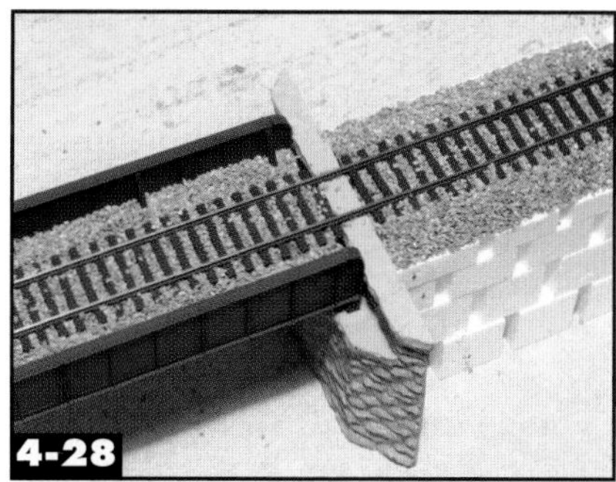

Ballast the bridge as with the layout. The stone abutment is from Chooch. *Jeff Wilson*

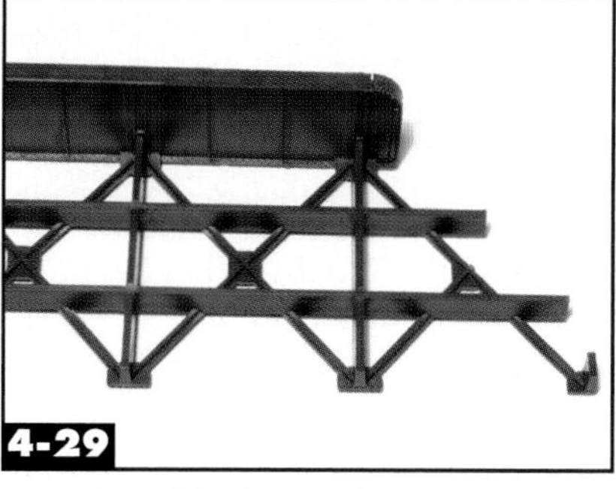

For a skewed bridge, cut the stringers and bracing as shown, then glue the floor assembly to one girder. *Jeff Wilson*

Skewed bridges

The cramped quarters of many model railroad layouts offer opportunities to follow the example of full-scale railroads and place bridges at angles other than 90 degrees. Skewed bridges can be modeled in either deck or through configurations.

One way to build a skewed through plate-girder bridge in HO scale is to use a Central Valley kit as a starting point, **4-29**. To do this requires one single-track bridge kit, plus an extra floor (stringer/floor beam) assembly.

I skewed my example by one floor-beam section, which worked out to a 45-degree angle. Shallower angles are possible, but the inner surfaces of the Central Valley girders have notches for the floor beams, so the inside of one girder would have to be modified.

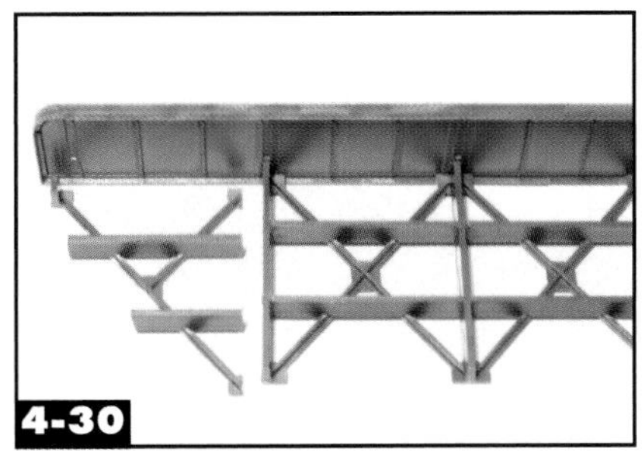
4-30

Cut an end from the spare floor section as shown at left, then glue it in place to the girder and main floor/beam section. *Jeff Wilson*

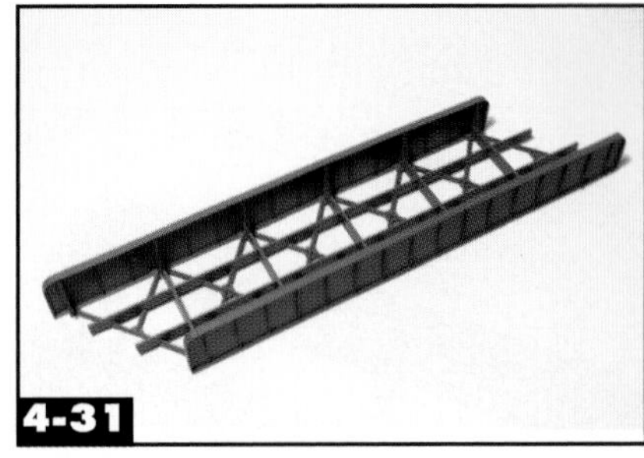
4-31

The finished skewed plate-girder bridge is ready for installation. *Jeff Wilson*

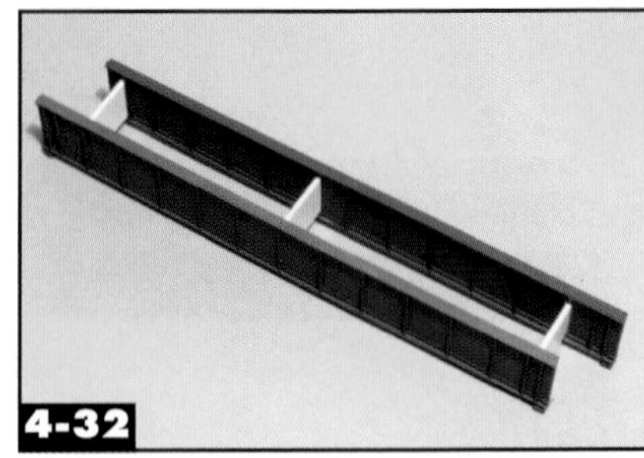
4-32

When making a skewed deck bridge, be sure the panels (stiffener angles) are even with each other. *Jeff Wilson*

Start by altering one end of the stringer/floor beam casting (see photo **4-29**). You'll need to trim away the end floor beam, then trim the stringers so that they'll extend to the pier or abutment as on a prototype bridge (see photo **4-11**, page 28). I used a chisel-point knife to cut through the parts; a razor saw would also work.

Glue one of the girders to the side of the stringer/beam piece (see **4-29**). Next, cut the spare stringer/beam piece, **4-30**, and add it to the main stringer/beam piece. Make sure the joint is square and that the stringers are aligned. Once that dries, glue the other girder in place, and your skewed bridge is ready to be installed on the layout, **4-31**.

The stringer extensions should rest on extensions of the abutment or pier, as the prototype photo in **4-11** shows. These might or might not be visible depending on the viewing angle of the model. If they can't be seen, they can be omitted.

Skewing deck bridges is a bit easier. Do it with a couple of Micro Engineering girders, using the same assembly techniques as described earlier for a square bridge, **4-32**. I used squares of thick (.080") styrene to space the girders after figuring out the skew angle I needed, keeping the spacers next to stiffener angles on each girder.

If the skew angle is slight, ties on the bridge and adjoining tracks are generally placed at angles near the abutment, as photo **4-2** (page 26) shows. If the angle is steep, the abutment's rear wall is usually squared to the track (photo **5-21** in Chapter 5 shows this on a skewed truss bridge).

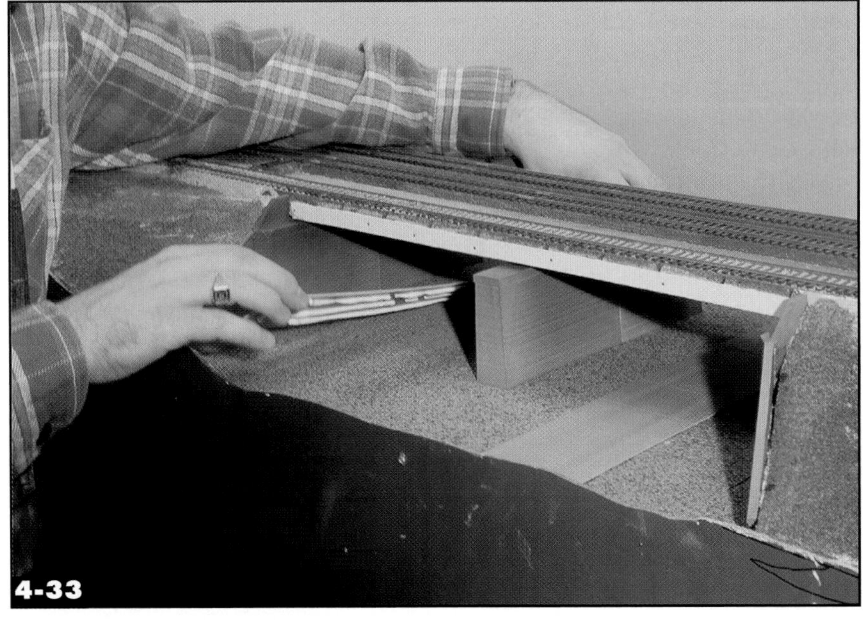
4-33

Girders glued to subroadbed

Another popular method of modeling plate-girder bridges is to glue the girders directly to the sides of plywood or foam subroadbed. This method has the advantage of not having to align separate bridge track with the track on the layout.

This is easily done with ballasted-deck through bridges, and works well as long as the underside of the bridge isn't visible. Make sure the subroadbed is cut to the proper width, with straight sides, for the length of the girders.

Photo **4-33** shows the roadbed ready for the girders, with the abutments and pier in place. Tacking styrene sheet to the edge of the subroadbed provides a good gluing surface for the girders. When gluing the girders in place, make sure the girders are level, the shoes rest firmly on the pier and abutments, and the girders completely cover the edge of the subroadbed, **4-34**.

Walkways

Many through and deck girder bridges have walkways along one side (see photo **1-2** in Chapter 1), sometimes on both. On deck bridges, these are made by extending some of the ties over the edge to support the platform

Model Railroader associate editor Cody Grivno modeled a girder bridge by first tacking sheet styrene to the edges of the plywood subroadbed, providing a smooth, easily glued surface for the girders. *Cody Grivno*

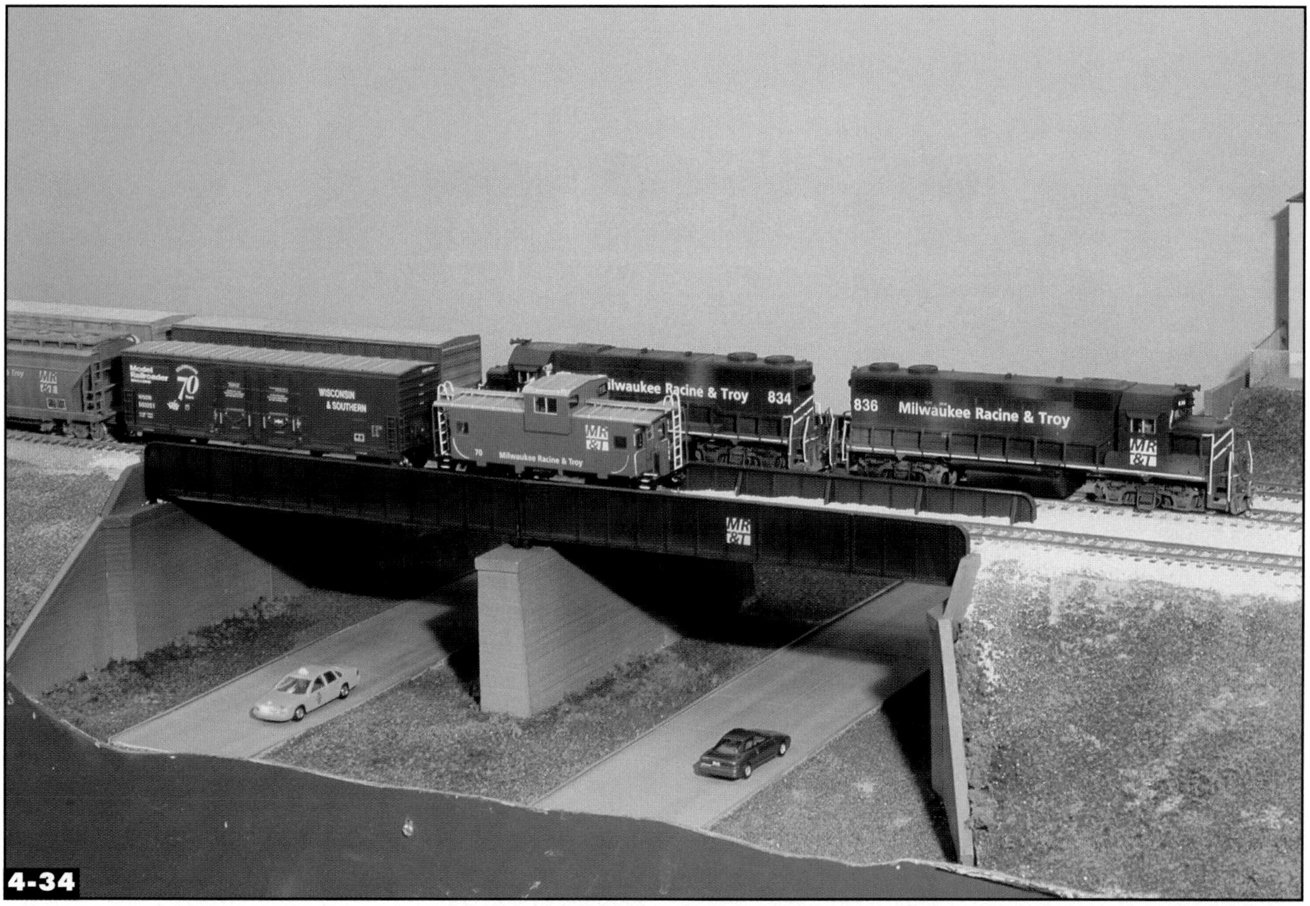

With the girders, scenery, and ballast in place, the technique used is invisible. *Cody Grivno*

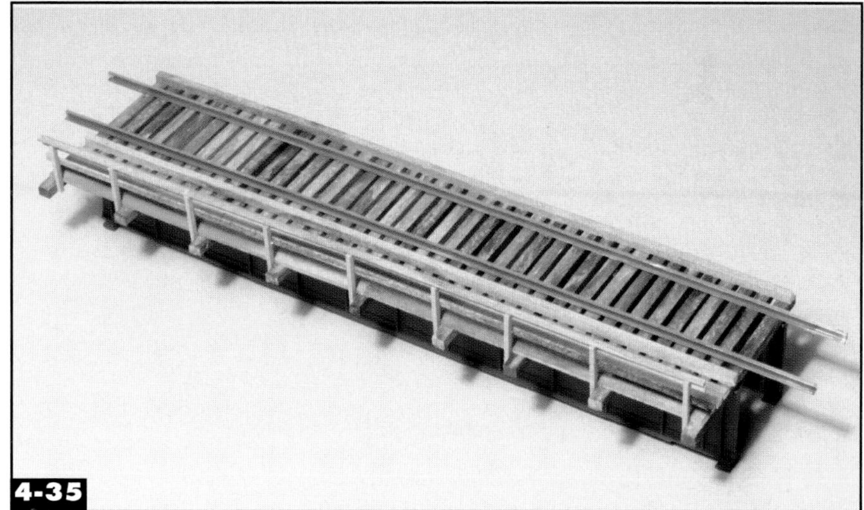

4-35

Add a walkway to a through or deck girder bridge by extending every third or fourth tie and installing the walkway floor, posts, and handrails made from scale stripwood. *Jeff Wilson*

for walkway planking. On some bridges, especially those where the walkway was added after the bridge was built, planks bolted to the ties extend outward to hold the walkway.

You can model this with real wood ties, placing a scale 14'-long tie every third or fourth tie (see **4-20**, page 31). Use scale 2 × 12 stripwood to create planking for the walkway. You can use single strips for the length of the bridge, but it will look more realistic if you use two or three pieces.

Glue vertical posts using scale 4 × 4 stripwood to the extended ties. The posts should be about 48″ long in scale. Next, make guard railings from scale 2 × 4 or 2 × 6 stripwood and glue them in place; your bridge is done, **4-35**.

Scale planking can also be used in a similar fashion over the open decks of through plate-girder or truss bridges to create a non-ballasted closed deck bridge.

Viaducts

The best way to model a tall viaduct is to start with a kit. Micro Engineering offers several complete kits in both N and HO scales. Separate components are also available; see the kit list starting on page 86. These kits can be combined to make structures of almost any length, and they can be modified with girders of various styles to match specific prototypes. Photo **4-36** (page 36) shows one of these viaducts installed on a layout.

Let's move to the next chapter and take a look at truss bridges.

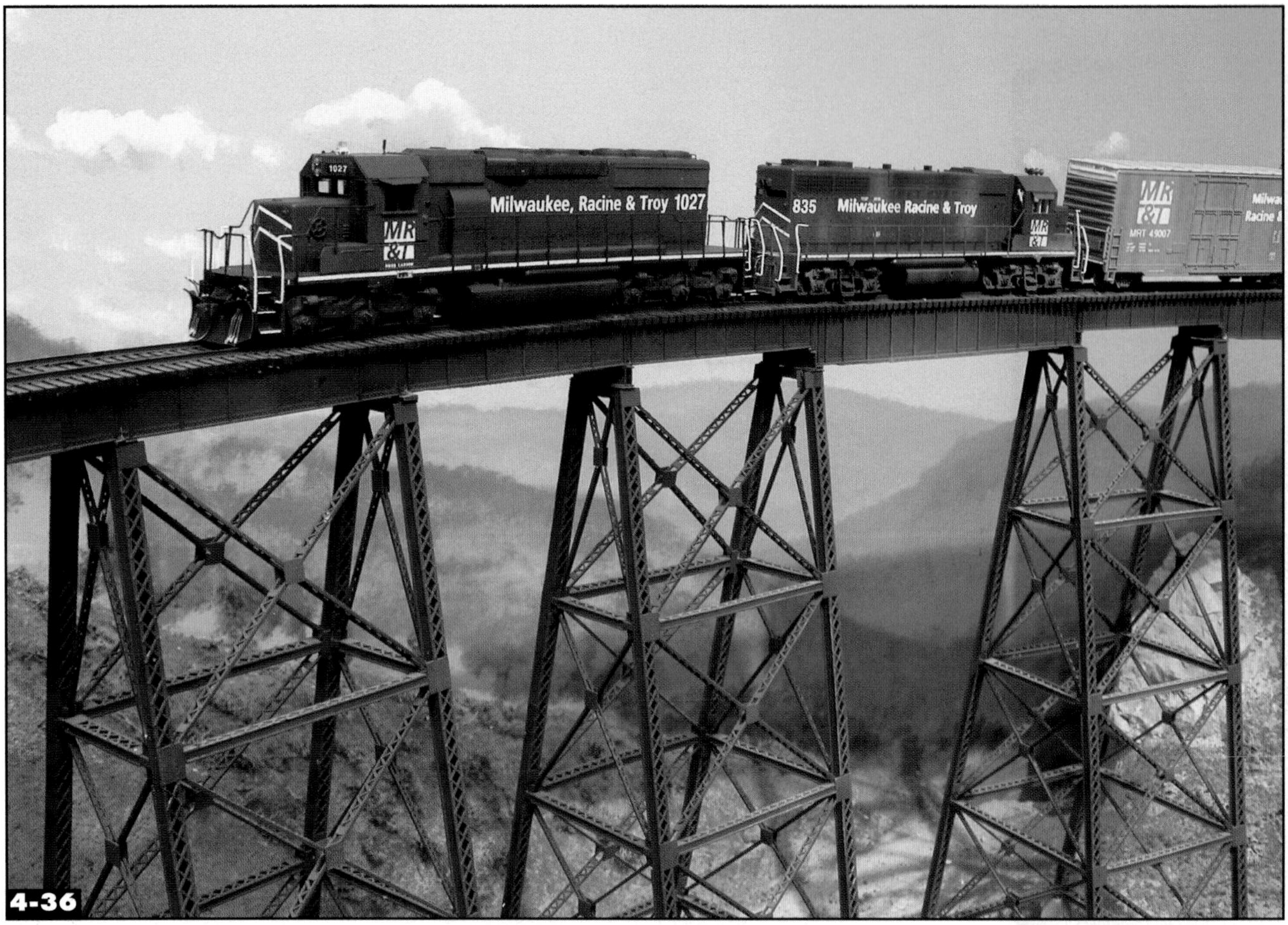

4-36

This viaduct on the Kalmbach club layout, the HO Milwaukee, Racine & Troy, was built using a Micro Engineering kit. *Tom Danneman*

Bridge track

Several companies offer bridge track, with its distinctive closely spaced ties (see photos at right).

In HO scale, Walthers track includes the running rails, guardrails, and guard timbers. If you need to adjust the track's length, cut a segment from the middle and join the ends together.

Central Valley bridge track is molded plastic with guard timbers, but doesn't include rail. Rail can be glued in place with super glue or Barge cement, with plastic spike heads pushed over the rail web to hold it in place.

Micro Engineering bridge track, available in N and HO scales (the HO track is shown in the photos at right), includes rails and is flexible. The guard timbers are separate plastic items that may be added after the track has been bent to shape.

Plastic bridge track needs painting to make it look realistic. I usually start with an airbrushed coat of dark gray or grimy black. Follow this by using a brush to highlight individual ties with black and various shades of brown and gray. Paint the sides of the rails dark brown, with black highlights.

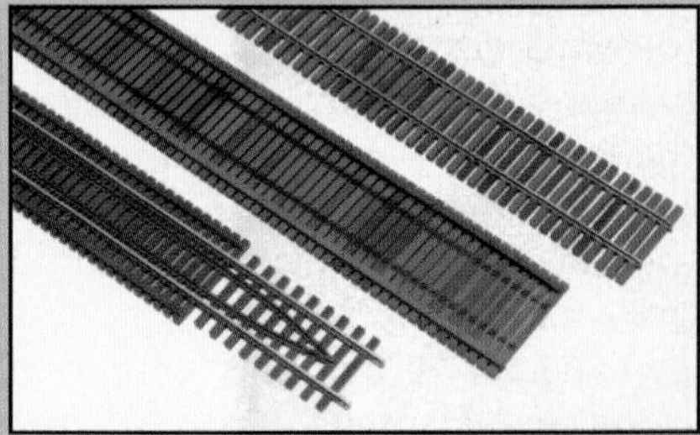

Commercial bridge track in HO scale includes Walthers, Central Valley, and Micro Engineering. *Jeff Wilson*

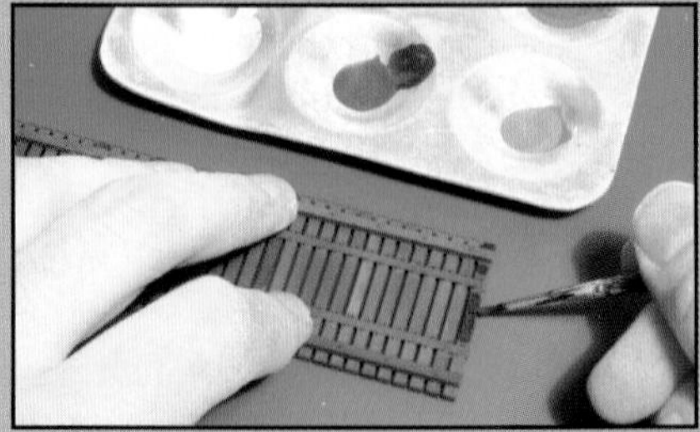

Variations of brown, gray, and black work well for painting ties. *Jeff Wilson*

Painting plate-girder bridges

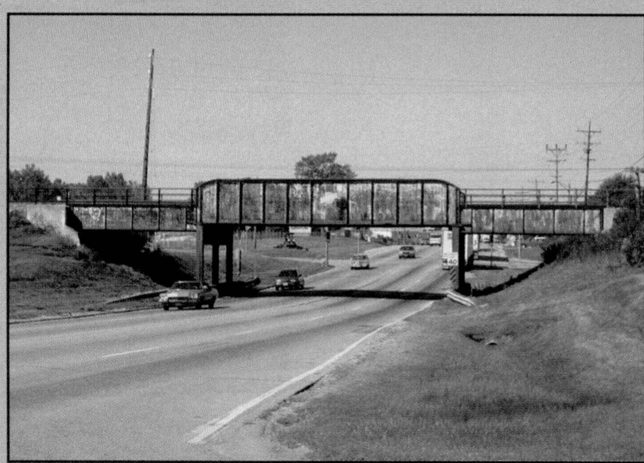

It's been a few years since this Chicago & North Western bridge has received a coat of paint. *Jeff Wilson*

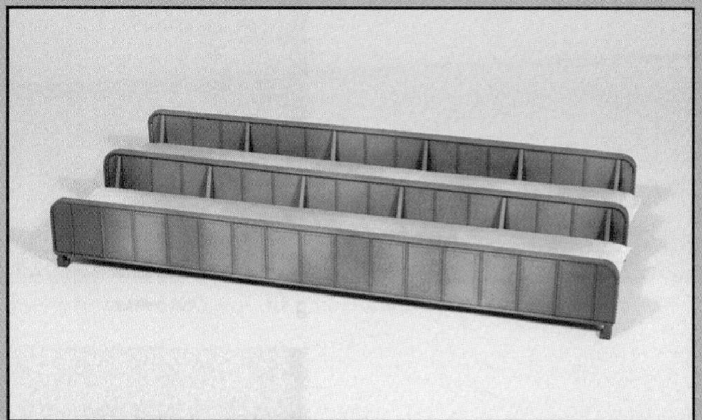

To replicate the weathered paint look, start by giving the bridge a base coat of brown and oxide red colors. *Jeff Wilson*

Plate-girder bridges may be painted any color, but the most common colors are black and silver. Bridges are usually kept in good repair, but if a few years pass between painting, patches of rust and accompanying weathered streaks often appear, especially on lighter-colored bridges like the old Chicago & North Western bridge shown here.

An airbrush or spray can will provide the best results in painting. If you're painting the bridge black, do it after the bridge is assembled. If you're painting it a lighter color, paint the girders separately from the flooring before assembly.

On the example in the photos, I created the effect of the primer coat showing through by first painting the girders with a mix of rust and oxide red colors. I then used an airbrush to apply the final silver color, using a vertical spray pattern and making sure I didn't completely cover the previous colors.

Streaks of rust are easy to create by dry-brushing. Start by dipping the tips of the bristles of an old brush in paint, then brush off most of the paint on a paper towel. Use the nearly dry brush (hence the name of the technique) to streak the paint onto the model. Use vertical strokes to match the effects that Mother Nature has on prototype bridges.

For additional weathering, use another brush to lightly dust on powdered artist's pastel chalks in various browns, reds, and black.

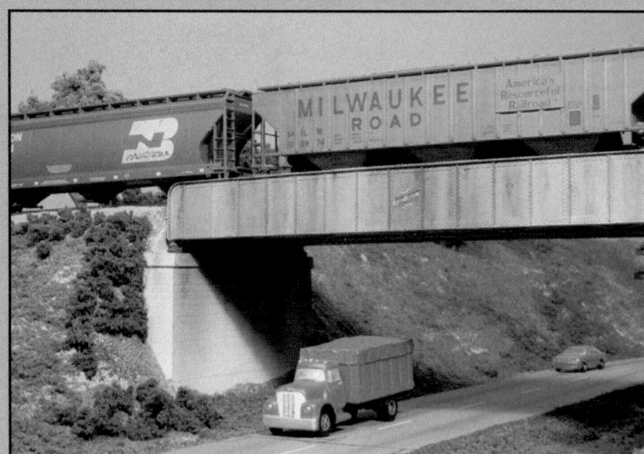

Finish by streaking the bridge with silver, letting some of the base colors show through. Dry-brushing and an application of artist's pastel chalk dust add some additional accents to both the bridge and the abutments. This is a Central Valley double-track bridge on a Walthers abutment. *Jeff Wilson*

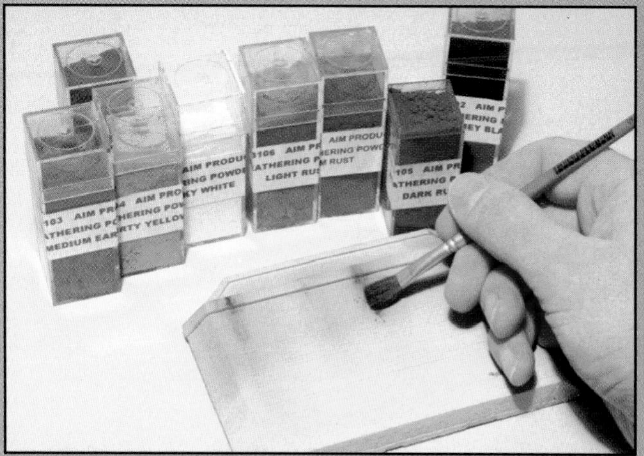

AIM Products offers this set of powdered chalks, with several rust and grime colors that are handy for weathering bridges and other structures. *Jeff Wilson*

Truss bridges

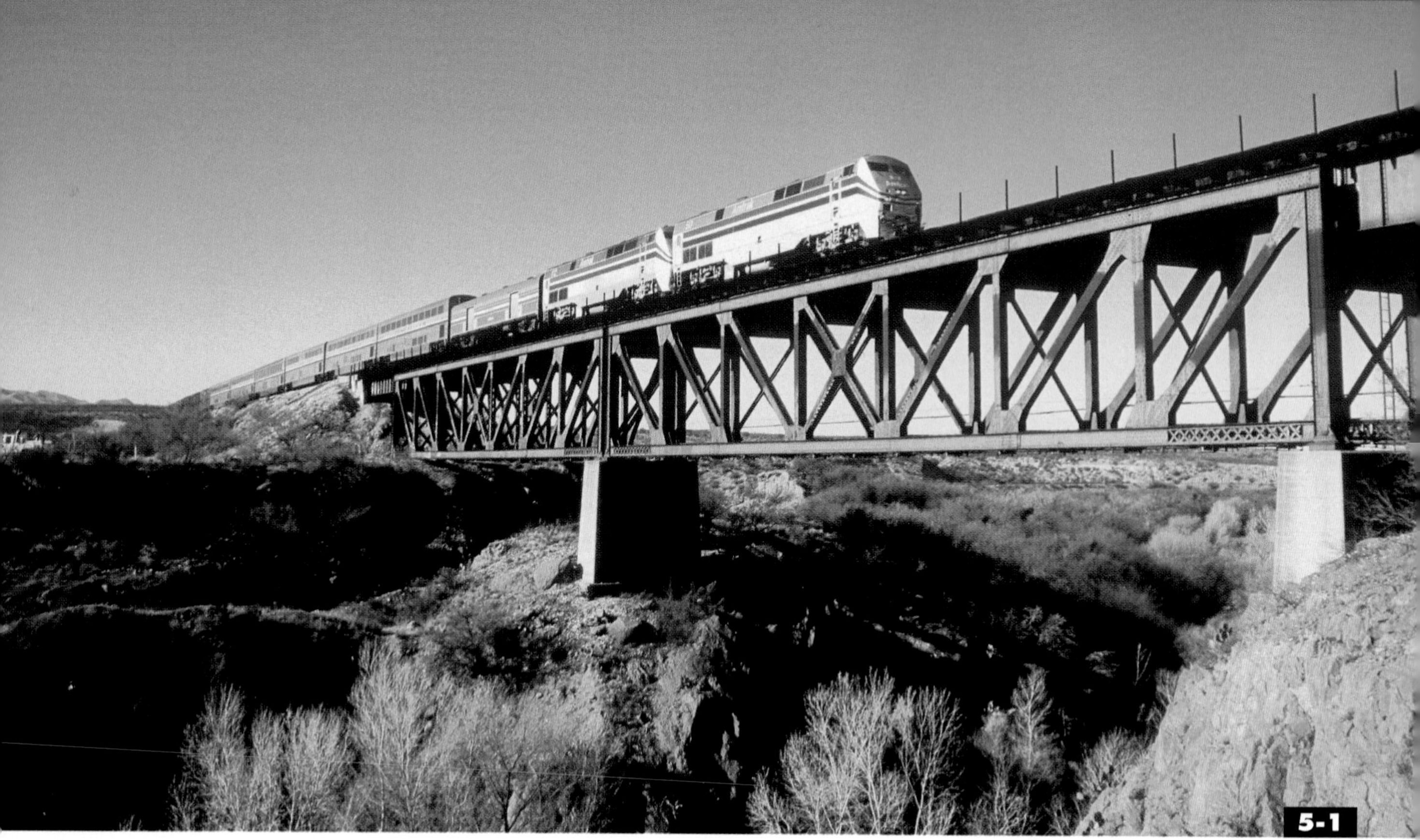

FIVE

Truss bridges are often used for long spans, as shown here on the former Southern Pacific main line near Vail, Arizona. The middle two spans are riveted Pratt deck trusses, with shorter plate girder bridges at each end. *Jeff Wilson*

In the early to mid-1800s, the wood truss span was the solution to the costly alternative of masonry bridges. As locomotive and car weights increased, bridge builders turned to metal—first iron, then steel—for greater strength in truss bridges.

Through the end of the 19th century, railroads built progressively longer spans using improved truss styles, then turned to continuous truss and cantilever bridges for long spans where intermediate piers would be difficult or impossible to use. Even though the heyday of truss bridge building peaked in the early 1900s, many long spans were built later. Many early truss bridges are still in use and can be seen along today's railroads, **5-1**.

Truss components

Truss bridges come in three basic styles: deck, with the supporting structure below the track, **5-1**; through, where the truss sides are above the deck and are connected by bracing across the top, **5-2**; and half-through, or pony, with shorter side trusses, the tops of which aren't connected.

Truss bridges use many different patterns or styles for their vertical and diagonal members. Illustration **5-3** shows many popular truss designs that have been used over the years.

Photo **5-2** also shows the basic parts of a metal through-truss bridge, in this case a Pratt. The top and bottom chords bear the weight of the load. The vertical members at the ends are posts; in the middle, they are hangers that can be in compression or tension

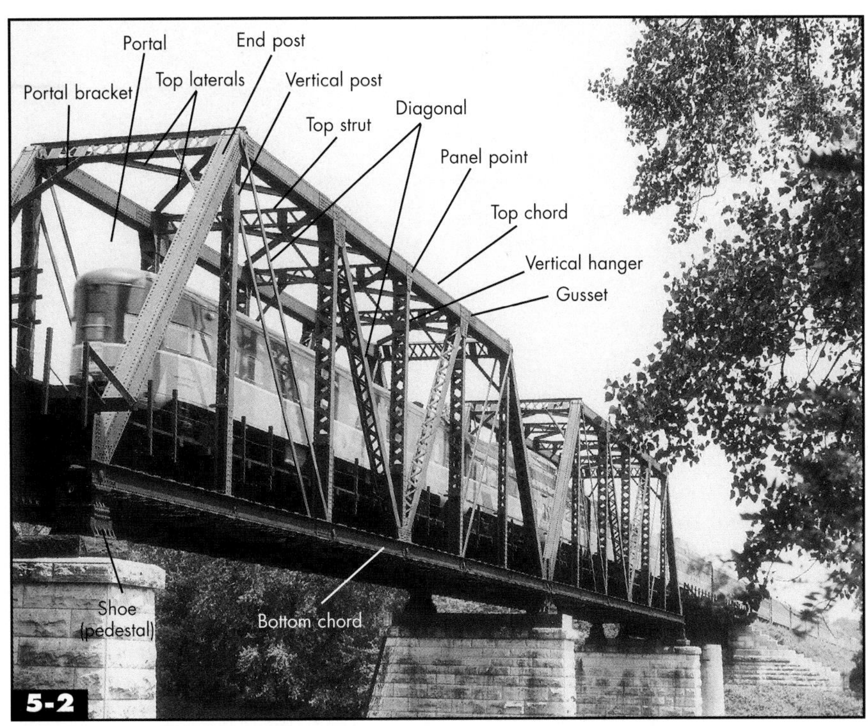

This Pratt through-truss bridge spans the Rock River on the Chicago, Burlington & Quincy line at Oregon, Illinois. *Jim Scribbins*

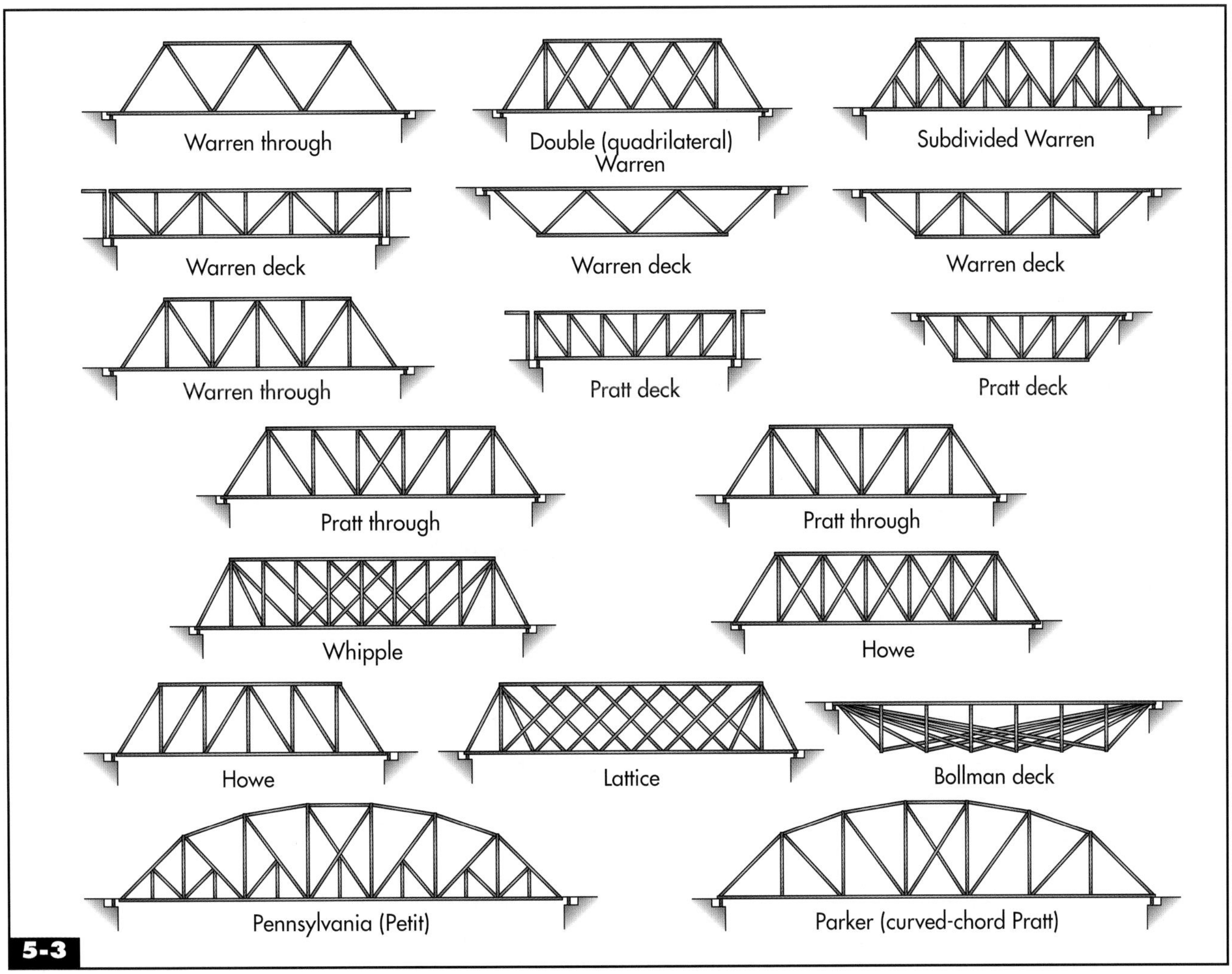

Warren through
Double (quadrilateral) Warren
Subdivided Warren
Warren deck
Warren deck
Warren deck
Warren through
Pratt deck
Pratt deck
Pratt through
Pratt through
Whipple
Howe
Howe
Lattice
Bollman deck
Pennsylvania (Petit)
Parker (curved-chord Pratt)
5-3

Truss bridges come in a wide variety of configurations: some simple, some intricate, and some quite beautiful. The Warren pattern is most common on modern bridges.

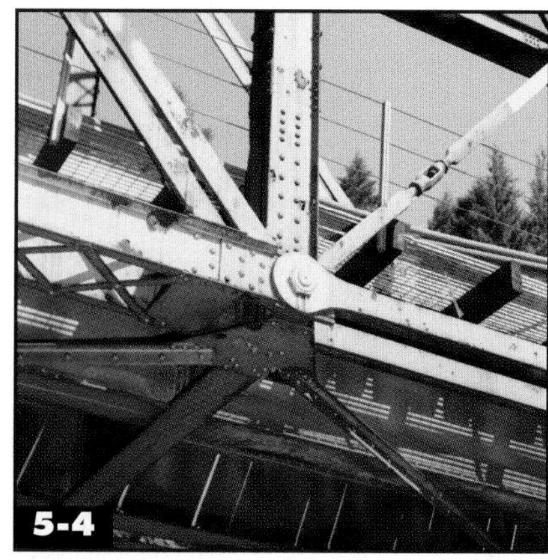

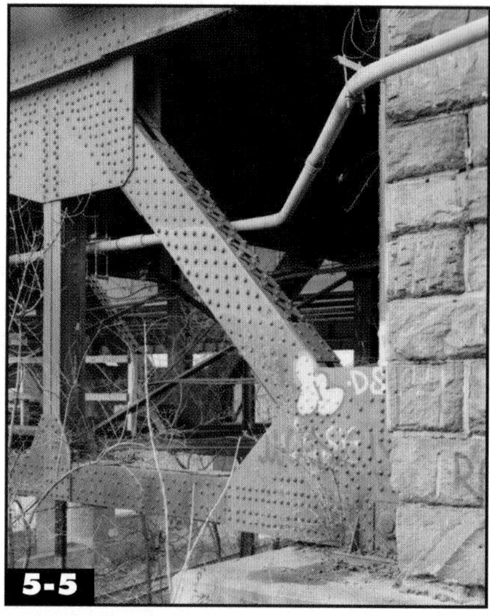

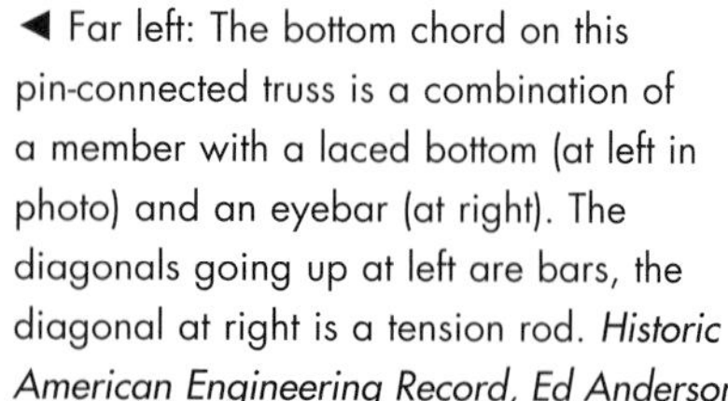

◀ Far left: The bottom chord on this pin-connected truss is a combination of a member with a laced bottom (at left in photo) and an eyebar (at right). The diagonals going up at left are bars, the diagonal at right is a tension rod. *Historic American Engineering Record, Ed Anderson*

◀ This Warren deck truss uses riveted connections. The vertical member at left is made from back-to-back channels; the diagonal is a box made of channels connected by lacing, with stay plates at top and bottom. *Historic American Engineering Record, Joseph Elliott*

depending upon the truss type. The diagonal members are indeed called diagonals, and the diagonals at the ends are the end posts.

All of these components are called truss members. Truss members can be made in several ways, with various components forming a box, I, or H cross section. The sides of the members—called segments—are generally channels, plates, or angles, and they are joined by lacing (steel straps at angles) or by steel plates. Double lacing has straps that cross in an X pattern; single lacing has non-crossing straps.

Small steel plates at the ends of laced members or spaced along a member are called stay plates; a plate that runs the full length of a member is a continuous plate. You'll see examples of all of these components in the bridge photos throughout this chapter.

The members on truss bridges were usually connected by pins (**5-4**), rivets (**5-5**), or a combination of the two. Modern bridges are bolted or welded together.

The tension members on pin-connected bridges are lighter than compression members and are made of rod or strap connected on the ends with eyebars. Popular into the early 1900s, pin-connected bridges could be easily assembled on site with unskilled labor. They are also easier to analyze mathematically than more complex designs. One drawback of pin-connected bridges is that they can suffer heavy wear at the pin joints.

Riveted designs, with gusset plates where members meet, are stronger. Improved rivet materials and installation equipment made riveted construction more common in the early 20th century, and riveting became the dominant practice soon thereafter.

Panel points are where the truss intersects with the floor beams, which run crosswise between the truss sides, **5-6**. The floor beams are in turn connected by the stringers, which run lengthwise underneath the track.

Bridges are described in length by panels, marked by the panel points, and the panels are equally spaced along the bridge.

On top of the bridge, the trusses are connected by top struts (going straight across) and top laterals (the angled X pieces).

The end opening of a truss bridge is called the portal. The opening must be at least 16′ wide and 22′ tall between the top of the rail and the bottom of the portal bracing.

As with girder bridges, trusses rest on pedestals and shoes of various configurations.

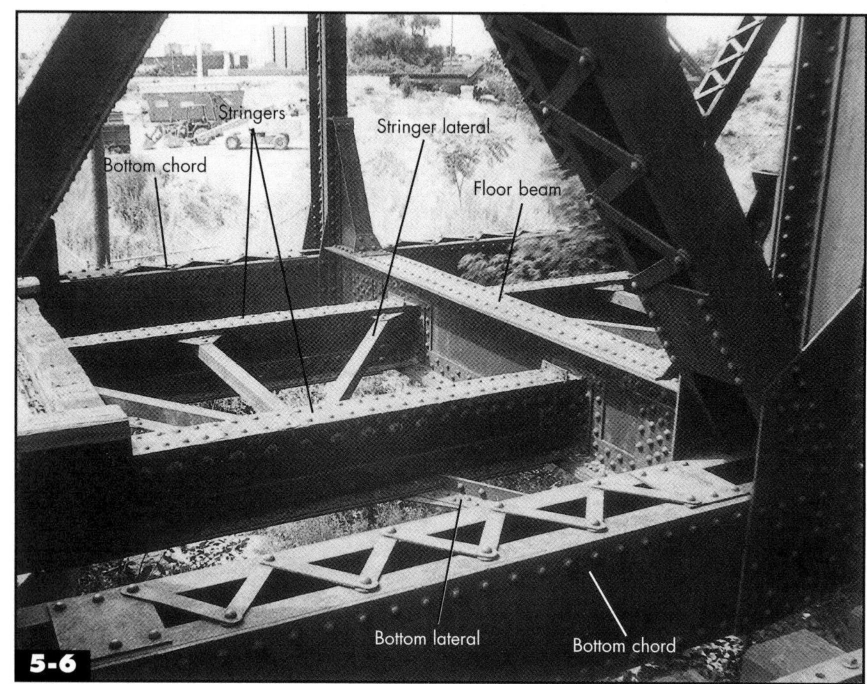

With the ties and rail removed, the parts of this Warren truss are in plain view. Note the laced-box lower chord and diagonal, as well as the riveted connections. *Harold W. Russell*

▶ Some Howe wood trusses survived well into the modern era. This pair of 161'-long spans, built in 1933, remained in service through the 1980s on the Union Pacific near Everson, Washington. *David P. Morgan Library collection*

▶ Below: Whipple trusses, like this one on the Boston & Maine, have diagonals that span multiple panels. The bridge at left is a Warren truss. *David Plowden*

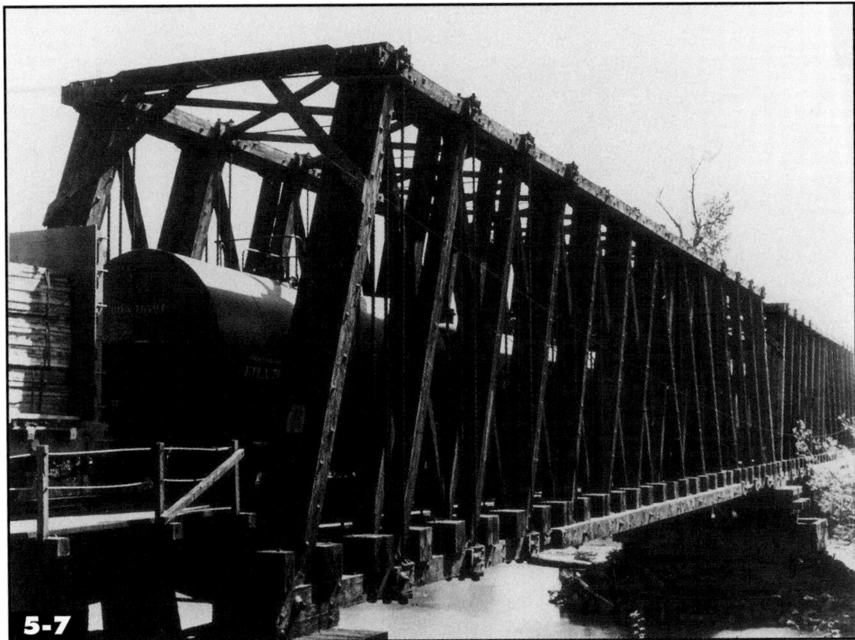

5-7

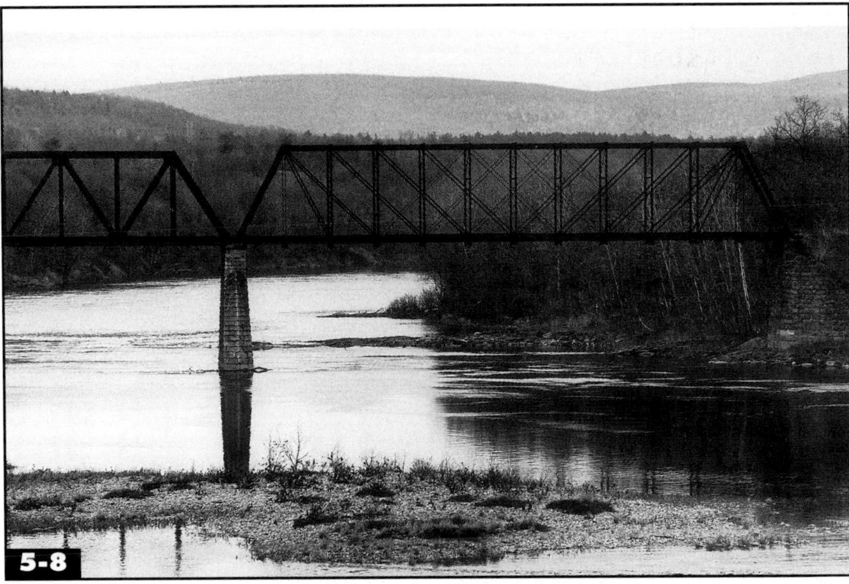

5-8

Truss designs

Each type of truss has its own distinctive pattern, and each has variations (see **5-3**, page 39). Being able to recognize the patterns will help you identify the prototype styles, making it easier to choose and build model bridges that are correct for your layout.

The earliest truss design commonly used on railroad bridges, around 1840, was the Howe, **5-7**. Revolutionary when introduced, the Howe design allowed builders to span long gaps with wood bridges. It played to the strengths of wood with diagonal members in compression and vertical members (iron rods) in tension.

Many wood truss railroad bridges were built well into the 1900s, although bridges made of iron and steel became the dominant in the late 1800s. The Pacific Northwest, with its ample timber resources, was a popular locale for wood bridges.

The Pratt truss (see **5-2** and **5-3**, page 39), which would eventually become the most widely used truss design for railroad bridges, was introduced shortly after the Howe in 1844 and was a modification of the Howe design. The pattern of the Pratt's diagonals is reversed compared to the Howe (see **5-3**). Vertical members in the Pratt design are heavy because they are in compression, with the diagonals in tension.

The Pratt truss was originally built with wood and iron components, but beginning in the 1850s, iron members with pin-connected construction became predominant. Pratt bridges were economical to build, using less metal for a given length and strength than comparable Whipple or Bollman trusses (discussed below). From the 1890s to the 1920s, the Pratt design was by far the dominant truss style for railroad bridges.

Another early truss design was the Whipple, introduced in 1847, **5-8**. This design used longer diagonals, most of which spanned two panels. The Whipple design was popular for wrought iron bridges, especially for spans longer than bridges built to the original Pratt design.

One of the earliest all-iron designs was the Bollman (see **5-3**, page 39). This design was short-lived and was used mainly by the Baltimore & Ohio (the design's developer, Wendel Bollman, was employed by the B&O). Although structurally sound, it required more material than contemporary metal Whipple and Pratt bridge designs. Though not widely used, the Bollman truss is credited with helping advance the development and use of all-metal bridges.

Patented in 1848, the Warren truss is still widely used today, **5-9** (page 42). The Warren truss relies on alternating diagonal members for tension and compression, with the diagonals in

5-9

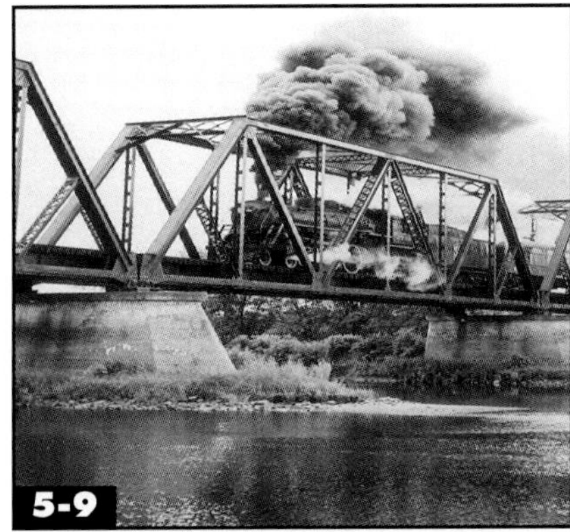

▲ Warren trusses, such as these Soo Line spans, are easy to identify, with diagonals in alternating directions in each panel. *Jim Scribbins*

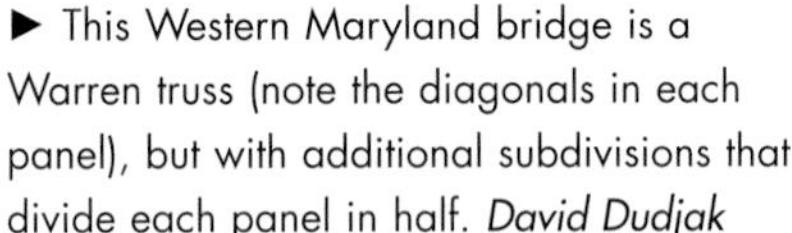

▶ This Western Maryland bridge is a Warren truss (note the diagonals in each panel), but with additional subdivisions that divide each panel in half. *David Dudjak*

7596
5-10

DO NOT WALK
NOR TRESPASS ON
THE BRIDGE
5-11

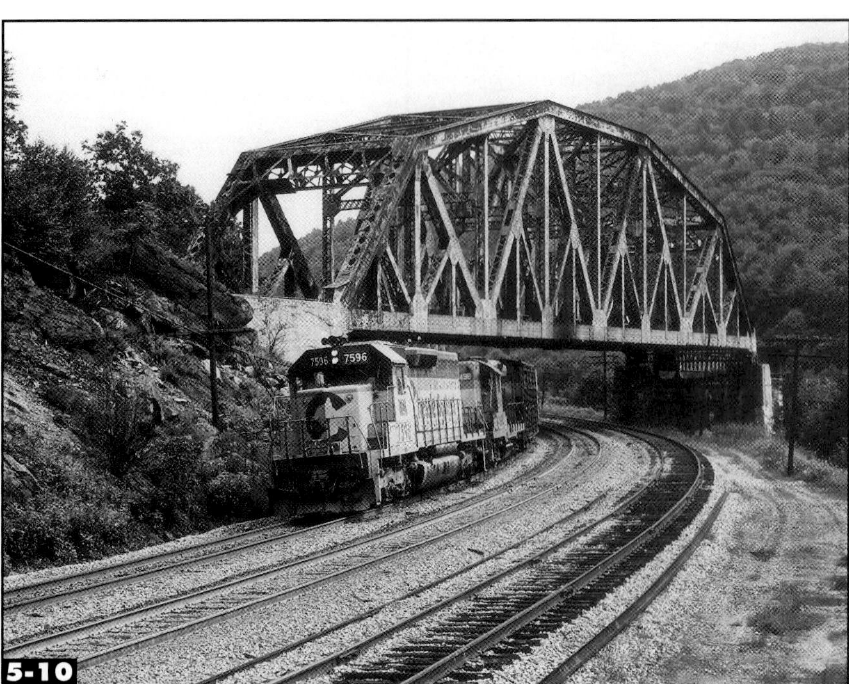

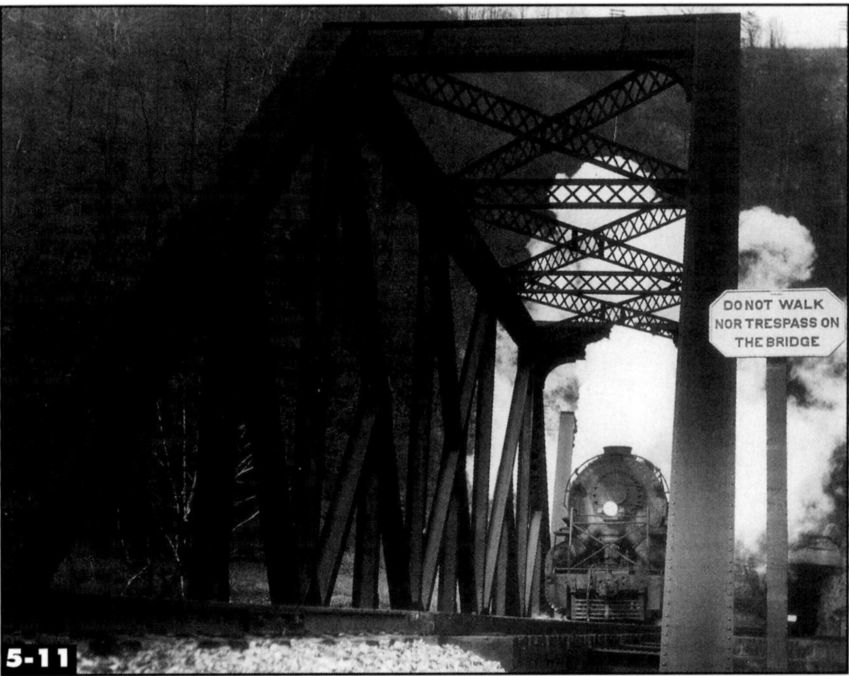

Baltimore trusses are a version of the Pratt (note the diagonals) with subdivisions. *Rusty Ball*

each panel reversed. This gives the bridge its distinctive "W" pattern. Its riveted-truss design is common on short spans and pony bridges, but it is often used for longer spans as well.

Some Warren bridges have only diagonals; others have vertical members at the panel points. A common variation is the subdivided Warren, which has vertical members where the diagonals connect to the top and bottom chords, **5-10**. Another variation, the double (also called quadrilateral) Warren, has an extra set of diagonal members (see **5-3**, page 39).

As bridges grew increasingly longer in the late 1800s, the Pratt and Warren designs eventually became dominant, as both—with their single-panel diagonals—were more rigid in long spans than the Whipple. From the 1920s on, the Warren became the dominant truss design.

A modification to the Pratt design was to add subdivisions to the panels with half-length diagonals. The result, developed in 1871, was the Baltimore truss, **5-11**. The subdivisions mark the additional floor beams not found on a conventional Pratt.

Another popular modification to the Pratt design, used for long spans, is the Parker, which is essentially a Pratt with a curved top chord, **5-12**. In general, standard Pratt designs are used for spans up to about 150′, with Parker trusses used from that distance to just over 300′.

The advantage of the Parker truss is that the curved top chord (actually a series of straight members angled to form an arc) provides great strength while consuming less steel than an equivalent conventional straight-top-chord bridge, which would have to maintain the extreme height over its entire length.

A further variation on the Pratt and Parker is the Pennsylvania or Petit truss, first used in 1875, **5-13**. This design resembles a Parker but has subdivided panels with half-length diagonals similar to the Baltimore. Pennsylvania trusses are the longest of the simple truss bridges, with lengths generally

► The Parker truss is a variation of the Pratt, with a curved top chord, used for longer spans. *Gordon Odegard*

► Below: The Pennsylvania or Petit design is used for the longest simple span truss bridges. The falsework under the bridge at left will be removed when construction is complete. *David P. Morgan Library collection*

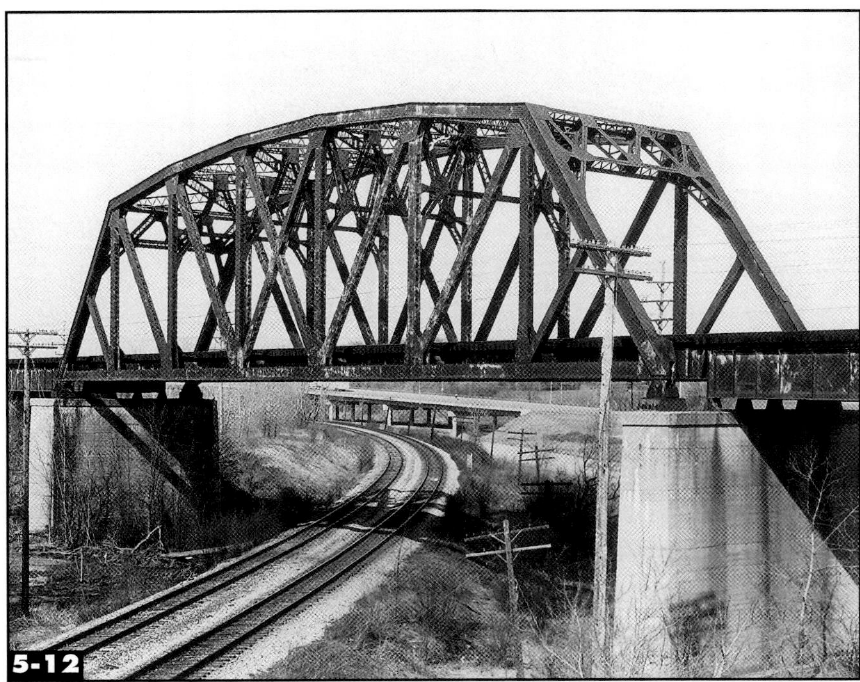

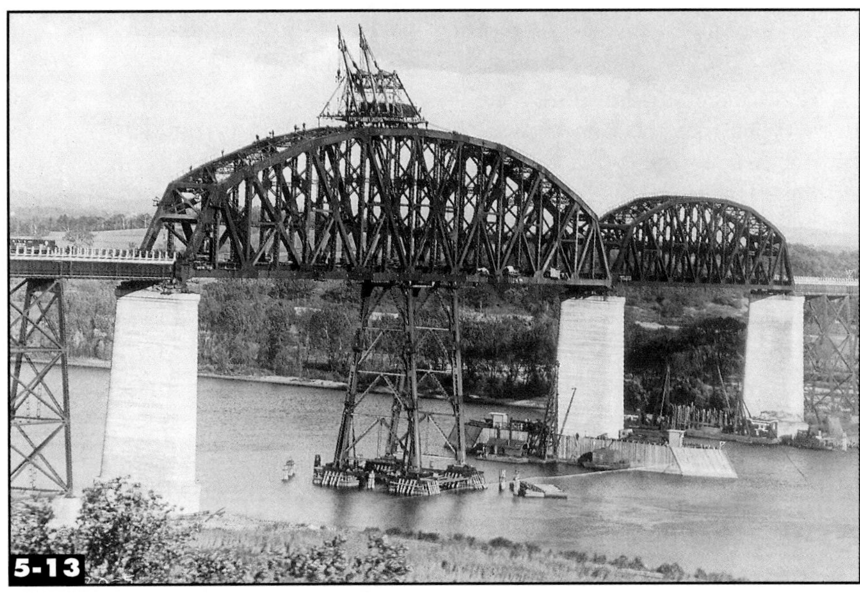

over 300′ and sometimes over 500′.

Although it wasn't as popular as the Pratt or Warren, the lattice truss design was used extensively by a major railroad—the Chicago & North Western, **5-14**. With its multiple diagonals, the lattice looks similar to the Whipple at first glance, but it lacks vertical members, except for end posts.

The steel plate-girder bridge came into use on longer spans in the early 1900s, replacing the common through truss, which was often employed in the 1800s and early 1900s for spans from 100′ to 150′. By the mid-1900s, most new truss bridges were long spans, including continuous trusses, cantilevers, long Pennsylvania through spans, and long Warren decks.

Variations

Although truss bridges fall into specific classes with common components, many spotting features differentiate them. Not all 130′ through Pratt bridges are created alike!

The most distinctive areas are the portals at each end. Some are plain in design as in photo **5-11**, while others have intricate bracing or decorative curved steelwork at the top of the portal. A common variation was to include the date of construction in the steel or iron work at the top.

Other spotting features include the style of the members (laced or plate), the type of construction

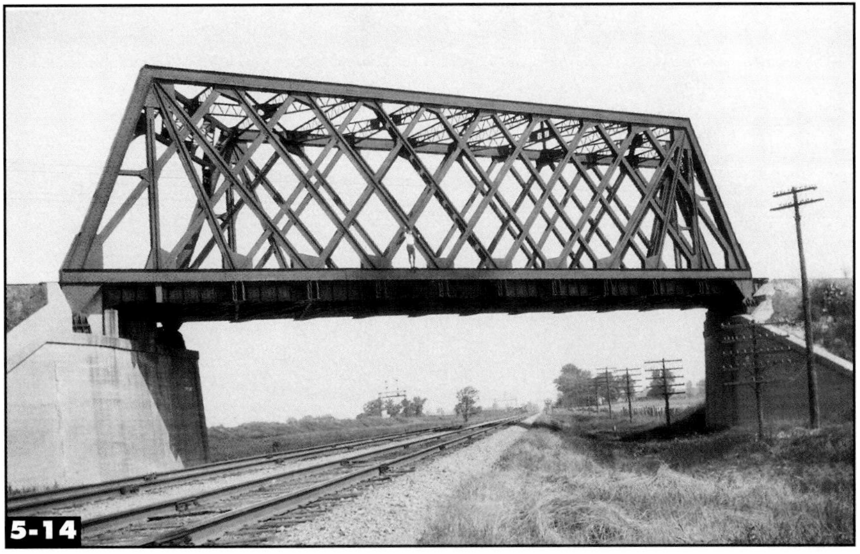

► The lattice truss, shown here on the Chicago & North Western, has diagonals spanning multiple panels, with no vertical members (except for the posts). *W. Christiansen*

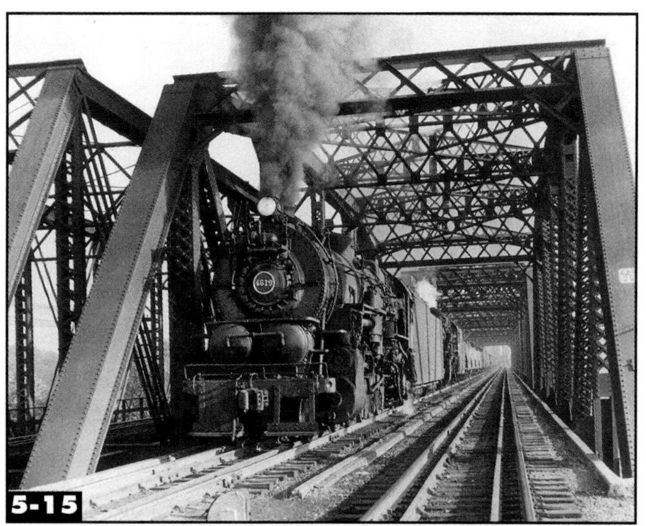

This double-track truss bridge on the Pennsy features a ballasted deck. The end posts are continuous-plate boxes, while the diagonals and hangers are double-laced. *Don Wood*

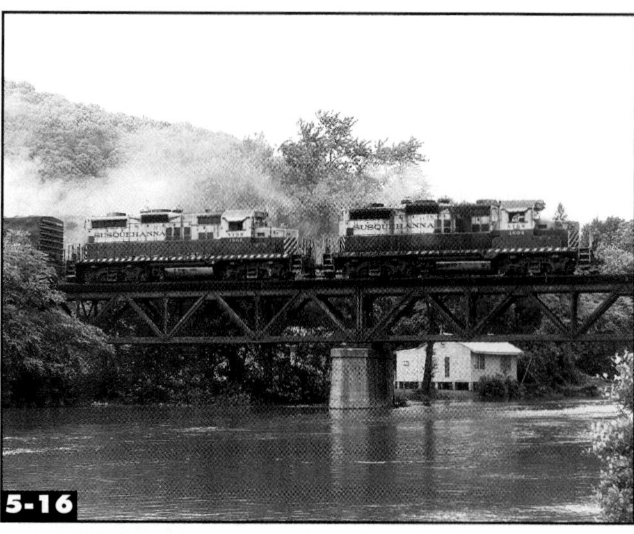

A pair of Warren deck trusses was used to span the Ramapo River on the New York, Susquehanna & Western. *Don Dorflinger*

(riveted, pinned, or combination), and the type of pedestals used (see Chapter 4 for more information on pedestals).

Most truss bridges are open-deck types like the one shown in photo **5-6** (page 40), with the bridge ties laid directly on the stringers. These decks are sometimes closed by adding wood planking or metal grating to create a deck for walking, similar to the plate girder bridge walkways discussed in Chapter 4.

Ballasted-deck trusses aren't as common as ballasted plate-girder bridges, but they do exist, **5-15**.

Double-track bridges, like the one in photo **5-15**, are another fairly common variation. They follow the same truss designs as single-track bridges, but the members are heavier to support the additional weight.

Deck and pony trusses

As with plate girder bridges, deck versions of trusses are used where below-bridge clearance isn't an issue. Most of the common truss patterns can be found in deck versions, and they can be spotted by the same diagonal patterns used on through-truss bridges. The illustrations in **5-3** (page 39) show how deck versions of truss designs have the same truss pattern as the through versions. In other words, you can't simply take the side truss and flip it upside down.

Most deck spans have the trusses squared off at the ends, with the bridge pedestals at the bottom of the structure as shown in the Pratt deck in **5-1** (page 38). Photo **5-16** shows a Warren deck as part of a multiple span.

Deck trusses may also have their end members angled, with the pedestals on extensions of the top chord, **5-17**.

On some deck trusses, the track is placed directly on the top chords, as in the Warren deck in photo **5-16**. In other cases, the stringers and floor beams are placed atop the top chords, **5-18**.

As with through trusses, the longer the span, the deeper the truss and the heavier the individual members must be. The Santa Fe multiple-span Warren truss bridge in **5-19** is a good example of a long deck truss.

Pony truss spans, **5-20**, were frequently used for highway bridges, but aren't nearly as common on railroads as through or deck trusses. Their shorter truss sides limit their length, meaning plate-girder bridges are generally used instead of pony trusses.

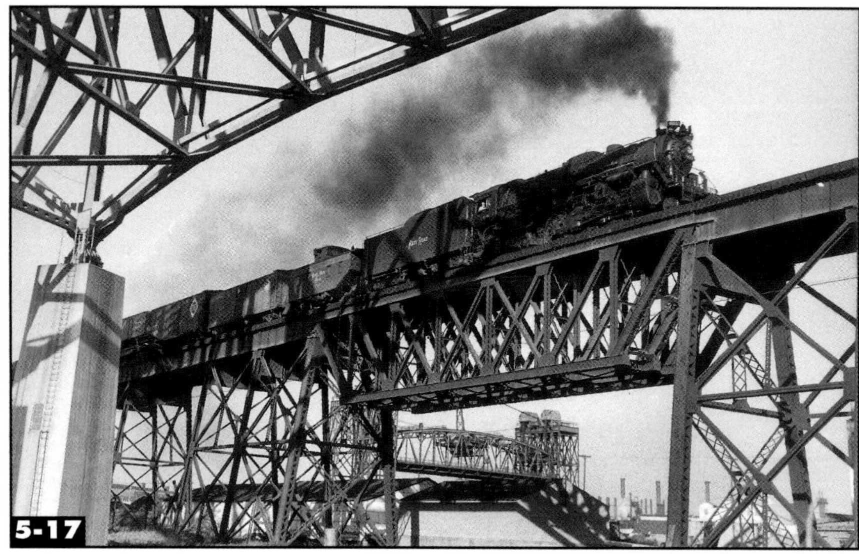

Some deck trusses have diagonal end posts, with the bridge pedestals on extensions of the top chord. This deck Pratt bridge on the Nickel Plate Road is one example. *Herbert H. Harwood, Jr.*

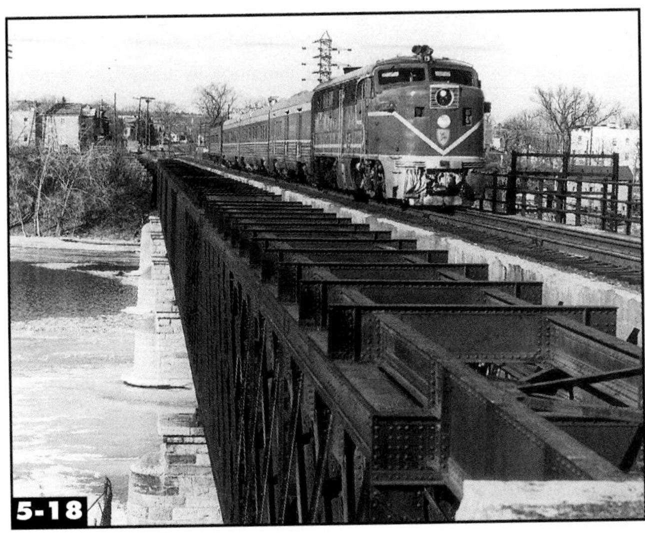

5-18

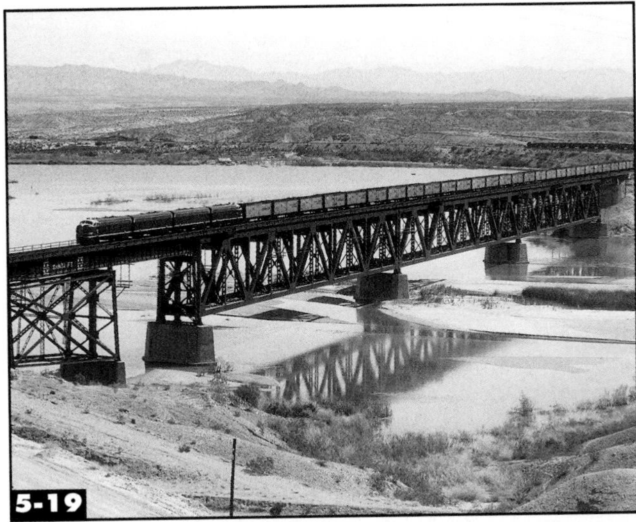

5-19

▲ This trackless deck truss bridge shows how the stringers and floor beams rest on the top chords. The floor beams are directly above the panel points. *Jim Shaughnessy*

Above right: The Santa Fe built these long (more than 300') Warren deck truss spans to cross the Colorado River at Topock, Arizona, in 1945. *Santa Fe Ry.*

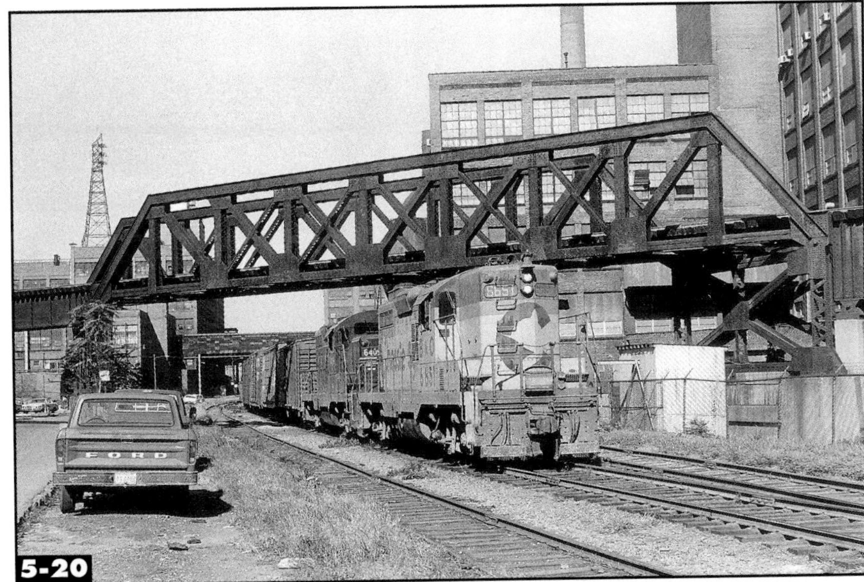

5-20

► A Chessie System train passes under a skewed pony truss bridge of the Akron & Barberton Belt RR in Akron, Ohio. *John Beach*

Skewed spans

Like plate-girder bridges, truss bridges are sometimes skewed where tracks cross rivers, highways, or other railroads at angles other than 90 degrees, **5-21**. As on skewed plate-girder bridges, the floor beams still run between trusses at 90-degree angles, with the ends of the stringers on blocks on the pier or abutment.

The panel joints in a skewed truss bridge still must be directly across from each other; the two sides of the bridge can't just be shifted off-line by a couple of feet. Because of this, the skew in a truss bridge will be off by one or more

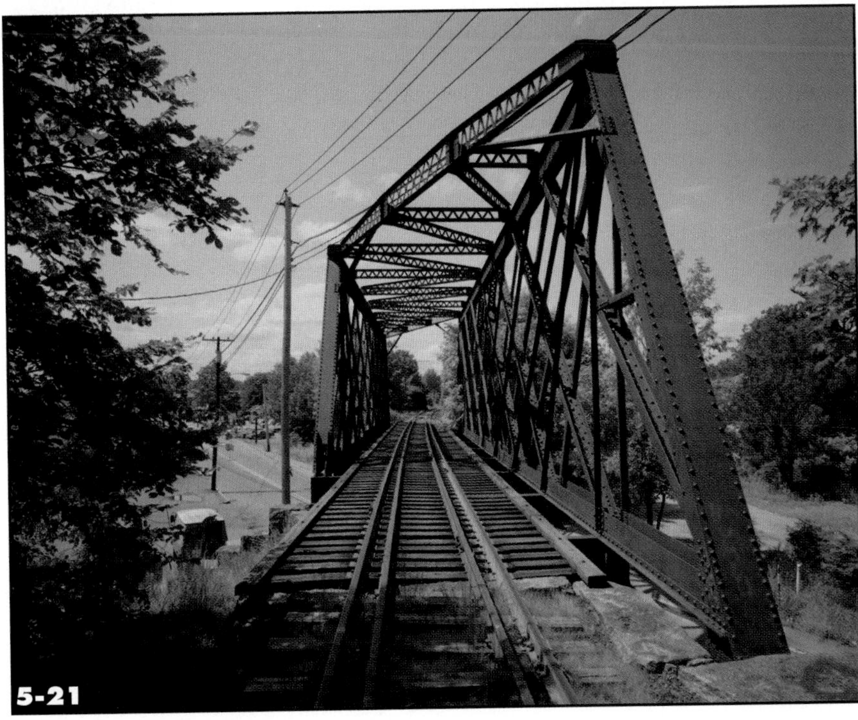

5-21

An extremely sharp skew is found on this lattice bridge, with the skew offset by three panels. Note how the abutment back wall is square to the tracks. The bridge, on the Boston & Maine in Waltham, Massachusetts, was built in 1894. *Historic American Engineering Record, Jet Lowe*

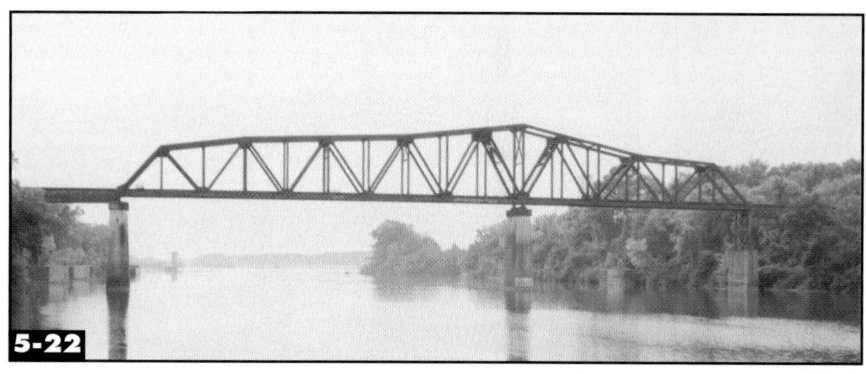

5-22

◀ Continuous truss bridges, used for long spans, have intermediate supports with a taller truss structure over the supports. This one, on the Gulf, Mobile & Ohio Warrior River crossing near Tuscaloosa, Alabama, was built in 1924. *Historic American Engineering Record, David Deising*

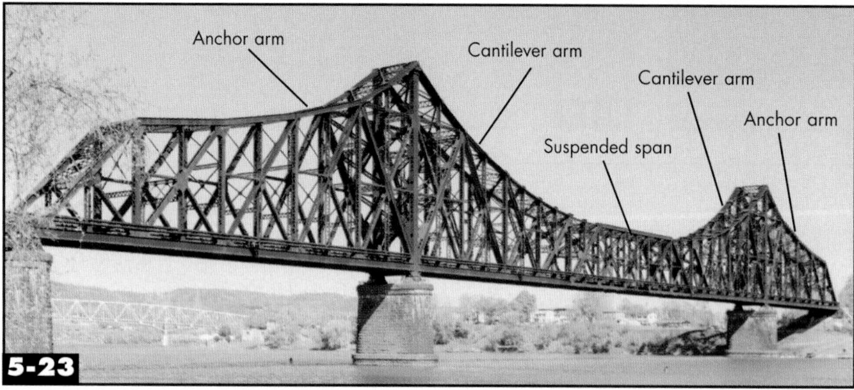

◀ Below: The Pittsburgh & Lake Erie used a cantilever bridge to cross the Ohio River at Beaver City, Pennsylvania. The total length of the cantilever is 1,400′, with 769′ between piers. *Historic American Engineering Record, Jet Lowe*

panel lengths. Subdivided bridges are often used for skew spans, and bridges may be skewed on one or both ends.

Other truss types

All of the above truss designs are simple spans, meaning they require support only at each end. A continuous truss design is sometimes used for exceptionally long spans, **5-22**. This design has an intermediate support (or supports) in addition to the end supports, but the bridge is a single structure.

Continuous trusses differ from a simple span by having deeper (taller) trusses over the intermediate supports (see **5-22**). Modeling a continuous truss by putting a support in the middle of a standard long truss would be incorrect.

Another modification of the truss design is the cantilever, **5-23**. The cantilever allows extremely long spans without a middle pier. Most such spans have a cantilever at each end, each of which is supported in the center with arms that reach to either side.

On each cantilever, the anchor arm reaches toward (and is anchored at) the shore, while the free arm—which is supported by its connection up and over the center to the anchor arm—reaches toward the cantilever on the other shore. Often the free arms hold a simple truss bridge between them like the bridge in **5-23**.

Cantilevers are complex and expensive to build, so their use is limited to locations where it would be impossible or impractical to build multiple piers in a waterway. The total span can be quite long: 1,400′, in the case of the bridge shown in **5-23**.

The steel arch is another bridge type used where intermediate piers aren't practical. A famous example is Hell Gate Bridge in New York, completed in 1917, **5-24**. Crossing the East River from Long Island to the Bronx, Hell Gate has a 977′ main span and, including its approach spans, a 17,000′ total length. It originally carried four ballasted tracks (one has since been removed).

Steel deck arch bridges can have single or multiple arches. A classic example of a deck arch is the Soo Line's multiple-arch bridge over the St. Croix River near Somerset, Wisconsin, **5-25**.

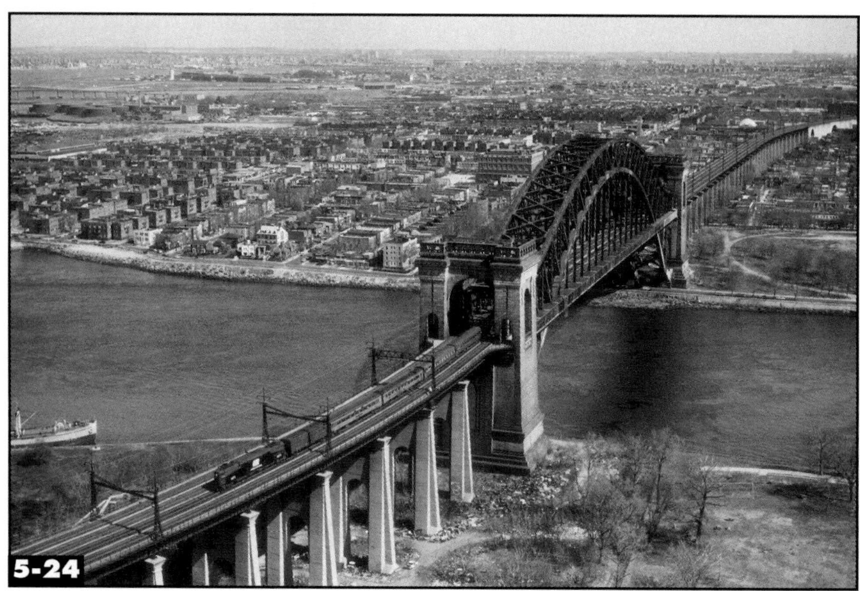

5-24

New York's Hell Gate is among the best known of the long steel arch bridges. It has a 977′ main span. *Victor Hand*

The Soo Line crosses the St. Croix River near Somerset, Wisconsin, on this impressive multiple-arch deck bridge. The bridge is 2,682′ long and 185′ wide. *William D. Middleton*

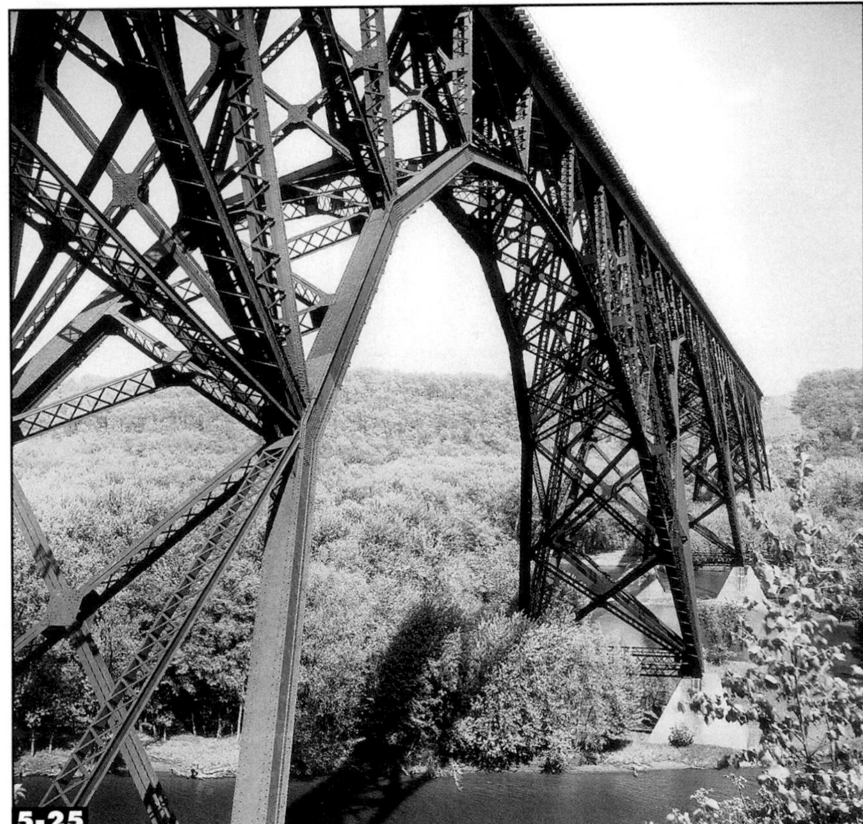

Materials

Wood truss bridges were popular through the mid-1800s and some were built well into the 1900s, especially in the Pacific Northwest and other areas where timber was plentiful. However, most wood trusses were replaced with wrought iron or steel spans by the early 1900s.

Cast iron was first used for bridges in the U.S. in 1845. The material was sufficient for highway bridges but proved too weak and brittle for railroad loads. Wrought iron was an improvement, and by 1860 it had became the material of choice for truss bridges and remained so through the late 1800s, when steel began to come into popular use. Although most wrought iron railroad bridges were replaced in the 1900s, some iron highway bridges have survived into the 2000s.

Through the first half of the 1800s, steel was far too expensive to use in bridge construction. However, by the 1870s, improved processes for making steel had driven the price down to a point where it became practical, and problems with quality and consistency had been solved.

Offering greater strength with less weight, steel's strength and durability made it superior to iron. However, it was still expensive, meaning many late-1800s bridges were a mix of steel (for critical components) and iron.

The first all-steel railroad bridge, a five-span Whipple truss, was completed in 1879 over the Missouri River at Glasgow, Missouri, on the Chicago, Alton & St. Louis. By the mid-1890s, steel had replaced iron on almost all new bridge construction.

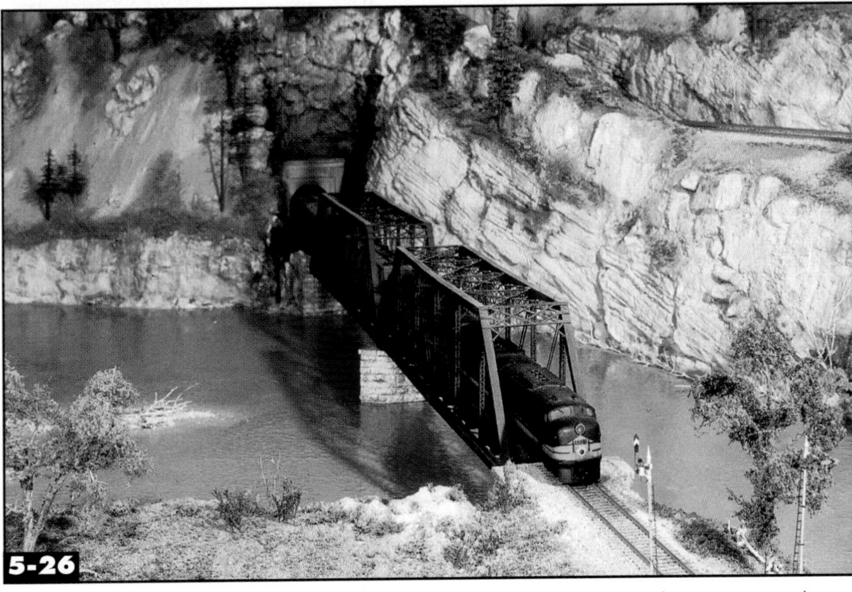

These HO scale Pratt through-truss bridges are made by Central Valley. The scene is on the Northern Pacific layout of Central Valley's owner, Jack Parker. *George Hall*

Modeling

Truss bridges are lacy and complex, and they make eye-catching models on layouts. Because of their multiple joints, sometimes-intricate laced members, and bracing, the easiest way to model a truss bridge is to use one of the many commercial models available in N through O scales (see the list of available kits beginning on page 86).

Two of the nicest models available are HO scale kits for through-truss bridges: a scale 150′ Pratt from Central Valley, **5-26**, and a 144′ Warren from Walthers, **5-27** (page 48). Walthers also offers a double-track version of its Warren bridge, **5-28** (page 48), based on

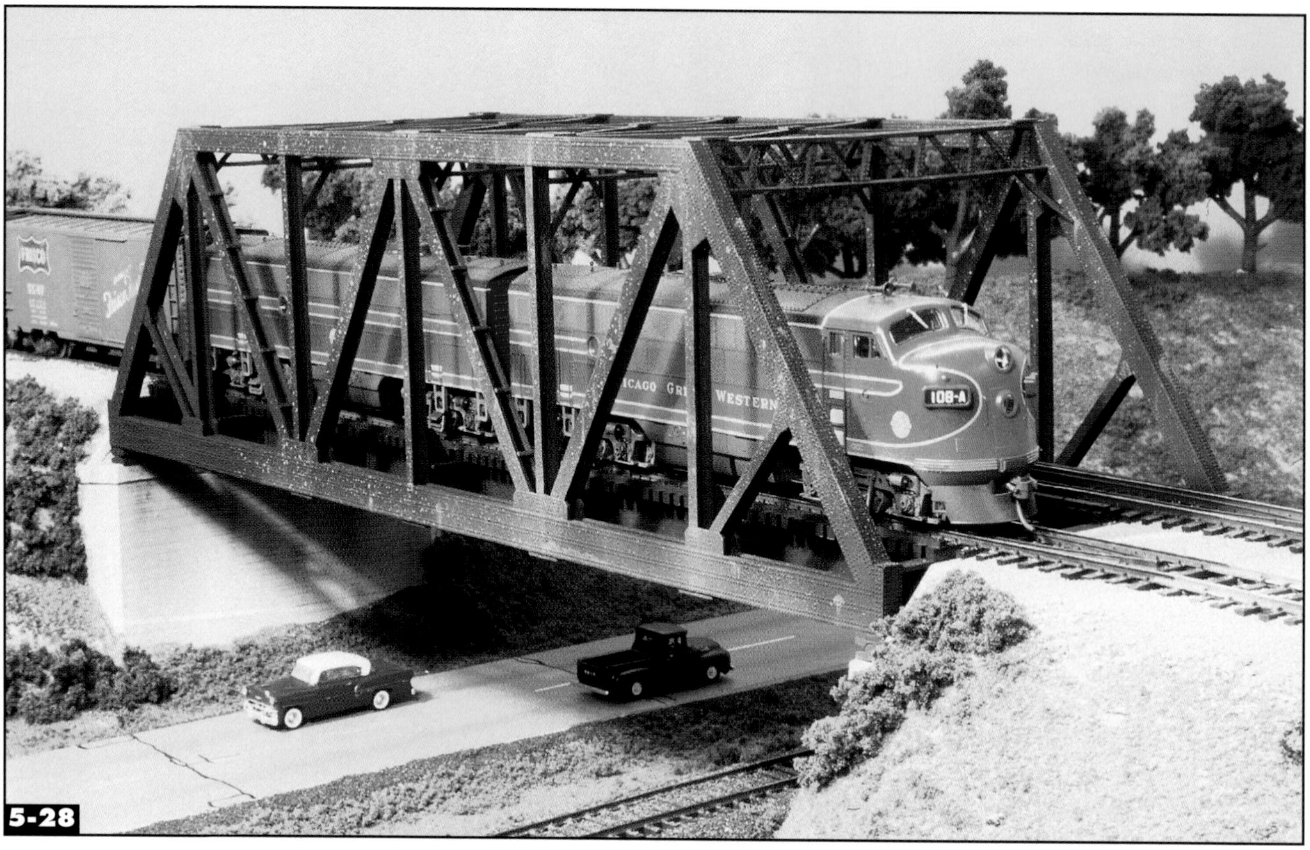

5-28

Walthers offers a kit for a double-track Warren truss in both HO scale (shown) and N scale. *Jeff Wilson*

the Nickel Plate Road's bridge spanning the Wabash River at Lafayette, Indiana.

In O scale, Atlas O offers single- and double-track versions of a 160'-long Warren truss, although Atlas O incorrectly calls it a Pratt. Atlas also offers a Warren pony truss in both N and HO scales, as well as short deck truss bridges based on the same design. The detail on these kits is limited, however, with no floor beams or stringers—just a molded bridge floor—and surface details only on the outside of the truss sides.

Kato makes an N scale single-track through Warren truss bridge. Although it's designed to be used with the company's Unitrack system, it can be modified to work with standard N scale track as well.

Parts are available for kitbashing or scratchbuilding, including trusses in a variety of sizes from Plastruct, **5-29**, and sets of members in lace and steel plate designs of various sizes from Central Valley **5-30**.

One of the best ways to create a unique bridge is to modify an existing bridge by swapping some of its members. For example, try substituting laced members for steel plate members.

If you're feeling adventurous, you can use the parts to scratchbuild a bridge. You'll need to follow original engineering drawings or published plans if possible. For through bridges, start with stringers and floor beams from one of the commercial kits and combine them to make longer spans if desired.

Now that we've explored truss bridges, it's time to move on to concrete and stone bridges.

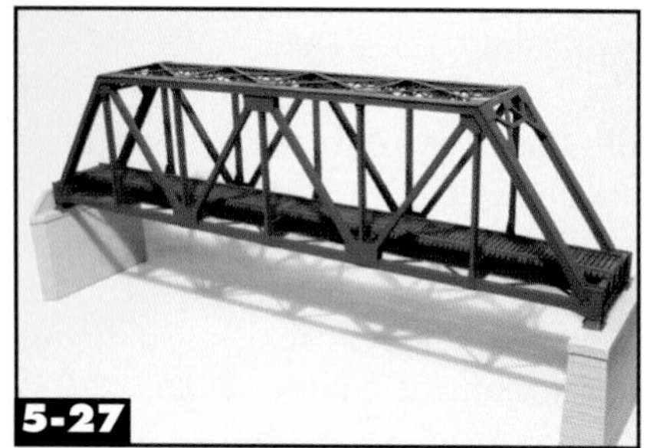

This HO scale Warren truss is an injection-molded kit available from Walthers. *Jeff Wilson*

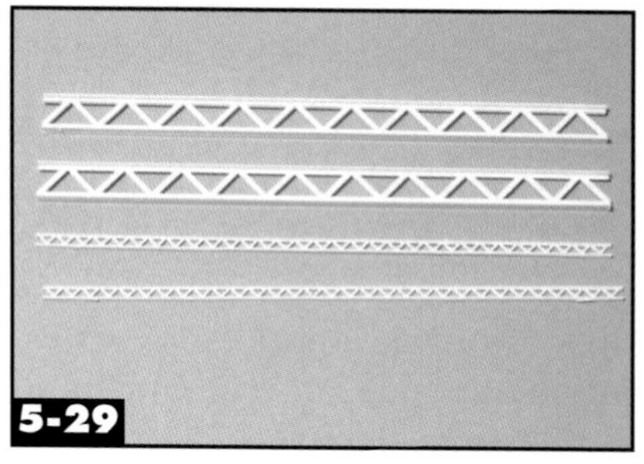

Plastruct offers injection-molded styrene trusses in various sizes. *Jeff Wilson*

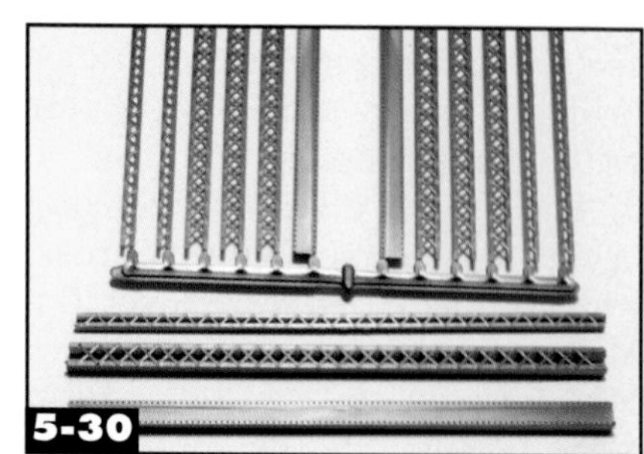

Central Valley offers its truss bridge members as a kit. The parts are ideal for scratchbuilding or kitbashing. *Jeff Wilson*

Covered wood bridges

Although you might not immediately think "truss" when looking at a covered bridge, that's exactly what they are: a wood truss bridge covered with sheathing. Covered railroad and highway bridges were common in New England, and many were also found in the Pacific Northwest, as well as in other areas of the country. A few of these bridges lasted into the late 1900s. The truss framework was covered by wood sheathing and a roof to protect the load-bearing members from the elements.

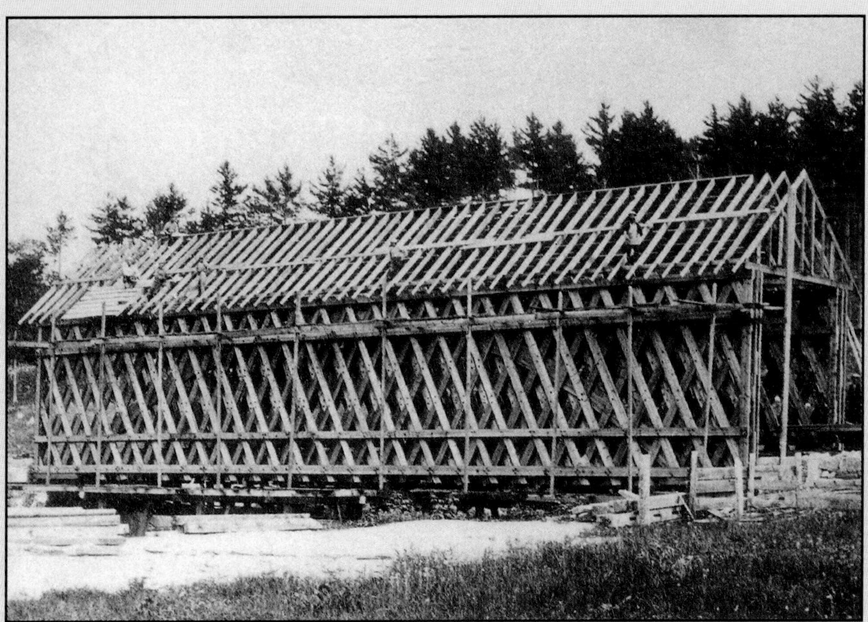

▲ Lurking under the sheathing of a covered wood bridge is a wood truss—a lattice in the case of this Boston & Maine structure. *Richard Sanders Allen collection*

▼ The St. Johnsbury & Lamoille County was a shortline railroad known for its covered wood bridges. It had several in service into the late 1900s. *Allen Collection*

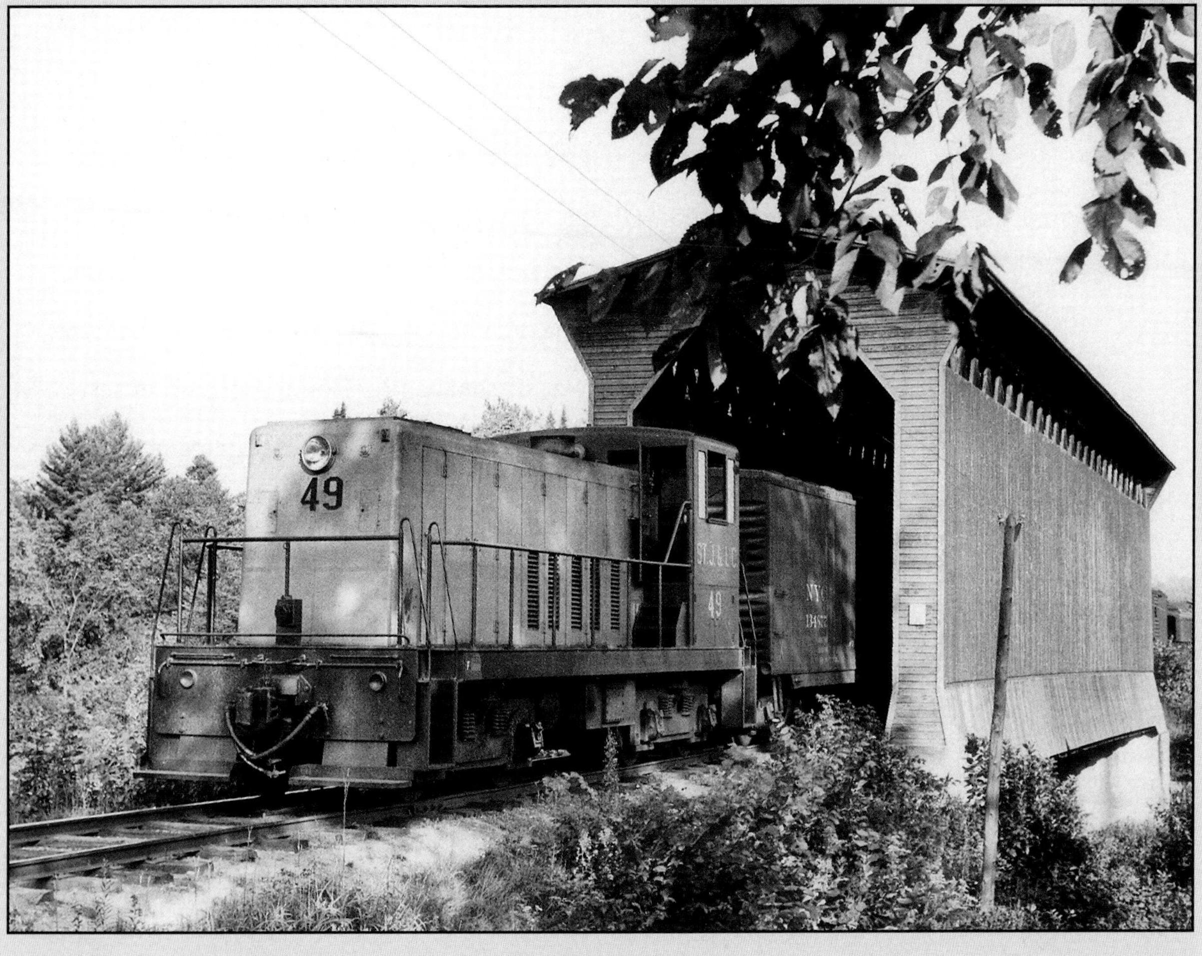

Stone and concrete bridges

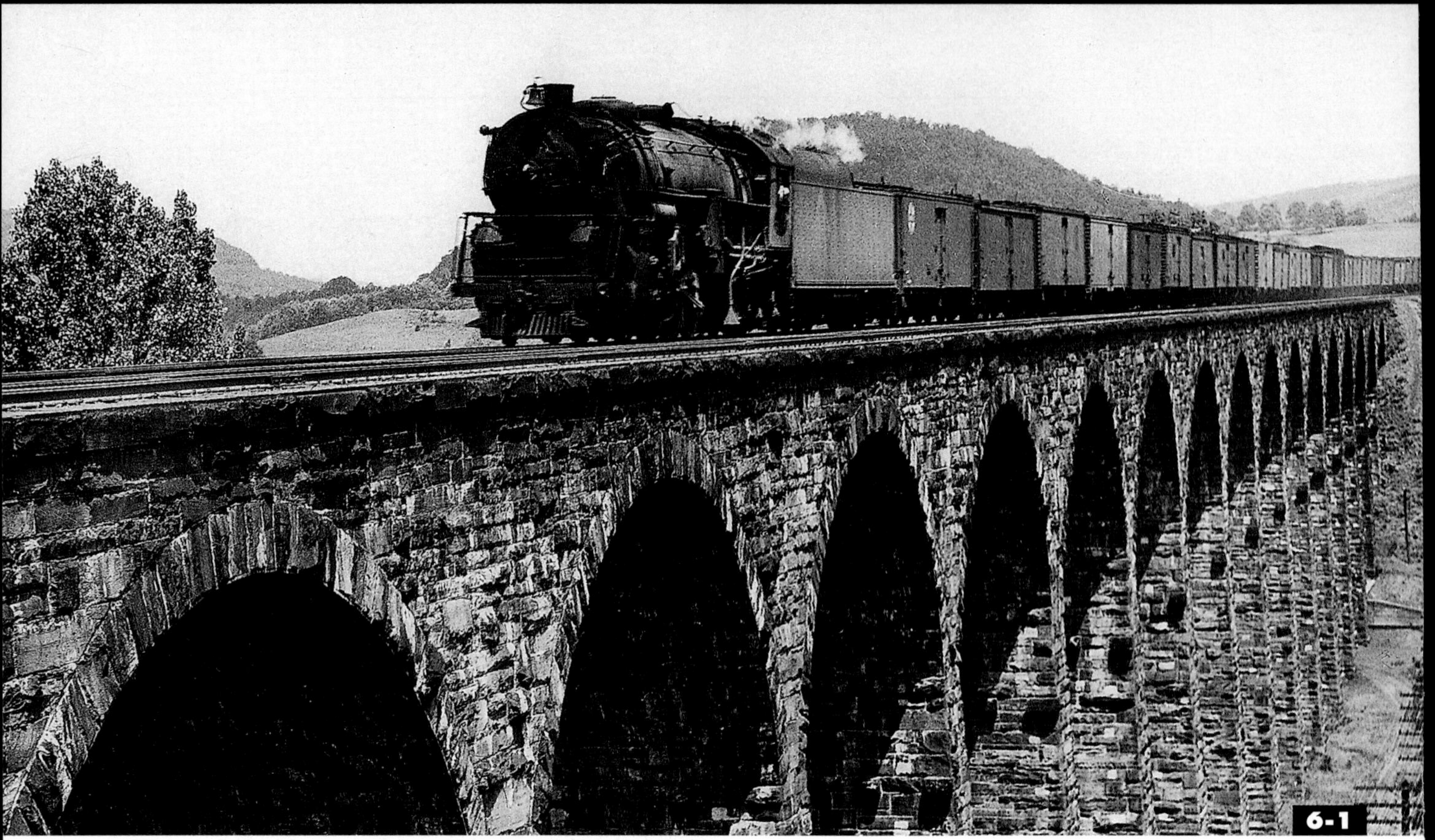

6-1

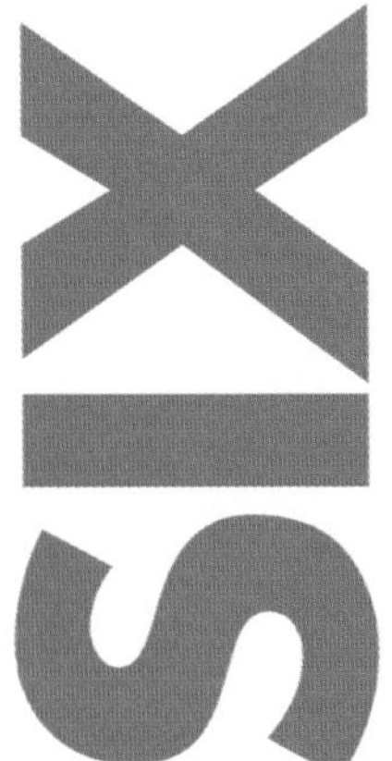

The Erie Railroad's Starrucca Viaduct, 1,200′ long and 110′ tall, was built in 1848 and remains in service today. *Charles A. Elston*

Some of the most dramatic railroad bridges are the oldest: stone-arch structures. This shouldn't come as a surprise, as masonry has been a staple of bridge construction for thousands of years. Many stone-arch bridges built in the 1800s—both large and dramatic as well as small and utilitarian—are still in service in the 21st century, carrying heavy loads the designers and builders could not have conceived of when the bridges were built.

Concrete has become the masonry material of choice for modern bridge installations and replacements. Like stone bridges, concrete bridges can be found in a vast array of sizes and configurations.

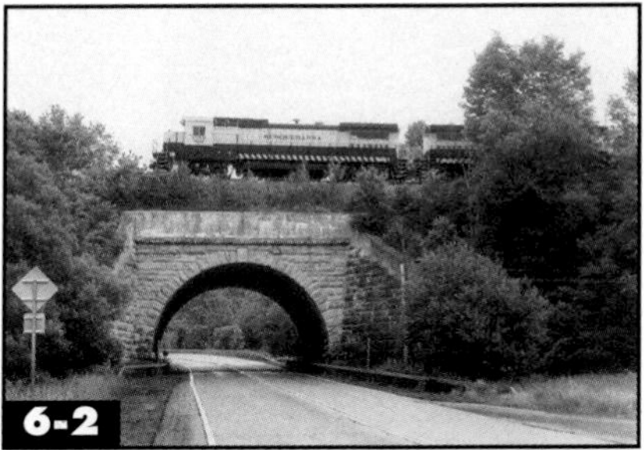

▲ Many small stone-arch structures remain in service, crossing highways, streams, and even other railroads. *J.J. Young, Jr.*

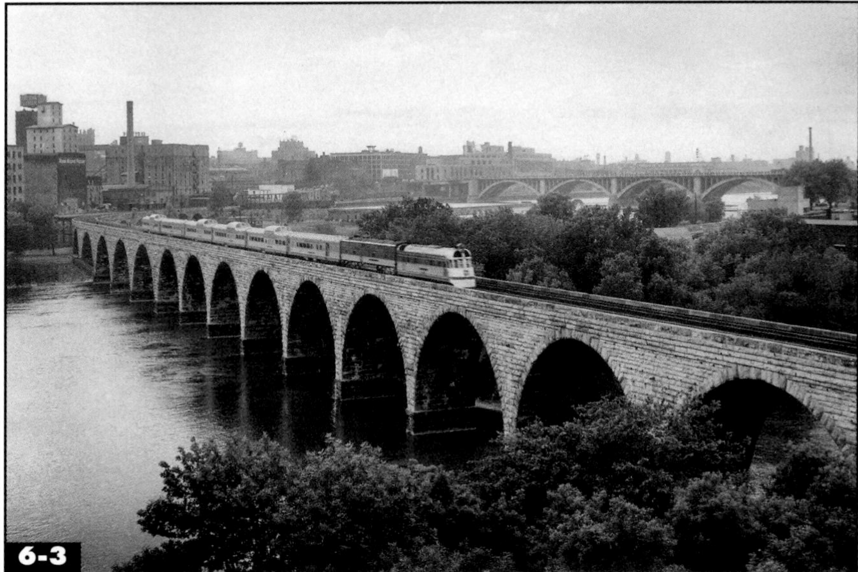

► The Great Northern's stone-arch bridge across the Mississippi is notable for being curved at one end (at left in the photo). *Chicago, Burlington & Quincy*

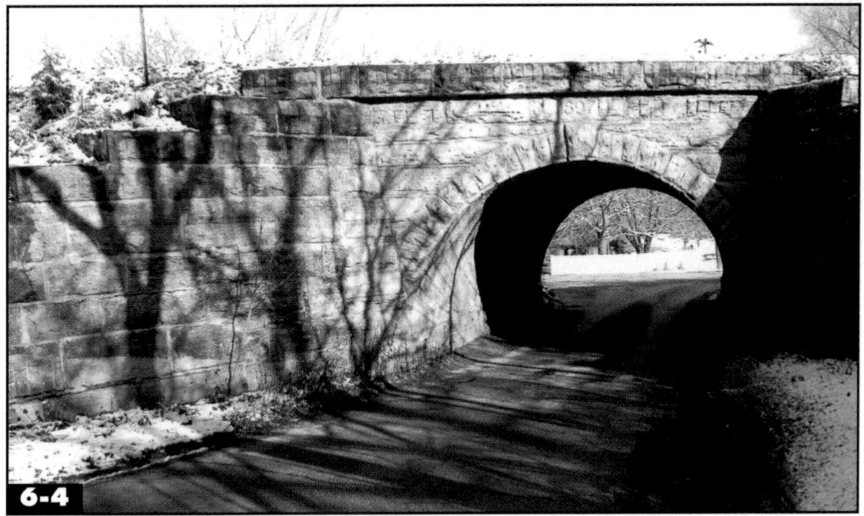

Built in 1897, this skewed stone Chicago & North Western bridge, is still in service and plenty sound. Modern vehicles passing under it are limited by tight clearances. *Jeff Wilson*

Stone-arch bridges

Some of the most famous and easily recognizable railroad structures are stone-arch bridges. The picturesque Starrucca Viaduct is perhaps the best-known stone-arch railroad bridge in the United States, **6-1**. Completed in 1848, the 1,200'-long, 110'-tall structure remains in use today, carrying trains far heavier than those of the era when it was built.

Multi-arch structures such as Starrucca are generally called viaducts. Far more common single-arch structures are usually just termed "bridges," **6-2**, and smaller ones are called culverts.

The basic principle of the stone-arch bridge is the use of gravity as an aid for strength. Stone is strong in compression. By assembling stones into an arch, the gravity pulling them down—with the weight of other stones and material on top—forces the stones together, eventually transmitting the load down to the abutments and piers.

The arch design results in a very strong support, which is why many stone bridges built in the 1800s are still in service when wood and light truss bridges of the same era have long since been replaced by more modern spans. The longevity of stone-arch structures also testifies to the skill of the masons who built them and the engineers who designed them.

The main drawback of stone construction is cost. Starting around 1900, concrete supplanted stone as the material of choice.

The key elements of these bridges are the stones that form the arch ("voussairs"), with the keystone at the top center. The key principle of the design is that all joints among the voussairs must point toward the center of the arch. Arches are often semicircular but can also be elliptical or pointed.

Arches can be placed on piers of almost any reasonable height, but they require substantial abutments at each end to hold the forces transmitted by the arches. Piers can be quite tall—as on Starrucca—or fairly low, as on the Great Northern's Mississippi River bridge, **6-3**.

When building an arch bridge, the piers and abutment are erected first. A temporary framework, called falsework, is then built between piers to hold the stones of the arch until they become self-supporting. Once all of the arch stones are in place, the remainder of the bridge structure is completed.

Stone bridges are not actually solid stone. The exterior walls are stone masonry, but the interior is either hollow or filled with sand, earth, rubble, or other material.

Stone bridges come in many shapes and sizes, from huge to

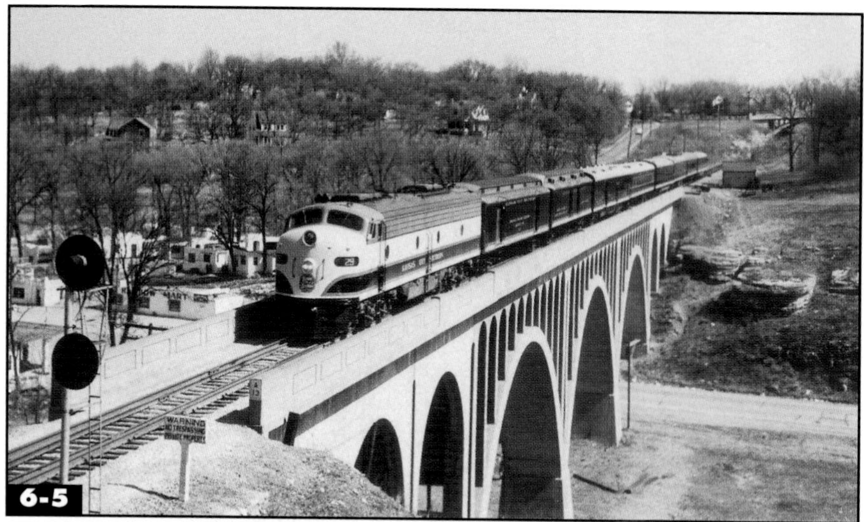
6-5

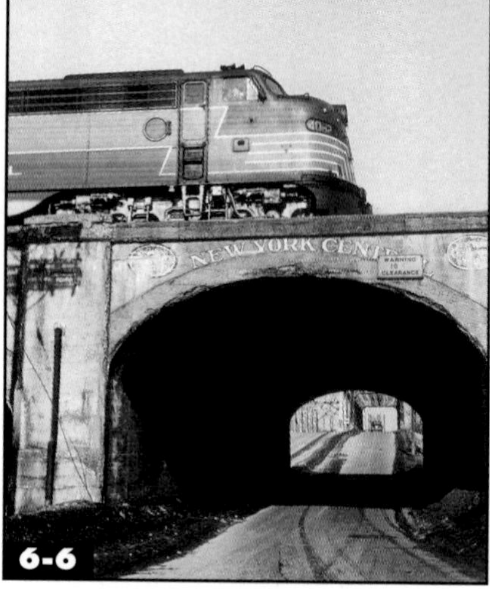
6-6

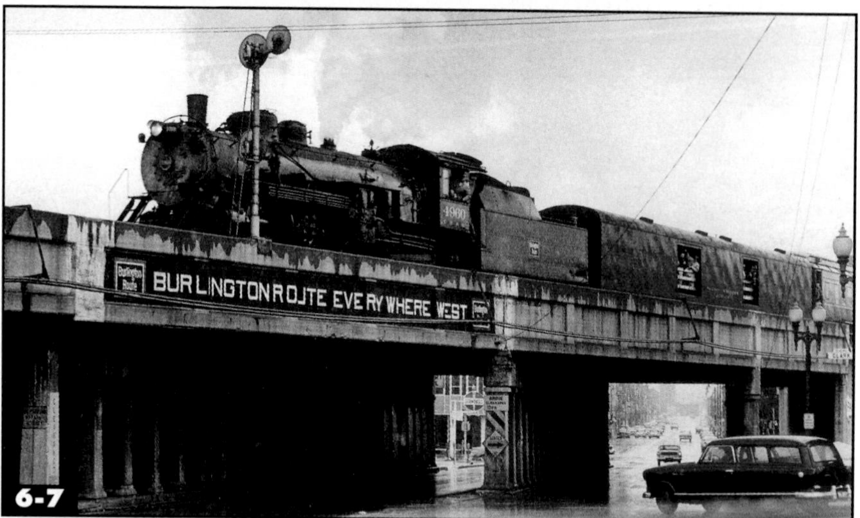

6-7

Above left: The Kansas City Southern built this graceful, impressive concrete viaduct outside Kansas City on its route to New Orleans. *Clarence T. Wood*

▲ This weathered concrete-arch overpass on the New York Central at Rome, New York, would make a great model on a gritty "working" model railroad. *Jim Shaughnessy*

◀ The Chicago, Burlington & Quincy's elevated line through Aurora, Illinois, features concrete construction. Note the multiple-pillar piers. *David P. Morgan Library collection*

small. Many of the small bridges over roadways, such as the bridge in **6-4** (page 51), are a paradox: Although old (100-plus years in this case), they remain more than strong enough to carry heavy modern rail traffic. However, their openings are quite small for today's cars and trucks. Because of this, many of these smaller bridges are on side streets and back roads.

Stone arches work best as straight spans. Although curved stone-arch bridges exist, they are comparatively rare because of the stresses involved in transmitting forces around a curve. The Great Northern bridge in **6-3** (page 51) is an example of a curved stone bridge. Built in 1883, the 23-arch double-track bridge is 2,100′ long, 76′ tall, and 28′ wide and has a six-degree bend at one end.

Stone bridges offer plenty of detail for the modeler. Many of them have intricately designed pilasters, railings (often of ornamental iron), and other decorative stonework on the bridge and surrounding walls.

The stone itself can be either cut or random stone, and it can be smooth or coarse cut. Colors vary greatly depending upon the type of stone used, as well as the age and weathering of the structure.

Maintenance is a key to long life for stone bridges. They are often repaired with concrete, and a common repair is to add concrete lining within the arch, resulting in a smooth finish.

Stone bridges are most common in the East, where most of the railroads were in the mid-1800s. They are found in the Midwest and scattered in other areas around the country. Due to their rigidity, stone bridges are rarely built in areas prone to earthquakes.

Concrete bridges

Early concrete-arch bridges followed many patterns, with varying arch designs. These feature closed or open spandrels, **6-5**. The design can also be much simpler, as in a road overpass, **6-6**.

Concrete has been used on railroad bridges since the mid-1800s. In fact, one of the first uses of concrete in the U.S. was on the Starrucca Viaduct, where the base portions of the piers and deck covering are concrete.

Other types of concrete bridges include beam bridges (covered in Chapter 2) and slab bridges, where a single slab of reinforced concrete is used, usually as a trough above beams or girders (see "Ballasted-deck bridges" on pages 33-34). Other bridges look like solid concrete but have steel I-beams encased in the concrete for strength. Multi-span concrete bridges are often used in towns over roads and other obstacles in the city scape, **6-7**.

Many art-deco styled bridges from the 1930s have what appear to be concrete girders, but these are merely facades, **6-8**. From below they appear to be concrete spans, but a view from above reveals that many are through plate girder spans, with concrete sides just for show, **6-9**.

Most masonry bridges have ballasted decks, as can be seen in photo **6-5**. This is the simplest method, with a shallow trough at the top to contain the track and ballast. As with other ballasted-deck bridges, standard track (not bridge track) is used.

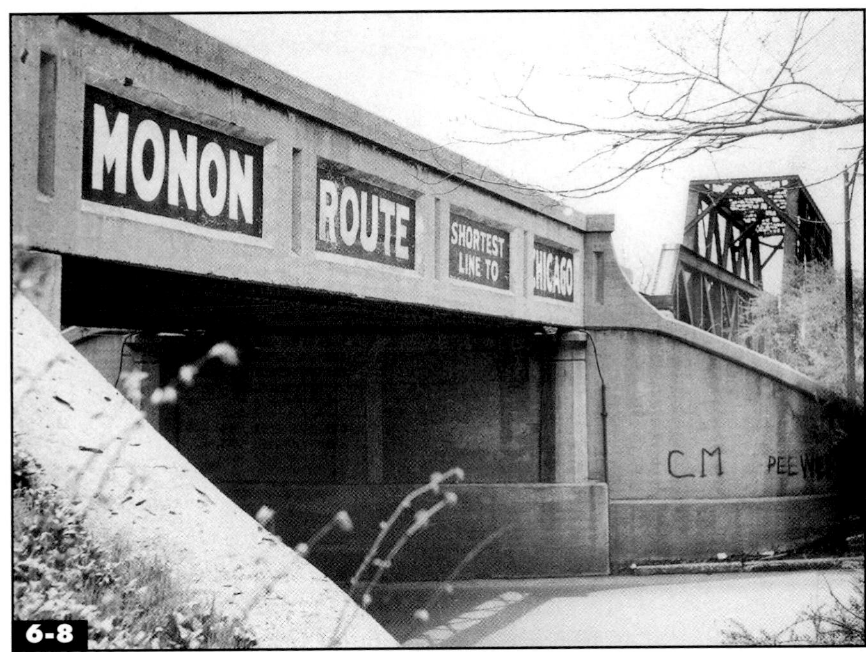

Many concrete bridges, such as this one on the Monon in Indianapolis, have interesting false facades and columns. *Linn H. Westcott*

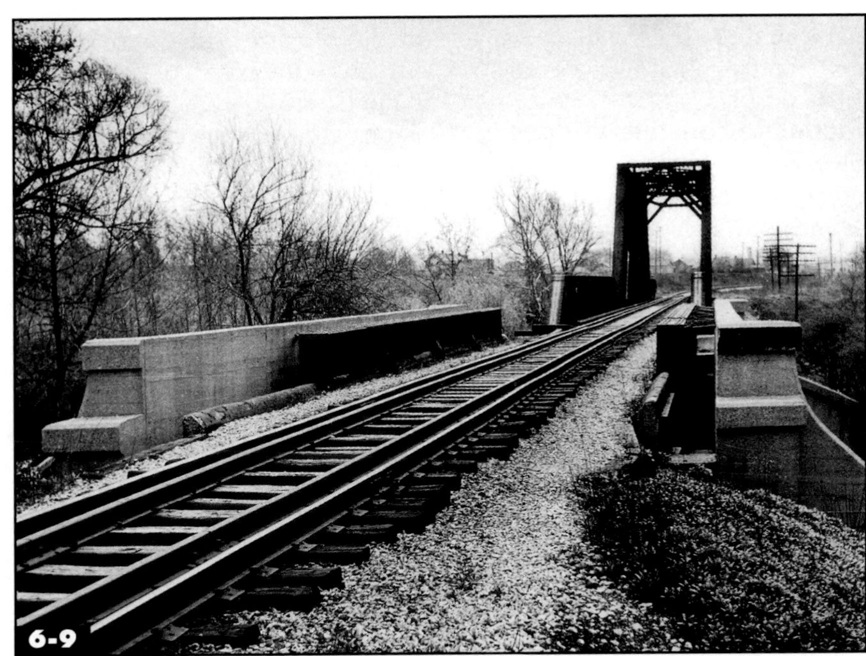

A view from above the Indianapolis Monon bridge reveals that the concrete girders are merely false fronts to a ballasted-deck plate girder span. *Linn H. Westcott*

Modeling stone bridges

The easiest way to model a stone bridge is to use a commercial model. There are many available (see the list of available kits starting on page 86), but be aware that some of them follow European designs and will look out of place on a layout set in North America. Many European models are also undersized. Check photos and dimensions on model company websites and other sources, such as the Walthers catalog. Compare the models to prototype photos.

Several companies offer textured styrene sheet to represent cut and random stone. Although these can be used as starting points for modeling, re-creating the appearance of a stone-arch bridge takes more than cutting an archway in a plastic sheet. You'll need to re-create the voussoirs around the arch opening, as well as the stonework inside the arch.

Photo **6-10** (page 54) shows a small HO scale Faller arch bridge. "De-Europeanize" models like this by removing the top track base and railing and replacing it with a plain styrene deck. Use styrene strips to represent concrete and beef up the edges.

Injection-molded plastic stonework always needs paint. One way to do this is to paint the whole surface flat medium or dark gray, painting a few blocks with various darker or lighter shades, and giving the whole structure a wash of yet another shade of gray, **6-11** (page 54). Chapter 10 will cover painting stone more fully.

The Faller arch bridge in **6-10** can be used on an HO layout as intended, but the deck is fairly narrow. It can be completed with N scale track and roadbed, and the proportions will look about right, **6-12** (page 54). Many models can be modified to make them wider or longer, or to alter the abutments or wing walls.

Rix and others companies offer stone-arch bridges and wing walls

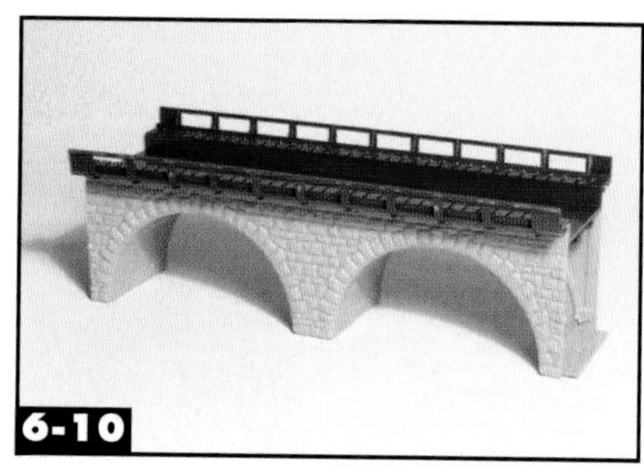

This HO scale Faller bridge has a very European-looking top, and the shiny orange plastic doesn't look much like real stone. *Jeff Wilson*

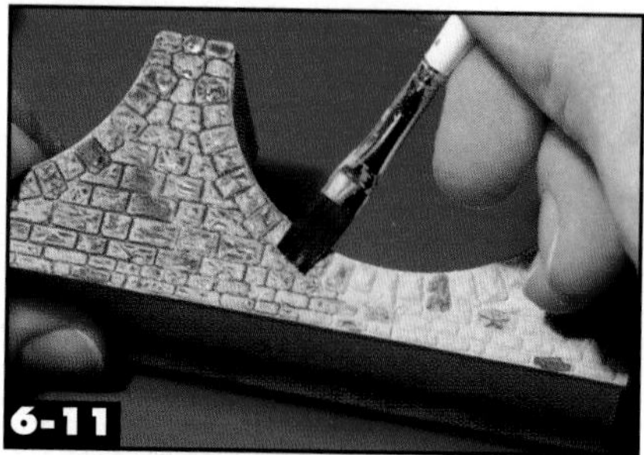

Painting the stonework gets rid of the unrealistic plastic shine. A wash of dark gray over the painted rocks helps vary colors. *Jeff Wilson*

that can be used to replicate simple prototype bridges like the one in **6-2** (page 51). One way to do this is to place the HO model below the level of the roadbed, **6-13**, and fill the gap between the top of the stonework and the track, with scenery. You can also secure the model to the roadbed, **6-14**, and the track will appear to run in a trough atop the bridge.

Modeling concrete bridges

Few commercial models of concrete bridges were available until Monroe Models recently released a couple of nice models of concrete overpasses, including an Art Deco span (see the list of available kits starting on page 86).

Concrete is easy to model with styrene strips and sheet. Styrene is easy to cut, shape, glue, and paint, and it can be layered to duplicate many concrete effects. I'll go step-by-step through a project, and you can use the same techniques to design your own bridge or duplicate a prototype bridge. (See Chapter 9 for additional information about modeling with styrene.)

I decided to build an HO model of Monon's concrete bridge and abutment shown in **6-8** and **6-9** (page 53). The bridge and surrounding concrete work are typical of bridges built in the 1930s.

I had no drawings to guide me—only three prototype photos of the Monon bridge—so I made my own drawings, **6-15**, using a pencil, scale rule, and graph paper. If you have to do this, guesstimate sizes based on known (or easy-to-estimate) dimensions. I figured a height of 14′ from the road surface to the bottom of the bridge was about right. I made the bridge itself 42′ long, judging its size from the road width and the sidewalk on one side.

I took the same approach to draw and re-draw the curved continuous wing walls until they looked right. Straight walls are much easier to model, but the curved walls lent a great deal of character to the structure.

Actual construction began with cutting out the main abutment wall. Transfer the outline of the wall to sheet styrene by photocopying the drawing, cutting it out, and using it as a stencil. I used .040″ sheet styrene, because it is stiff but still fairly easy to cut and work with.

Next, I added a strip of .100″ × .375″ styrene to the bottom of the rear of the wall to make a base, **6-16**. To curve the wall, I cut two pieces of .060″ styrene to the desired curve contour. Using liquid plastic cement to glue these on the back of the wall, I first glued down one end, clamped it, and let it dry. Then I glued and clamped the other ends, **6-17**, making sure the contour piece stayed aligned parallel with the bottom edge of the wall (if it doesn't, the curve will not be correct).

Cutting the raised trim along the curved contour of the wall requires care. I used a pencil to trace the wall contour onto a piece of .060″ plastic, **6-18**. I needed two of these pieces (front and back) for each side. With a sharp hobby knife, I scored this line using light pressure at first, then applying heavier pressure as the groove became deeper.

I traced another line a scale 12″ inside of the first line. This is the width of the trim piece. After scoring this line to sufficient depth, I carefully flexed the plastic at the marks until it snapped along the line.

The trim pieces were glued to the curved edge of the wall, **6-19**. As with the curved braces, I didn't try to glue an entire piece at once.

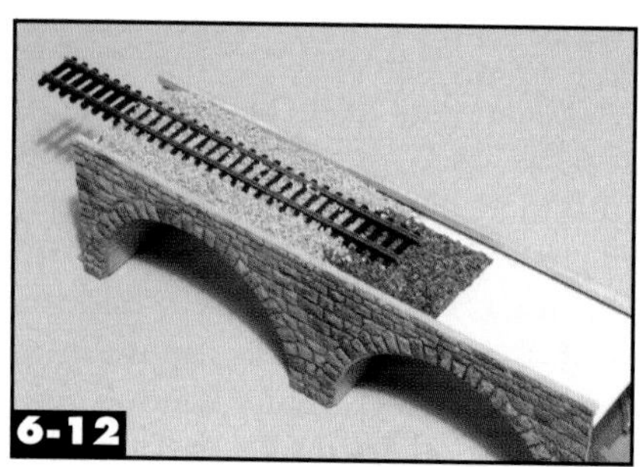

This view shows the new styrene deck and the styrene trim inside the top edges. The N scale track (on cork) looks right at home on this structure. *Jeff Wilson*

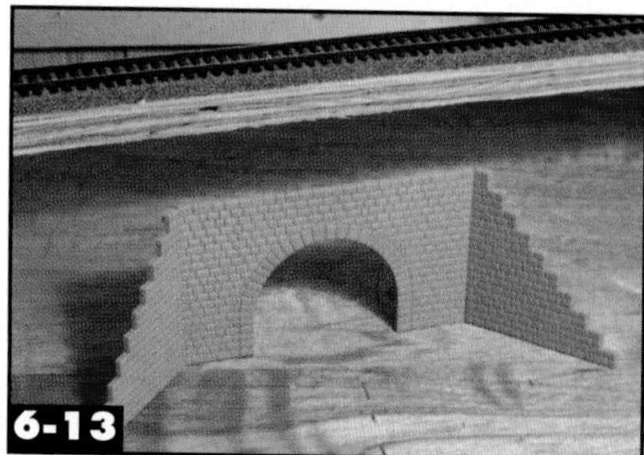

The Rix culvert can be positioned on the layout below track level, with earth fill above it. *Jeff Wilson*

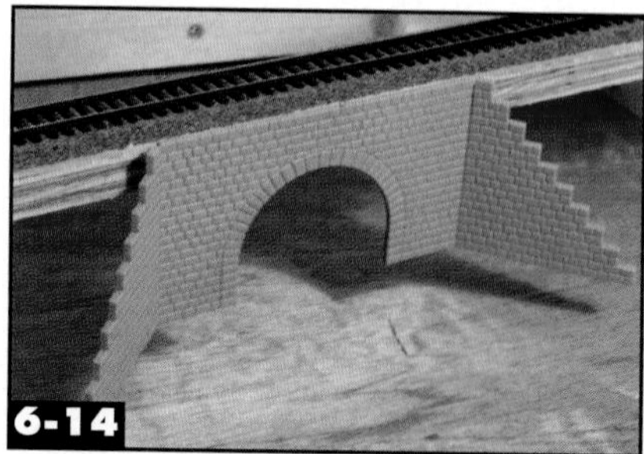

The Rix structure can also be placed at roadbed level for a different look. *Jeff Wilson*

Instead, I glued and clamped one end, making sure it was properly aligned, and let it dry. I moved around the piece one section at a time until it was glued in place. To ensure the realistic appearance of the finished structure, the trim must be glued securely to the wall with no gaps. The column base across the base of the face of the abutment should be made from heavier .100″ styrene, as photo **6-14** shows.

The columns take a bit of work. I wasn't sure if I could duplicate them precisely, but I wanted to capture their overall look. I beveled the edges of a .125″ × .375″ styrene strip with a miniature router made from a hobby knife blade stuck into a scrap board, **6-20**. I then pulled the plastic strip under the blade repeatedly to scrape off material—don't try to take off too much material in a single pass. If you go slowly, the cut will be relatively consistent.

I contoured the top caps for the column by hand, using a hobby knife to shape two pieces of plastic. You certainly don't have to go to this level of detail to have a nice model; omit details like this if you don't feel comfortable doing them or if the results aren't what you're looking for.

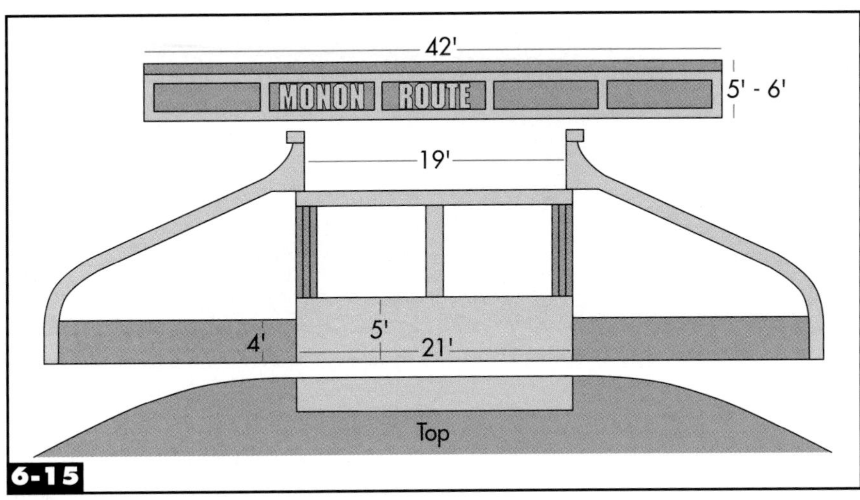

If you don't have prototype drawings for a bridge, you can make your own, as the author did for his HO scale copy of the Monon bridge in photos 6-8 and 6-9.

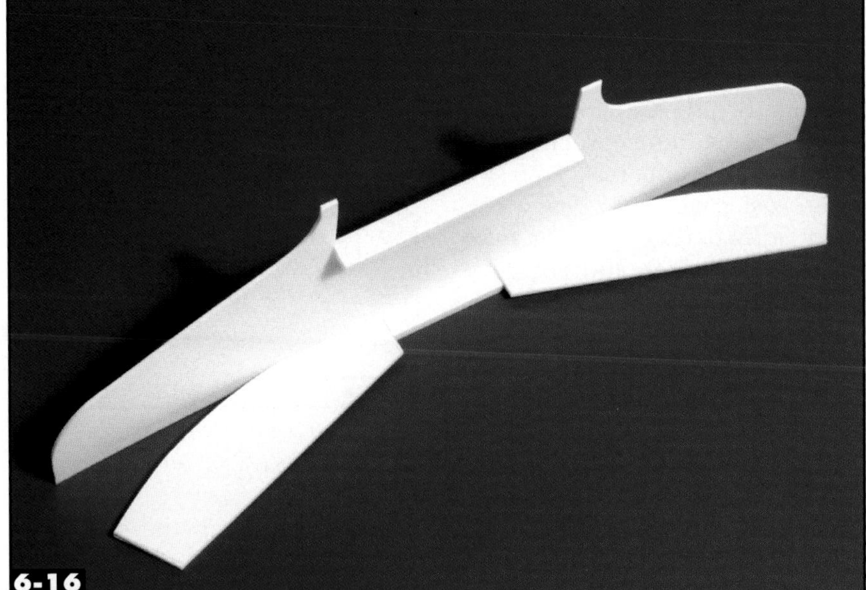

◀ The rear of the abutment wall shows the base and the contour pieces that give the abutment its curved wings. *Jeff Wilson*

▼ To get the shape you want, clamp the contour pieces in position until the glue dries. *Jeff Wilson*

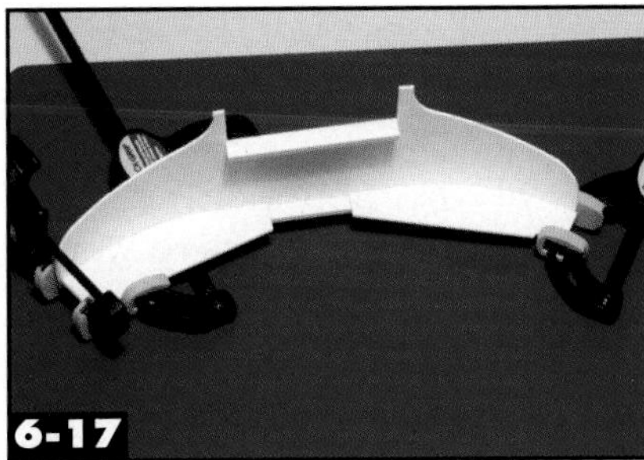

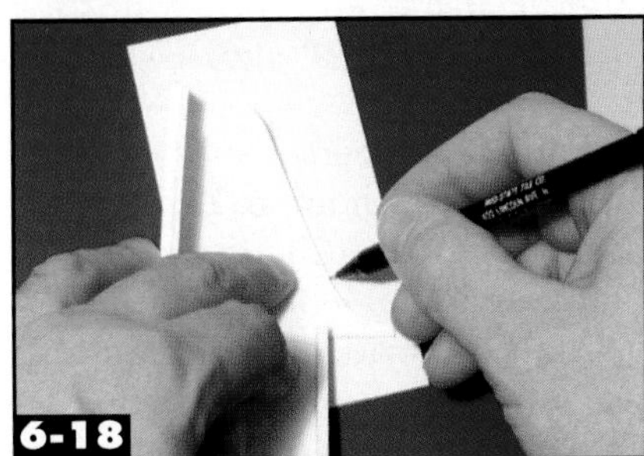

Trace the outline of the abutment onto a piece of .060″ styrene sheet to make the trim pieces. *Jeff Wilson*

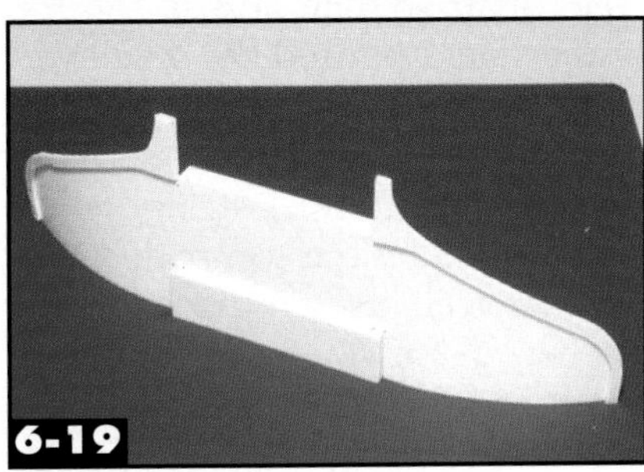

Here, the curved trim pieces have been installed, as have the .10″-thick base for the columns. *Jeff Wilson*

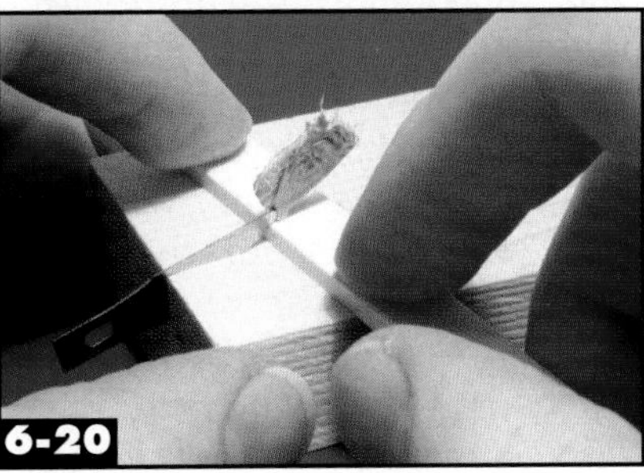

Pull strip plastic across a knife blade to bevel the edges. For safety's sake, make sure the blade tip is covered. *Jeff Wilson*

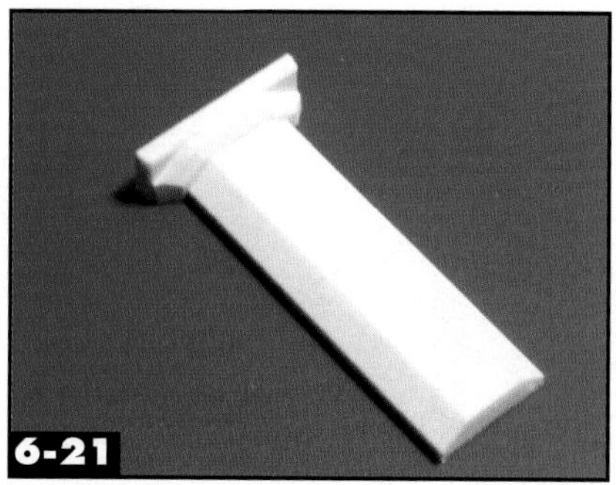

Two pieces of plastic—one contoured by hand—serve as a cap for the column. *Jeff Wilson*

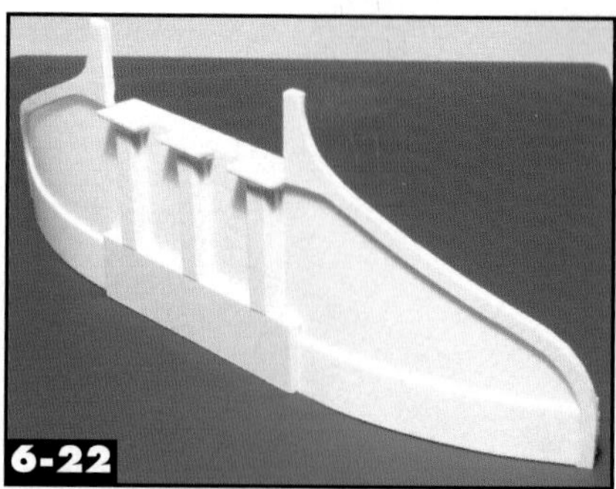

The completed columns are glued in place, as are the last .040″ base pieces along the bottom of the wall. *Jeff Wilson*

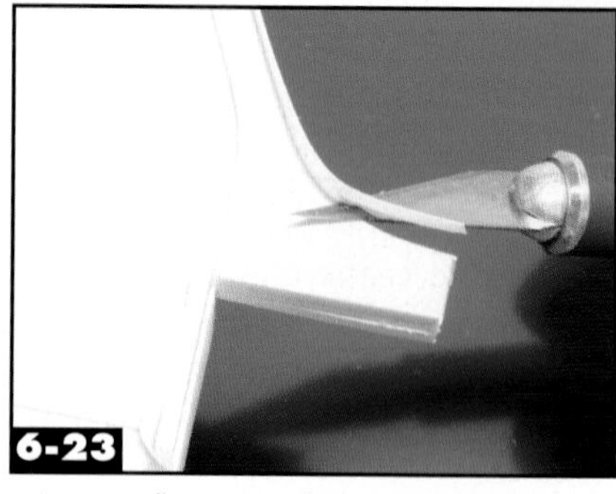

Glue .005″ sheet styrene to the edges (top and sides) of the abutment wall. Trim the plastic once the glue is dry. *Jeff Wilson*

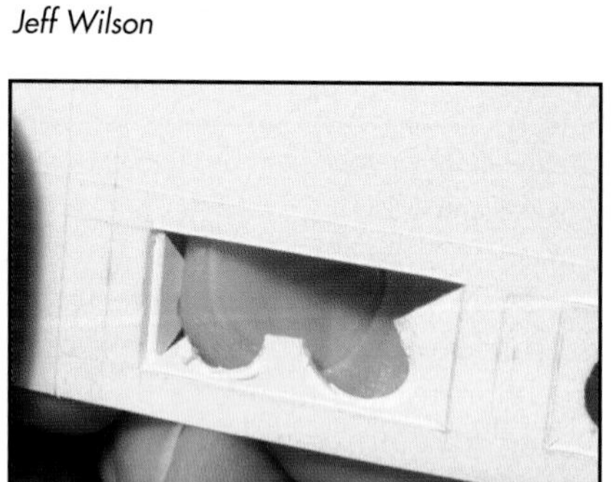

Drill holes in each opening, and cut lines to the corners. Each piece will then snap out easily. *Jeff Wilson*

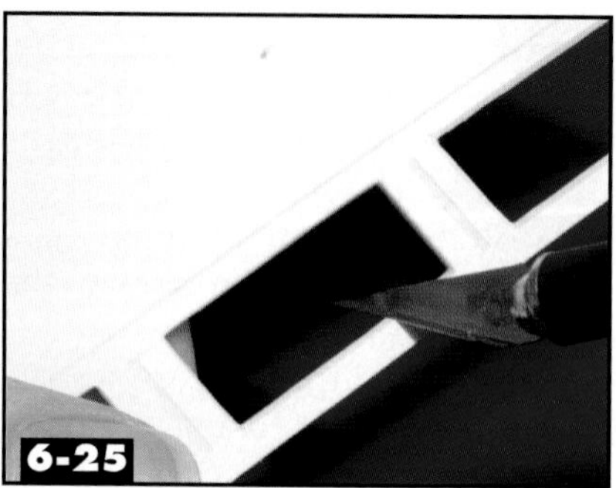

Scrape the openings with a knife to create a 45-degree bevel. *Jeff Wilson*

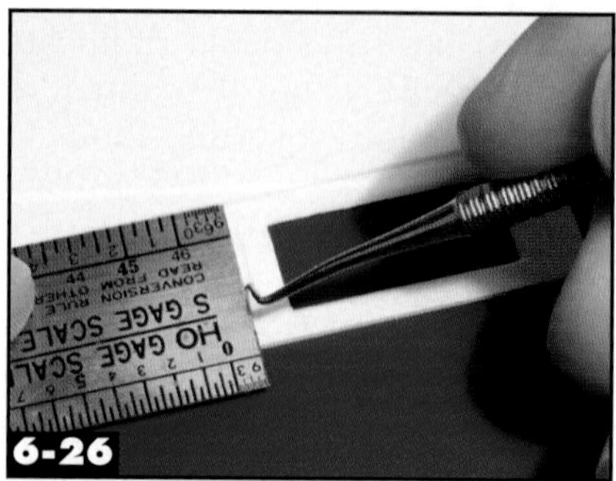

A dental tool works well for removing waste material from the vertical slots between the larger panels. *Jeff Wilson*

The completed column was ready to be glued in place, **6-21**. The columns must butt firmly against the large base at the bottom while clearing the opening for the bridge at top, **6-22**. The final base piece of .040″ styrene runs from the middle base to each end of the abutment.

Use a knife to scrape along the edge of the abutment wall to smooth the areas where you've glued three layers of plastic together. If the lines between the pieces are too visible, glue a layer of .005″ styrene on the edge, **6-23**. Once the glue dries, trim it with a hobby knife.

Mark and score the outside dimensions of the bridge side on a sheet of .040″ styrene, but don't break the side from the larger sheet. Leaving the sheet intact makes it easier to work with. Use a pencil to mark the outlines of the rectangular depressed areas. Score the outlines of all the openings using a hobby knife and a straightedge. Keep scoring the plastic until the cuts go all the way through. Be prepared for this to be a time-consuming process that results in sore fingers.

An easier way is to drill a couple of holes in each opening, **6-24**, then use a chisel-point blade to chop through the plastic from the holes to each corner. You can then bend and snap each piece out.

Use a hobby knife to clean and straighten the cuts. The prototype bridge's depressions have beveled edges. I used a hobby knife to scrape each edge at an approximate 45-degree angle, **6-25**.

Glue the top cap of .030″ × .150″ strip styrene across the top of the side. I figured the small vertical "slots" were too small to try to cut out, so I settled for scribing them deeply. A steel straightedge, held in line by the top trim piece, worked well as a guide for the scriber, **6-26**. A dental tool with small paddle-shaped blades is the best tool for simultaneously scribing and removing material because it cuts away the waste rather than merely pushing it to the side like many scribers.

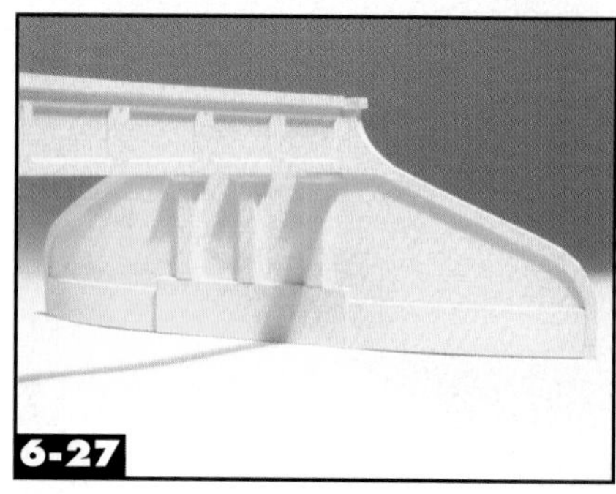

The finished model captures the overall look of the prototype bridge. *Jeff Wilson*

Bend and snap the side from the larger sheet of plastic. Apply liquid cement to the rear of the cut-out piece and press it to a piece of plain .040″ sheet. The side is now complete.

Paint the pieces concrete color and assemble them, **6-27**. You can use these techniques to model many styles of concrete railroad or highway bridges. You can also use styrene to model concrete-arch structures, **6-28**.

So far, we've looked only at bridges that are stationary. In the next chapter, we'll take a look at bridges that move.

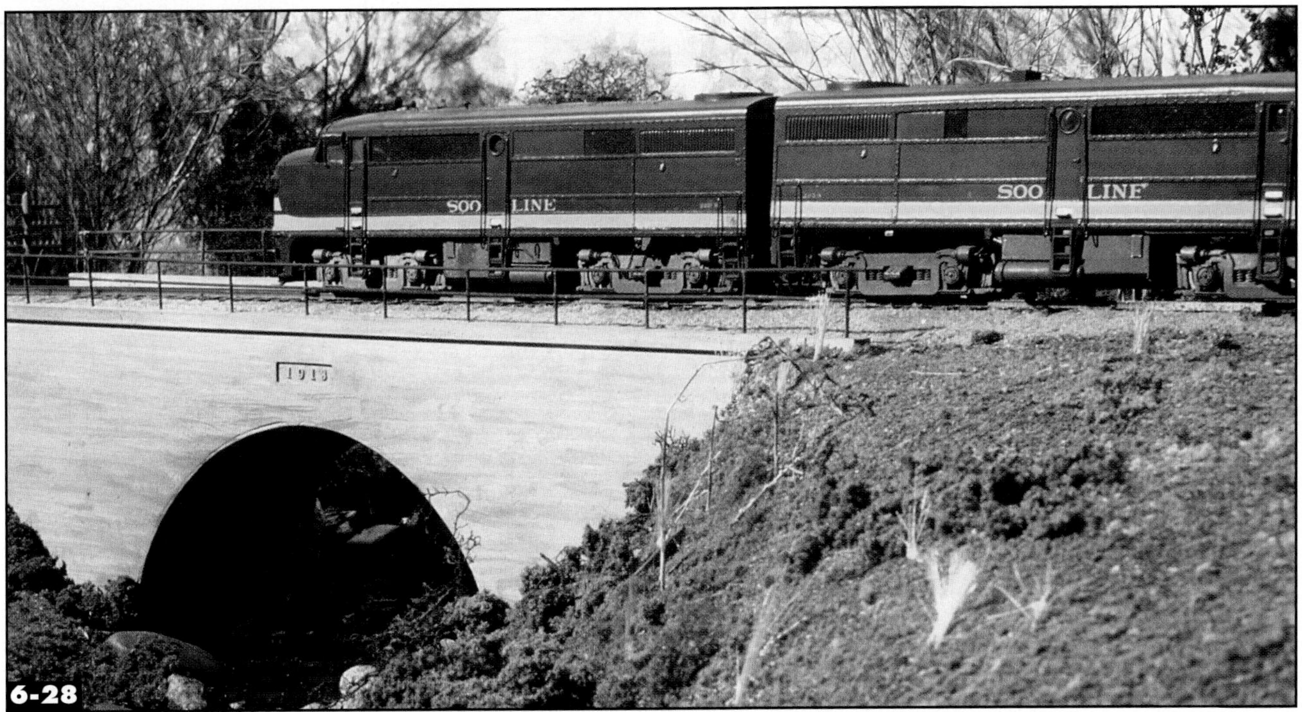

John Proebsting scratchbuilt this HO model of a concrete-arch bridge to match a Soo Line prototype. *John Proebsting*

Working with styrene

Styrene plastic is one of the most versatile modeling materials available, and it's particularly useful for simulating concrete. For large structures such as abutments, bridge sides, and piers, use Evergreen and Plastruct sheet styrene in .005", .010", .015", .020", .030", .040", .060", .080", .100", and .125" thicknesses. Standard sheets are 6" x 12" (Evergreen) or 7" x 12" (Plastruct), but for large projects Evergreen also offers larger sizes, including 8" x 21", 11" x 14", and 12" x 24".

If you have a really big project (or just need a lot of styrene), commercial plastics suppliers offer styrene in sheets up to 4' x 8'. Most medium-size to large cities have dealers—check the Yellow Pages under "plastics."

Strip styrene is available in dozens of sizes, and is also made in rods, tubes, beams, angles, channels, and other structural shapes.

The best way to cut sheet styrene is the score-and-snap method: Score the cut line with a sharp hobby knife. One pass is usually enough for styrene .020" and thinner; use multiple passes for thicker material. Bend the styrene at the scored line, and it will usually snap cleanly.

Scrape ragged or uneven edges with a hobby knife to clean them up (a large file also works well). Clean smaller cuts with a NorthWest Short Line True Sander.

Guide your cuts with a metal straightedge. Use a combination square or machinist's square to guide your blade on precise right-angle cuts.

You can cut strip material with a hobby knife, but a handy tool for cutting large quantities of strip is the NorthWest Short Line Chopper. (See photo **3-13** in Chapter 3).

Glue and paint

Use liquid plastic model cement for strip and sheet styrene. This cement dissolves the plastic on the mating surfaces and effectively melts the pieces together, resulting in a very strong joint. Super glue (cyanoacrylate adhesive) works well for bonding styrene to materials such as metal and wood.

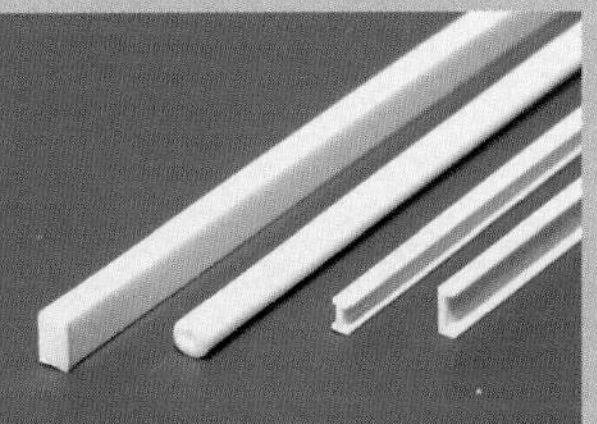
Styrene comes in many shapes, including channels, I-beams, tubing, and plain strips. *Jeff Wilson*

Most modeling paints can be used on styrene without problems, although I prefer acrylics like Polly Scale and Badger Modelflex. Airbrushing gives the smoothest finish, as do spray cans, but styrene can be easily brush-painted as well.

Movable bridges

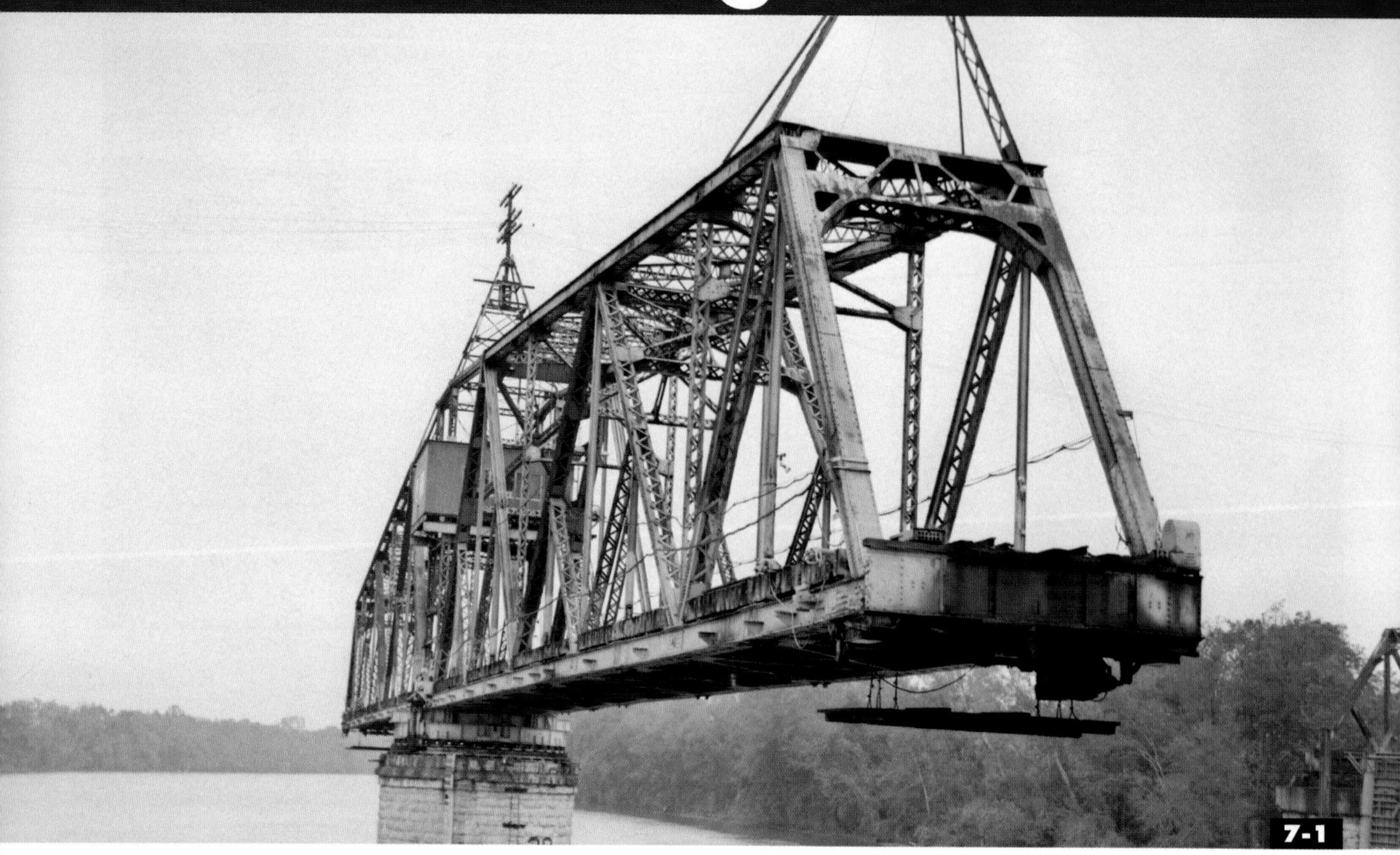

SEVEN

Movable bridges, like this Warren through-truss rim-bearing swing bridge, let railroads cross waterways at low levels, while still allowing water-borne traffic to pass. This 364′-long span was located near Bridgeport, Alabama, where the Louisville & Nashville crossed the Tennessee River. *Historic American Engineering Record; C.N. Beasley*

Movable bridges are used where railroads cross navigable waterways at low levels, especially in cities where tracks must serve nearby industries. Such bridges are also used where it would be impractical to build a bridge tall enough (or have approaches long enough) to clear ship and boat traffic.

Railroads began using movable bridges in the mid-1800s to clear the then-extensive system of canals and navigable rivers in the Northeast. Movable bridges are still in service all over the country. They come in many sizes and three basic types: swing bridges, lift bridges, and bascule bridges.

▶ A Great Northern passenger train crosses the Northern Pacific's swing bridge over St. Louis Bay between Duluth, Minnesota, and Superior, Wisconsin. A long fender surrounds the pivot pier and protects it from water-borne debris and possible collisions with shipping. *William D. Middleton*

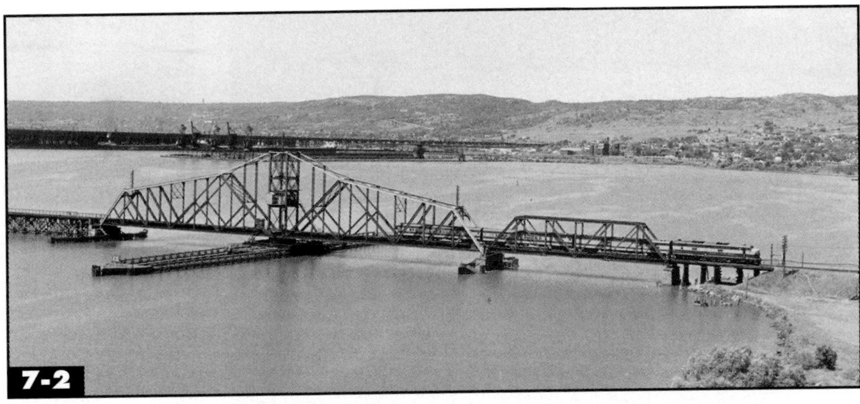
7-2

Below right: A PA-powered Delaware & Hudson passenger train crosses a center-bearing plate girder swing bridge on the Canadian Pacific at Lachine, Quebec. *Tom Nelligan*

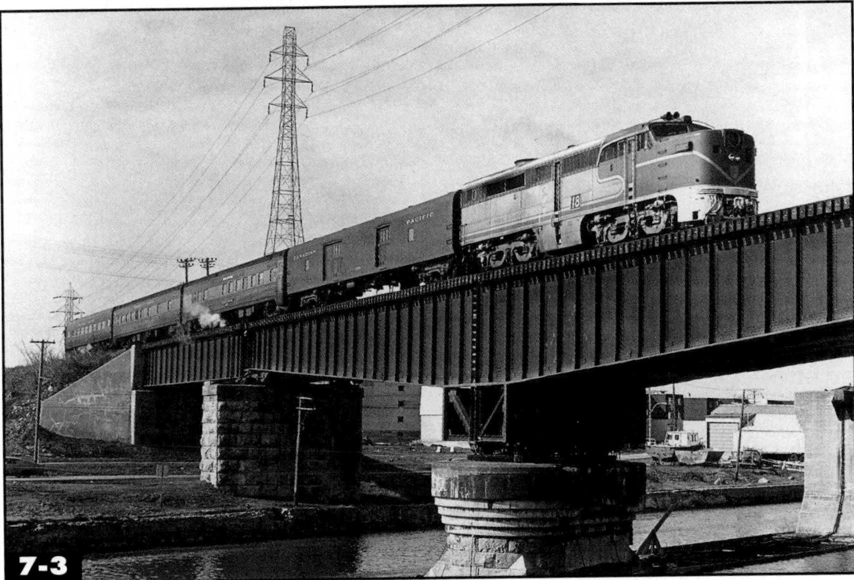
7-3

Swing bridges

The earliest type of movable bridges used by railroads were swing bridges. Swing bridges are located on a pier and open by pivoting, or swinging, horizontally to clear a path for water traffic. Photo **7-1** shows a swing span in the open position; **7-2** shows a closed span. The center support pier is often long, and often has an additional structure—a fender—made of pilings with cribbing at each end to protect the pier from floating debris or wayward boats, ships, and barges.

The main disadvantage of a swing bridge is that the pier the bridge pivots upon is a channel obstruction that can also alter river currents noticeably. The bridge doesn't provide a clear channel, but instead leaves two narrow channels, one on each side of the pivot. Another disadvantage is that the bridge must be swung open all the way regardless of the height of the vessel passing through it.

Swing bridges can be either plate-girder, **7-3**, or truss designs, **7-1** and **7-2**, with trusses generally

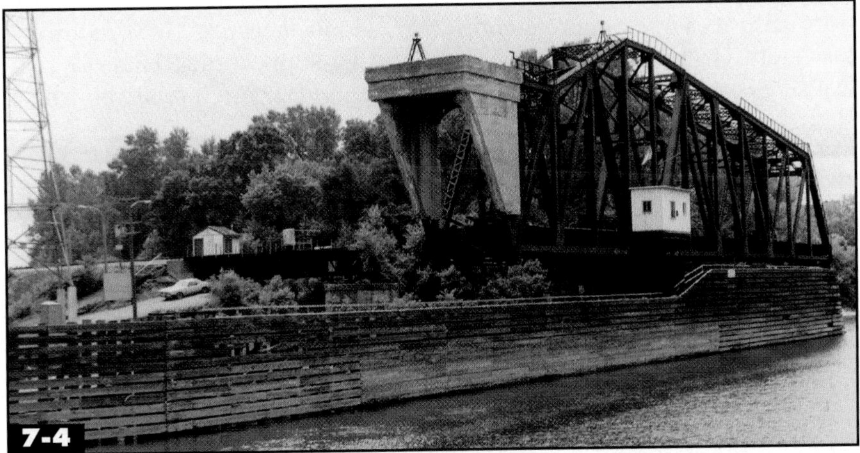
7-4

Above right: Offset swing bridges, such as this Chicago & North Western span, have a counter-weight on the short end. The bridge is on the Mississippi River in the Twin Cities. *Jeff Wilson*

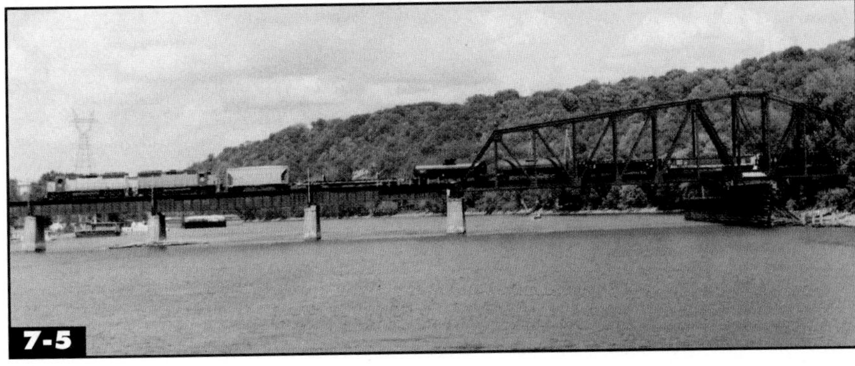
7-5

▶ Offset swing bridges provide a much wider clear span for river traffic compared to a centered bridge of the same length. *Jeff Wilson*

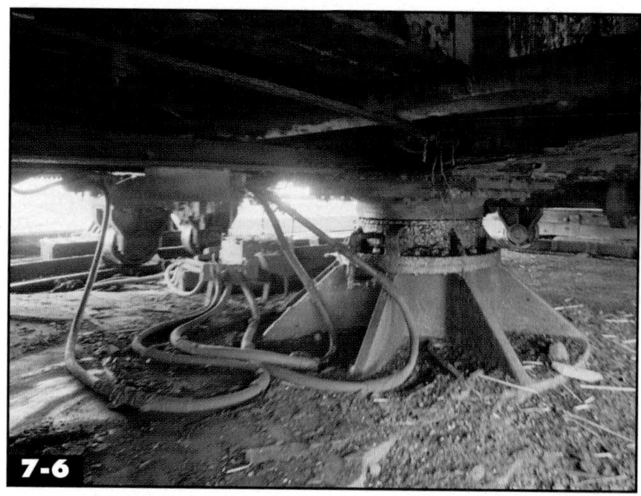

On a center-bearing bridge, the center bearing supports the entire weight of the bridge structure. The small wheels at the outside help balance the bridge as it pivots. *Historic American Engineering Record; Wm. Barrett*

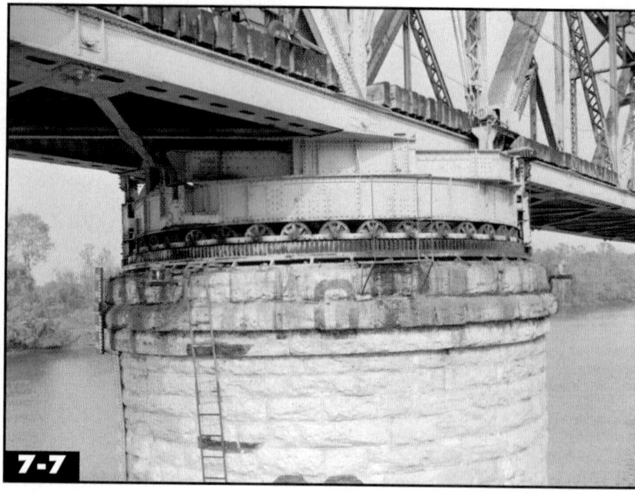

Large wheels on a track support the weight of a rim-bearing bridge. This bridge (the same as shown in photo 7-1) is supported by forty 20″-diameter wheels on a 25′-diameter track. *Historic American Engineering Record; C.N. Beasley*

used for spans over channel widths of 50′ or more. The bridges used for the movable spans are usually symmetrical, with the pivot at center (see **7-1**, **7-2**, and **7-3**). However, to provide a larger waterway channel, bridges are sometimes longer on one end, with a counterweight on the other end to make up for the size difference. Photo **7-4** (page 59) shows an offset bridge in the open position, with its large concrete counterweight visible; photo **7-5** (page 59) shows the same bridge closed. Swing bridges range in length from 50′ up to 400′ or 500′.

Swing bridges are center bearing, rim bearing, or a combination of the two. Center-bearing bridges swing on a pivot bearing that holds the whole weight of the bridge. A series of balance wheels on a circular track stabilize the bridge, **7-6**. Center-bearing bridges are simpler in design than rim-bearing bridges and use fewer construction materials because they require a smaller support pier. They are typically used where a relatively short, lightweight bridge (under 250′) is required.

Rim-bearing bridges are supported by a series of rollers around a rim that is usually as wide as the bridge itself, **7-7**. These bridges have wider bases, with a more complex structure between the bridge and pier. Rim- and combination-bearing bridges are more common on longer spans.

To move a swing bridge, an operator sits in a shelter either on the bridge structure itself or on the shore, controlling the bridge movements. As the bridge swings into place, contacts (wedges) on the ends of the swing span slide and lock into slots on the piers at the permanent track ends, **7-8**.

Rails on the bridge span are beveled to mate with rails on the adjoining track, **7-9**. They are raised when the bridge is open, allowing them to swing over the stationary adjoining rails as the bridge is moved to the closed position. They then drop down and lock into position.

Swing bridges started to fall out of popular use shortly after

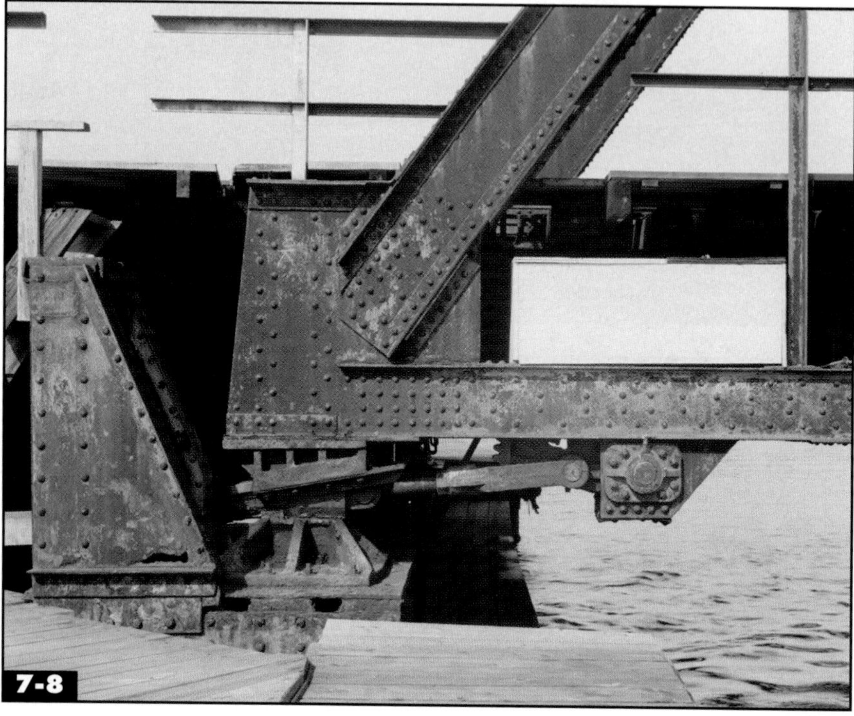

Wedges are remotely driven from a center-bearing bridge into a cross-girder at the end pier to support the live load. *Historic American Engineering Record; Wm. Barrett*

the beginning of the 20th century, as new technology came into use for bascule and lift bridges.

Bascule bridges

Bascule bridges have one end hinged, with the track bridge rising into the air from the hinged end, **7-10**. Although this basic type of bridge has been used since the days of castles with moats, it wasn't until the 1890s that the challenges of counterbalancing a heavy railroad span were met, allowing electric motors to efficiently drive the mechanisms. The bascule bridge quickly became popular for railroad use.

Bascule bridges offer several advantages over swing bridges, including speed of operation and the absence of a center pier to interfere with water traffic. Where a swing bridge must be opened completely to let water traffic pass, a bascule bridge need not be raised to its full height to clear water traffic.

The bascule design is also compact, allowing it to fit into cities and other areas where side clearances are tight, especially where there are neighboring bridges. They are common sights in crowded areas where multiple bridges cross narrow waterways.

Bascule bridges for roadways are often "double-leaf" bridges, with a pair of bridges (leafs) that meet in the middle of the span. The complexities of rail alignment and the support strength that would be required at the joint preclude this for railroads, so railroad bridges are almost all the single-leaf style.

There are several types of bascule bridges, **7-11** (page 62), but they follow two basic patterns. The first type in wide use, shown in photo **7-10**, is the rolling lift bridge. As the name implies, it rolls backward on curved extensions of the bridge girders, **7-12** (page 62). As it does this, the leaf rises and the counterweight drops. The counterweight makes this very economical to operate.

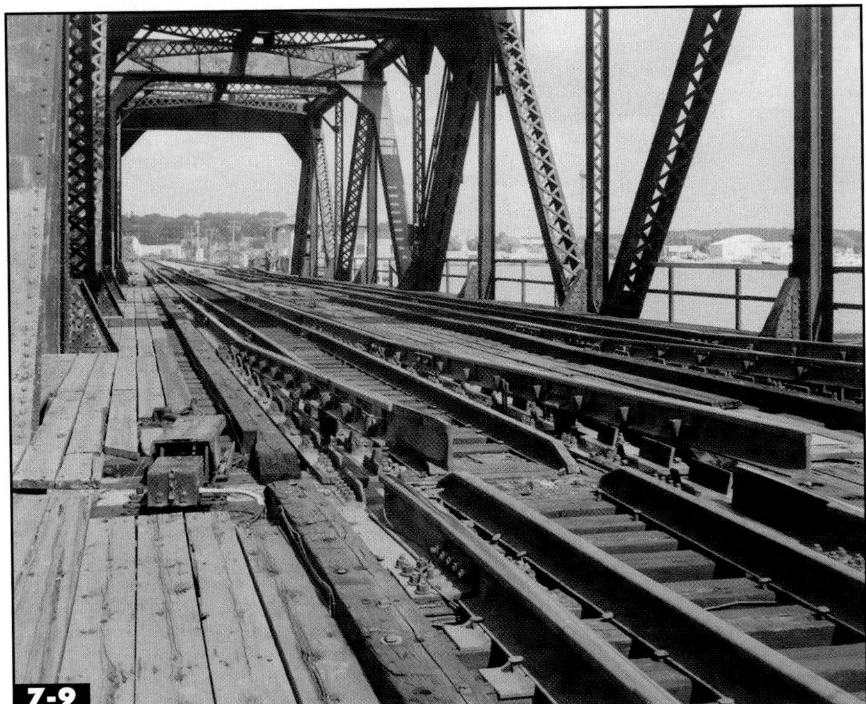

Rails, tapered at the ends, are hinged on the typical swing bridge. They are lowered to mate with the land-side rails once the bridge is closed and locked in position. *Historic American Engineering Record; Wm. Barrett*

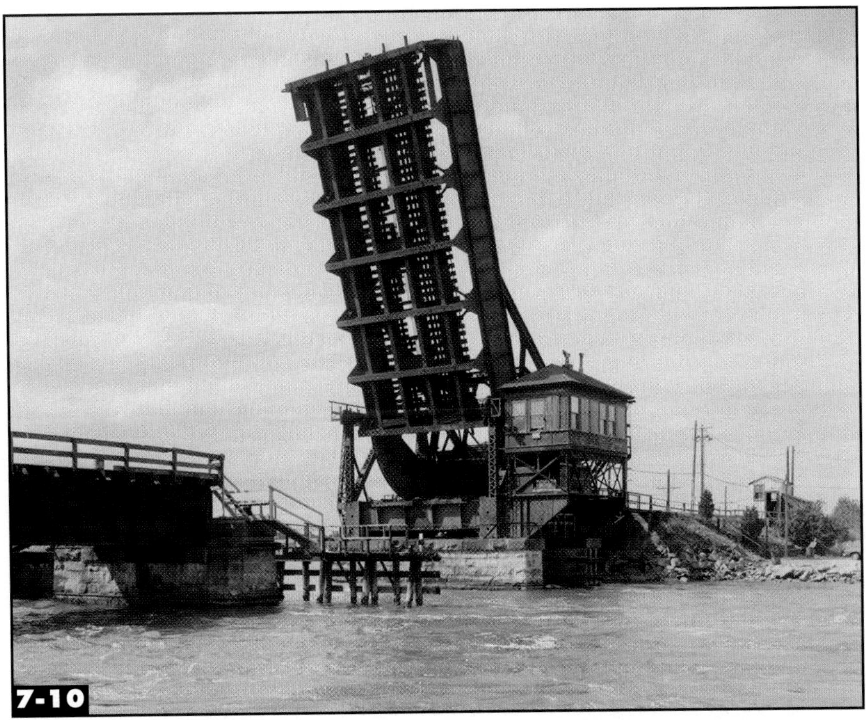

This double-track Scherzer rolling lift bridge was built on the New York, New Haven & Hartford near East Lime, Connecticut, in 1907. *Historic American Engineering Record; Wm. Barrett*

The Scherzer design is perhaps the most-common counterweight bascule design (see photo **7-10**).

The hinged or trunnion bridge eventually became the most common bascule type. A trunnion bridge has a heavy counterweight mounted on a frame at the fixed end of the span, **7-13** (page 63). The bridge rotates around a fixed pivot point. As the leaf is raised, the counterweight swings down. There are several variations of the trunnion bridge, including

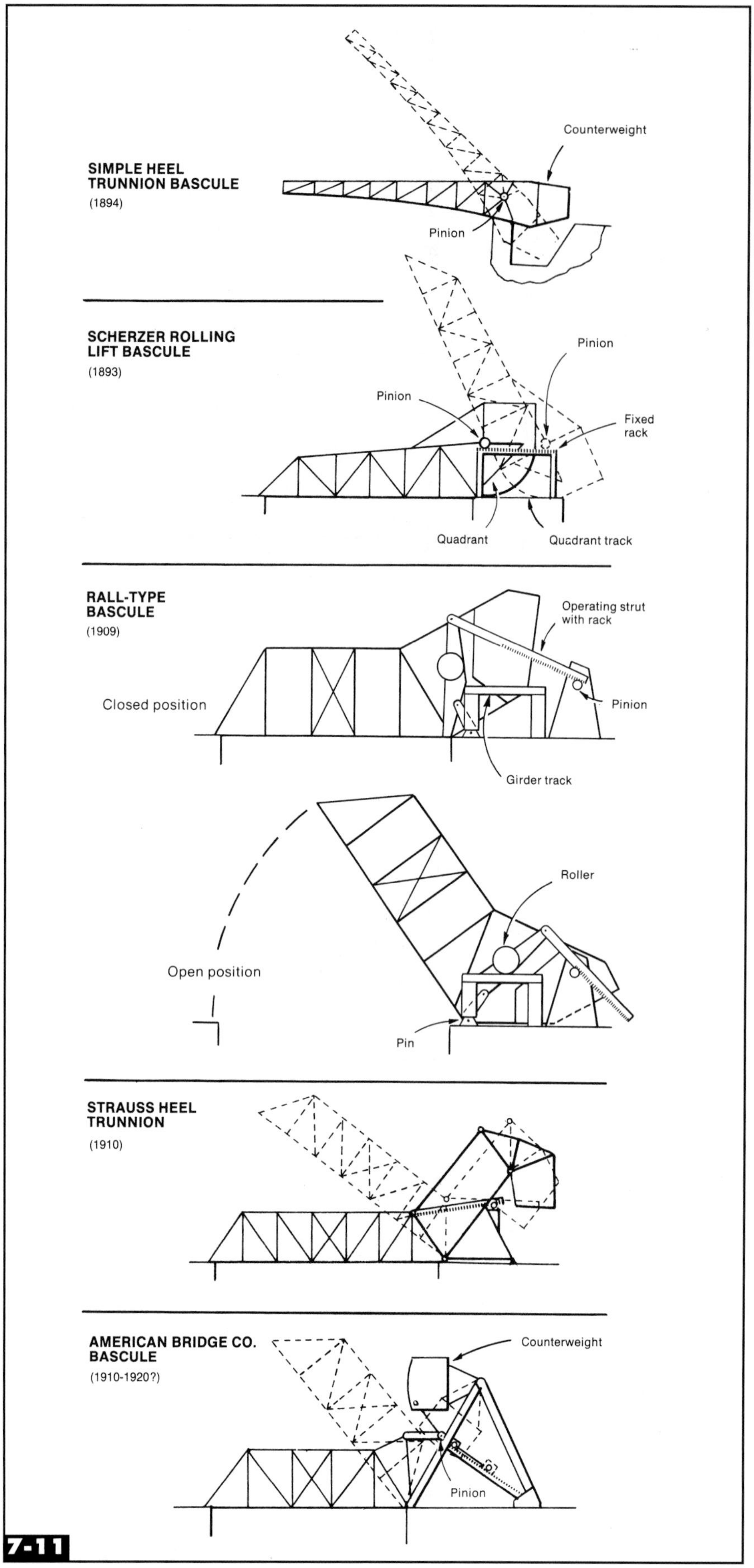

SIMPLE HEEL TRUNNION BASCULE
(1894)
Counterweight
Pinion

SCHERZER ROLLING LIFT BASCULE
(1893)
Pinion
Pinion
Fixed rack
Quadrant
Quadrant track

RALL-TYPE BASCULE
(1909)
Operating strut with rack
Closed position
Pinion
Girder track
Roller
Open position
Pin

STRAUSS HEEL TRUNNION
(1910)

AMERICAN BRIDGE CO. BASCULE
(1910-1920?)
Counterweight
Pinion

7-11

Bascule bridges were built in a number of different configurations, but they all operate on the same basic principle of being hinged at one end so the bridge deck can pivot upward.

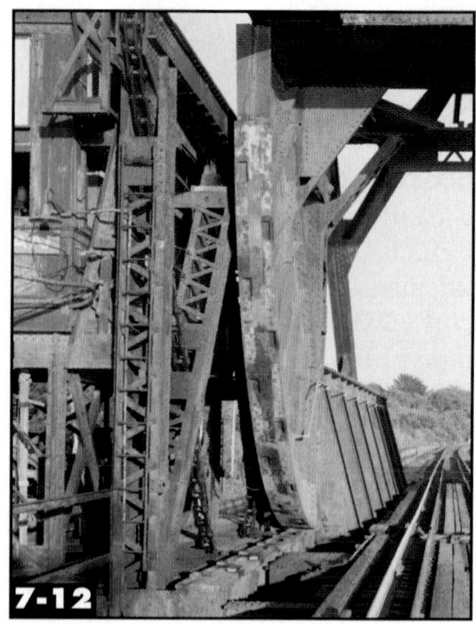
7-12

Rolling lift bridges live up to their name, rolling backward on rounded extensions of their sides. *Historic American Engineering Record; Wm. Barrett*

the Strauss, American Bridge Co., and Rall designs.

Lift bridges

The most modern—and the most impressive-looking—type of movable bridge is the lift bridge, **7-14**, which began to see wide usage in the early 1900s. The span of a lift bridge remains horizontal but is raised at both ends, sliding up on guides in tall towers at each end of the moving span. Large counterweights within each tower balance the weight of the moving span, making lift bridges energy efficient and quick to operate.

Like bascule bridges, lift bridges need to be lifted only far enough to let the vessel pass. One disadvantage is that the bridge doesn't provide a completely clear vertical opening as do bascule and swing bridges. They are also expensive to build and maintain. For this reason, the towers are built only as tall as needed for the waterway.

Because it provides a wider waterway opening compared to other types of moving bridges, the vertical lift has become the movable bridge of choice for long spans, with many exceeding 500′, **7-15**. In general, the longer the span, the larger and more substantial the towers.

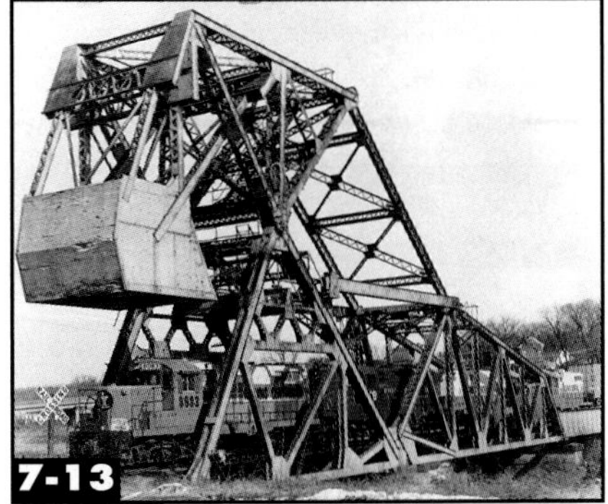

▲ The Illinois Central used a Strauss heel-trunnion bridge to cross the Galena River at Galena, Illinois. *W.C. Millhouse*

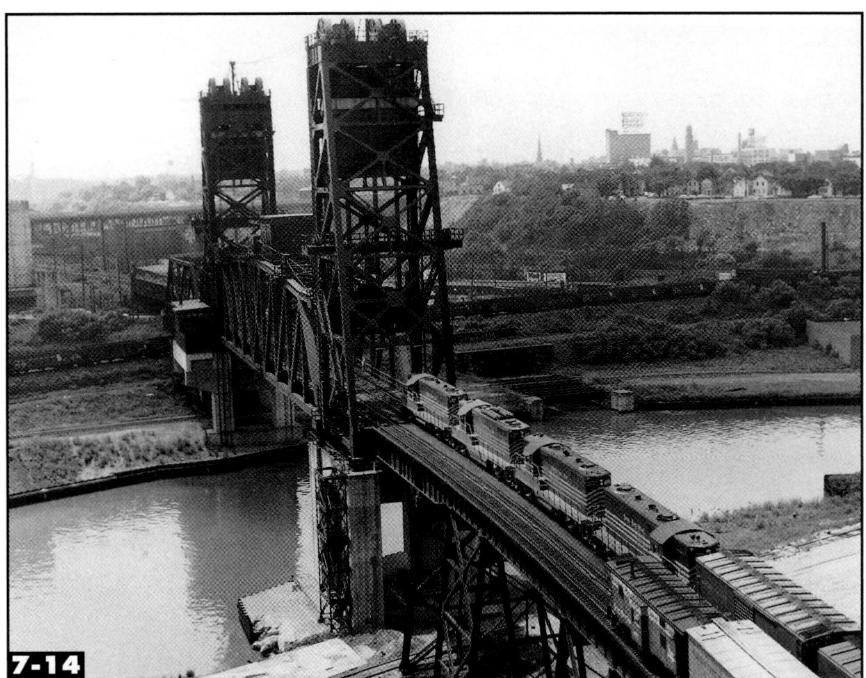

► This double-track lift bridge carried the Nickel Plate Road across the Cuyahoga River in Cleveland. With the bridge down, the counterweights are high in the towers at each end. *Herbert H. Harwood, Jr.*

Rail-highway bridges

Some moving bridges combine both roadways and railroads, **7-16**. Lift bridges were the most common type employed in these dual-use applications, but others were used as well, **7-17** (page 64). The rail line is usually below the roadway, so the rail portion of the bridge, which generally sees less traffic, can be lifted. The roadway portion stays in place, only to be raised when necessary for especially tall vessels.

To avoid disrupting highway traffic, many of these bridges have been replaced by taller highway spans.

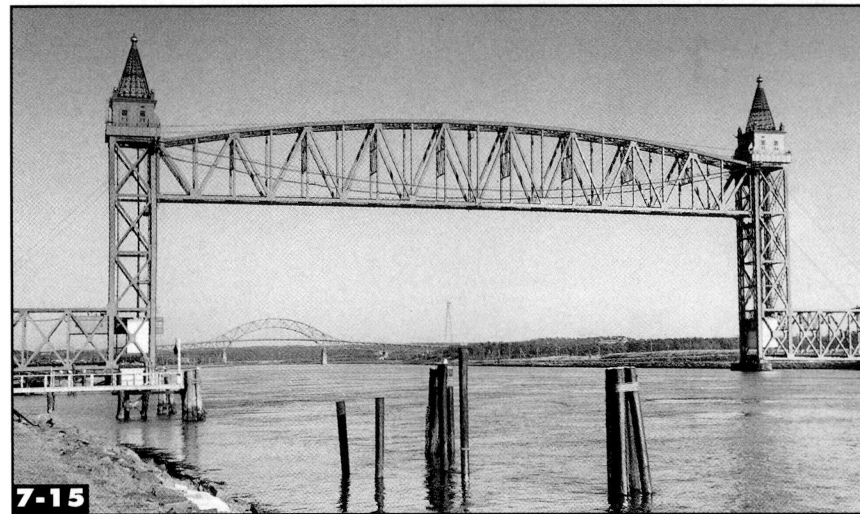

This 544′-long lift bridge carried the New Haven across the Cape Cod Canal at Buzzards Bay, Massachusetts. The bridge provides a 130′ high clearance. With the bridge up, the counterweights are just above track level. *Edward Ross*

Modeling

Detailed modeling descriptions for these complex bridges are a bit beyond the scope of this book. I recommend starting with one of the commercial models (see the list of available kits starting on page 86).

Modelers in HO scale have the most choices: Walthers makes a kit for a 27′-span double-track swing truss bridge. This Warren-truss bridge includes a concrete center pier, abutments, and an operator's cabin. A motorizing kit is also available.

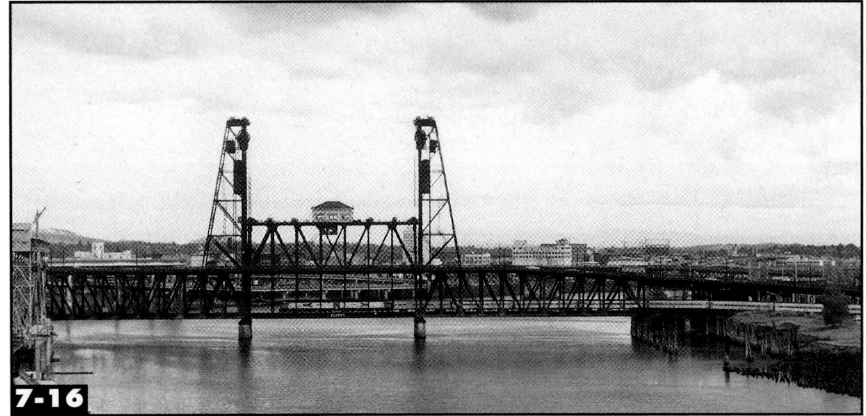

Portland's Steel Bridge is an example of a rail-highway lift span. The lower (rail) level can be lifted without disrupting highway traffic; the highway portion can also be raised for tall vessels. *John C. Illman*

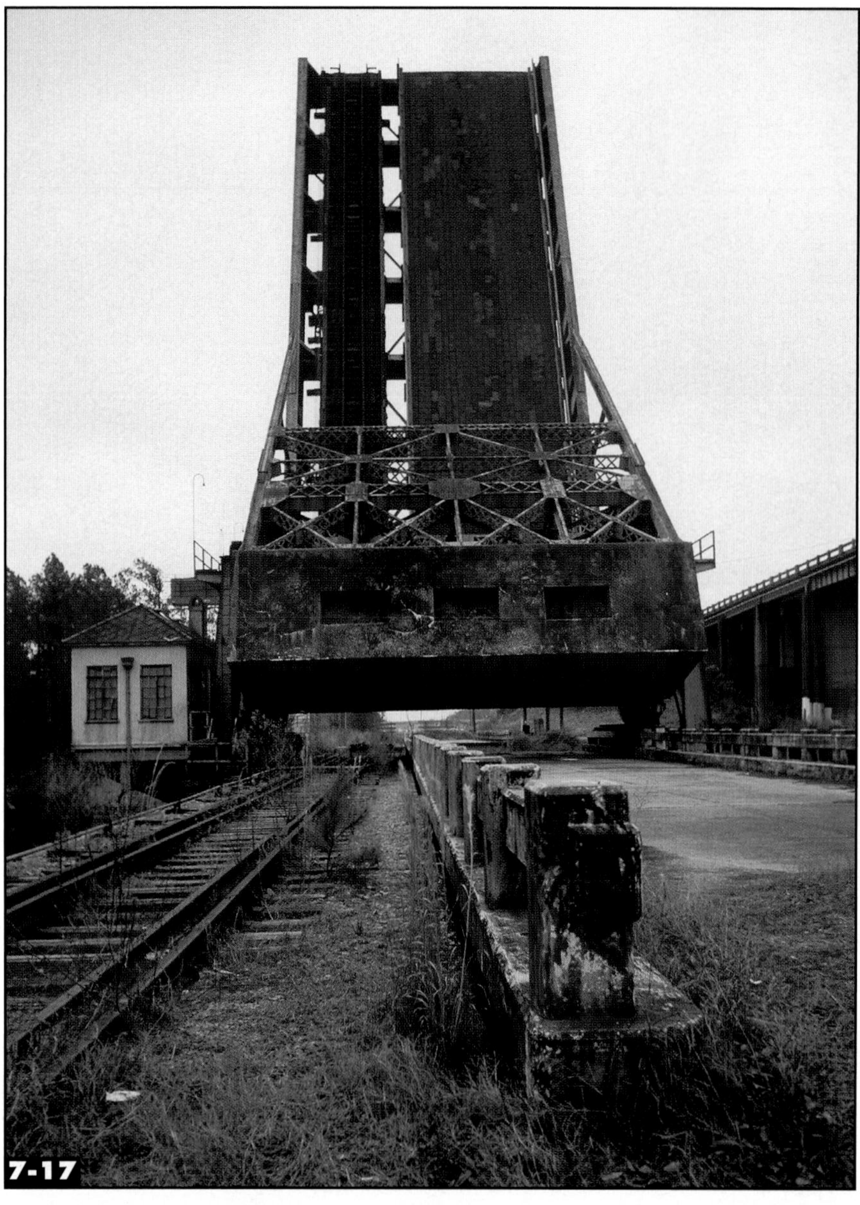

This out-of-service rolling lift bridge once carried highway traffic as well as Atlantic Coast Line trains over the Intercoastal Waterway into Myrtle Beach, South Carolina. *Jeff Wilson*

Two bascule bridges are available in HO scale. Walthers makes a single-track Warren-truss bascule bridge with a 21" span. The kit includes an operator's shanty, interlocking tower, abutments, and motorizing kit. Faller offers a rolling plate-girder bascule bridge in HO scale with an 18" total length and an N scale version with an 11" length. Each includes a motorizing kit.

Start with any of these models, then combine them with available simple-span bridges, bridge kits, or components to change the appearance to follow a specific prototype. You can also build your own, **7-18**.

Although working models are impressive, you don't have to build an operating bridge to have a realistic model. Many prototype moving bridges—including several substantial ones—were never (or seldom) opened after they were built. Constructed in the late 1800s and early 1900s, these bridges were built when engineers needed to allow for river traffic that either never materialized or dwindled away.

One way to enhance the visual variety and detail of a layout is to model a dummy bridge that is left in the open position. This could be another railroad bridge next to an active bridge in a metropolitan area, or it could be a background detail.

Operations could include simulated river traffic, which—since it has the right-of-way over rail bridges—can disrupt your scheduled trains, giving engineers and dispatchers an additional challenge during operating sessions.

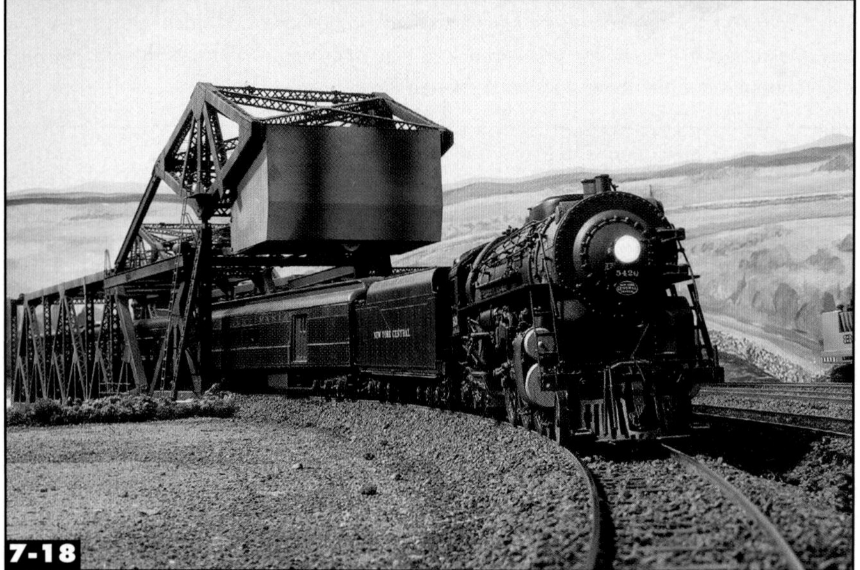

Harry Roberts scratchbuilt this impressive O scale model of a trunnion-style bascule bridge from brass and other components. *Paul Dolkos*

Highway bridges

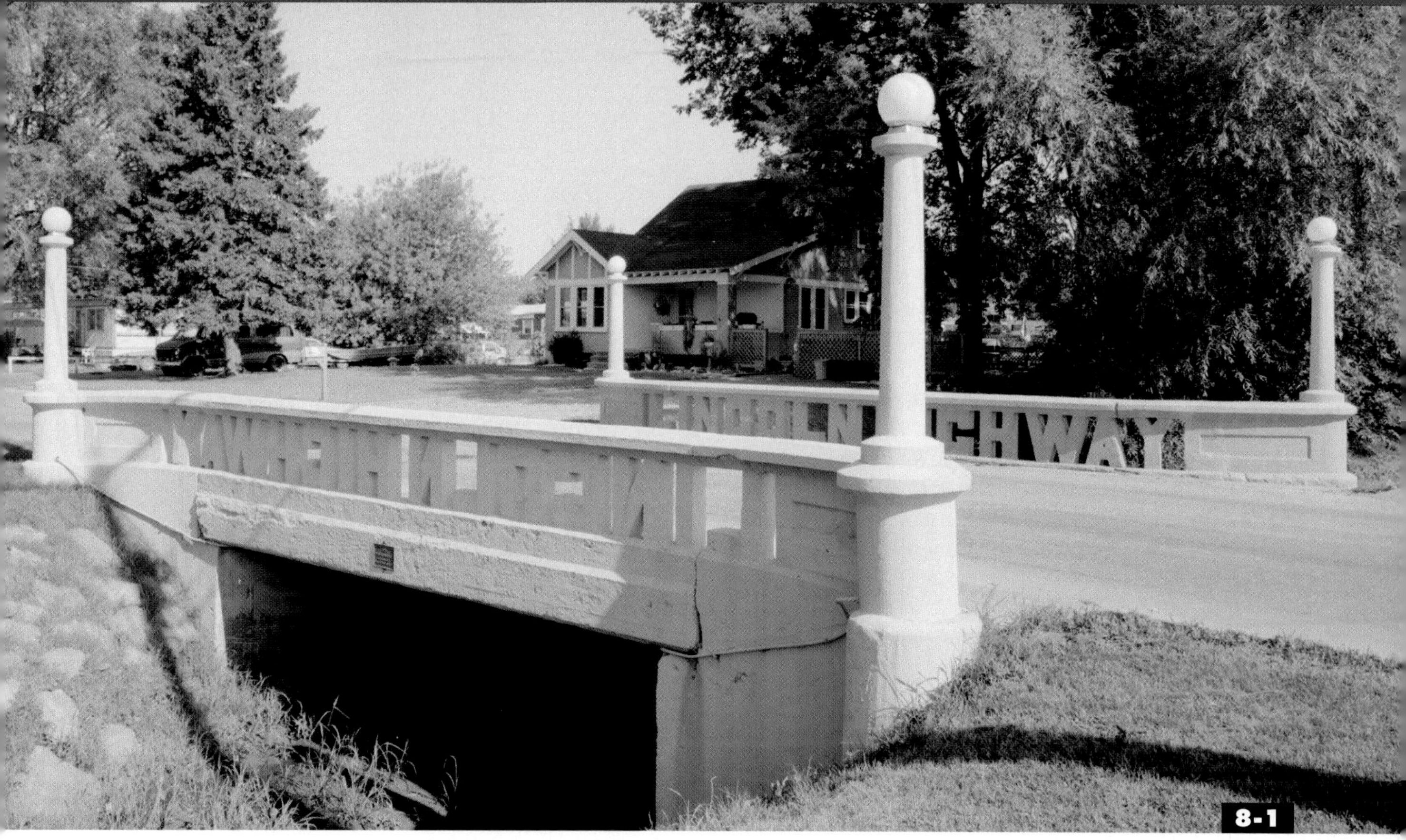

8-1

Modelers often don't take highway bridges as seriously as railroad bridges. After all, roads and highways are usually secondary to a scene—just passing through—while railroad bridges are typically the focal point of a substantial area on a layout.

Nevertheless, fascinating prototype road and highway bridge styles abound, **8-1**. Many of these, including early wood designs, truss bridges in various styles and sizes, and concrete and masonry structures with intricate railings, can be attractive additions to a layout.

Highway bridges, especially older ones, have unusual design features that lend themselves to modeling and add variety to a model railroad layout. The city of Tama, Iowa, built this concrete bridge for the then-new Lincoln Highway in 1914. The bridge still exists and has been restored. *Historic American Engineering Record*

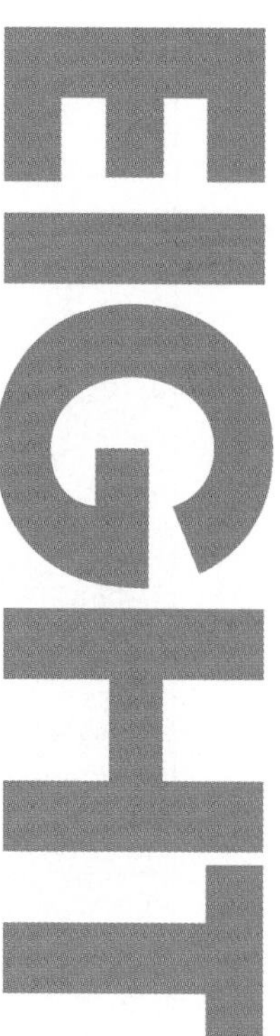

Prototype highway bridges

Many highway bridges, particularly iron and steel trusses, follow the same basic designs as railroad bridges. Many of the same considerations that apply to railroad bridges also apply to highway bridges, but highway bridges are generally lighter and lacier, since they carry much lighter live loads than railroad bridges, **8-2**.

Modeling highway bridges is largely a matter of era. You might find a bridge built on a highway in 1925 still in use today, but if it is, the road is probably now a secondary route. As on railroads, major routes have newer, heavier, wider bridges, while older iron and steel truss bridges, and even wood overpasses, still survive on secondary roads.

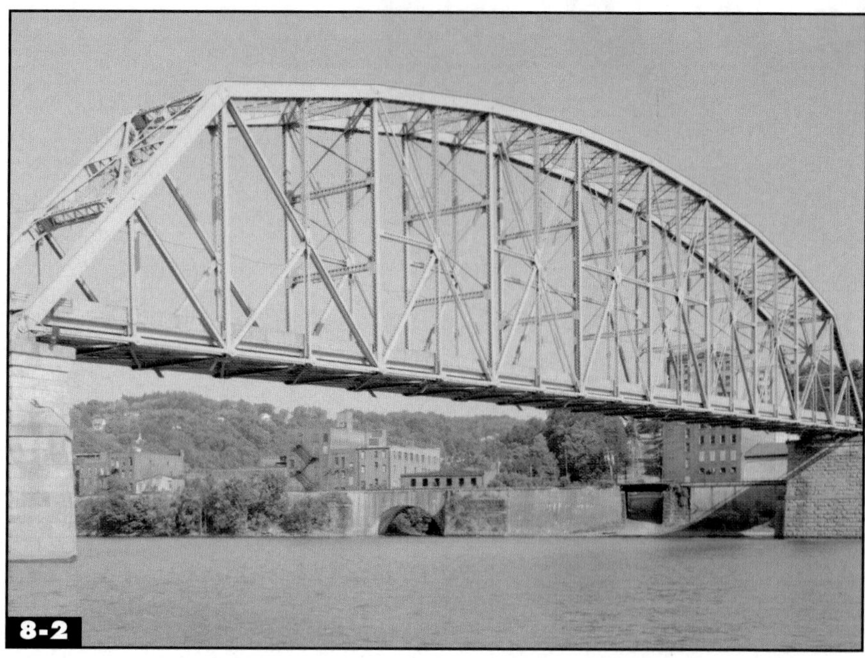

8-2

The construction of this 519'-long Pennsylvania-truss highway bridge at Brownsville, Pennsylvania, is much lighter than what would be required for a similar-sized railroad bridge. *Historic American Engineering Record; Joseph Elliott*

Types of road bridges

The wood highway bridge was probably the most commonly used bridge on early roads, especially for fairly short spans like crossings over railroad tracks. Common designs included the king post, a simple truss with each side frame member meeting at a peak in the middle, **8-3**. For longer bridges, the queen post design was often used, **8-4**. This design followed the basic design of a king post, but had a horizontal top chord to make a longer span.

Other wood designs were also used, some using only beams without the king or queen posts, **8-5**. These were commonly built for railroad overpasses, so they should be of particular interest to model railroaders. Most of these bridges used wood frame or pile bents with wood or concrete bulkheads or abutments. They were often used to get roads up and over railroads, with approaches much steeper than those found on

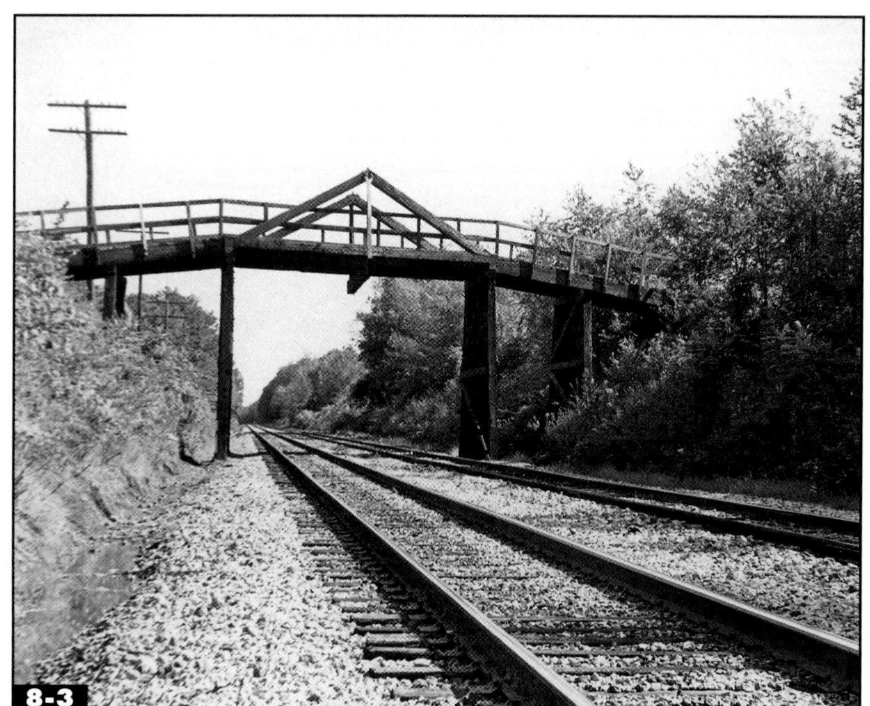

8-3

King-post bridges are simple trusses with a peak in the middle. *Harold Russell*

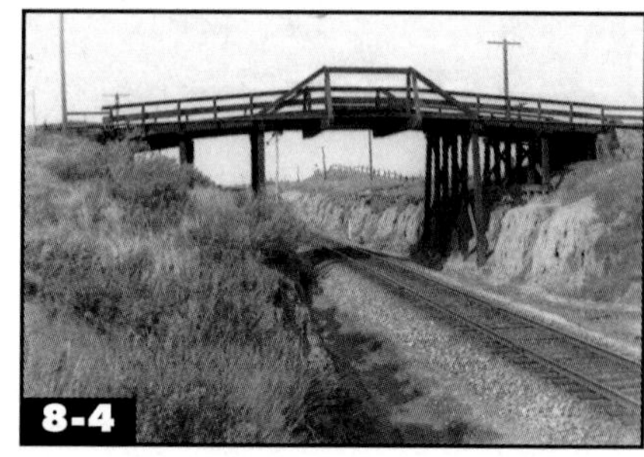

8-4

Queen-post bridges have a straight top chord with vertical hangers at each end. *F.H. Bartholomew*

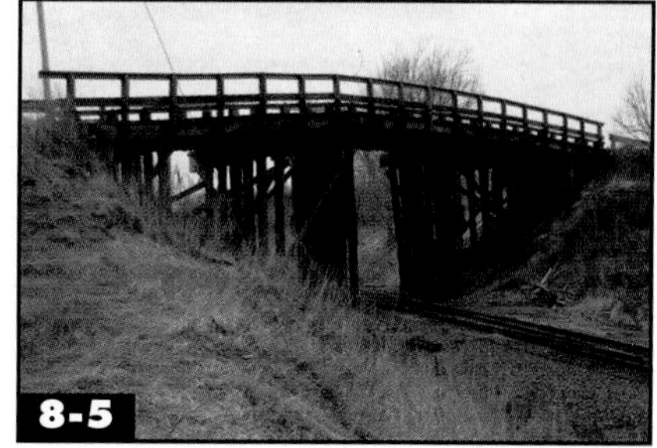

8-5

Some wood bridges used beams only, without king or queen posts. *Jeff Wilson*

► This single-lane wood-deck Pratt through-truss bridge was built in 1900. *Jeff Wilson*

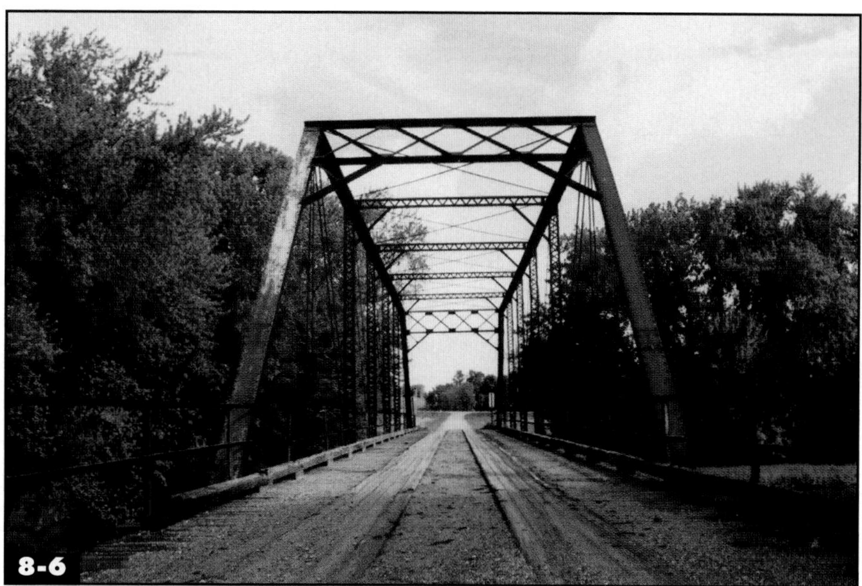

Below right: Pony (half-through) trusses were commonly used for highway bridges. This Warren truss rests on a wood-pile pier. *Jeff Wilson*

highways today. Some of these wood bridges are still in use, mainly on gravel country roads, but their numbers are dwindling.

Wood bridges almost always have wood-plank decks because other materials would be too heavy. Most have posted weight limits in the 4- to 8-ton range.

Iron and steel truss designs were also commonly used for highway bridges between the late 1800s and the 1920s. Depending on the length of the spans needed, longer bridges were usually through Pratt (**8-6**), Warren, Parker, and Pennsylvania (**8-2**) trusses. The big difference from comparable railroad bridges of the same length and truss style is that highway trusses required lighter members.

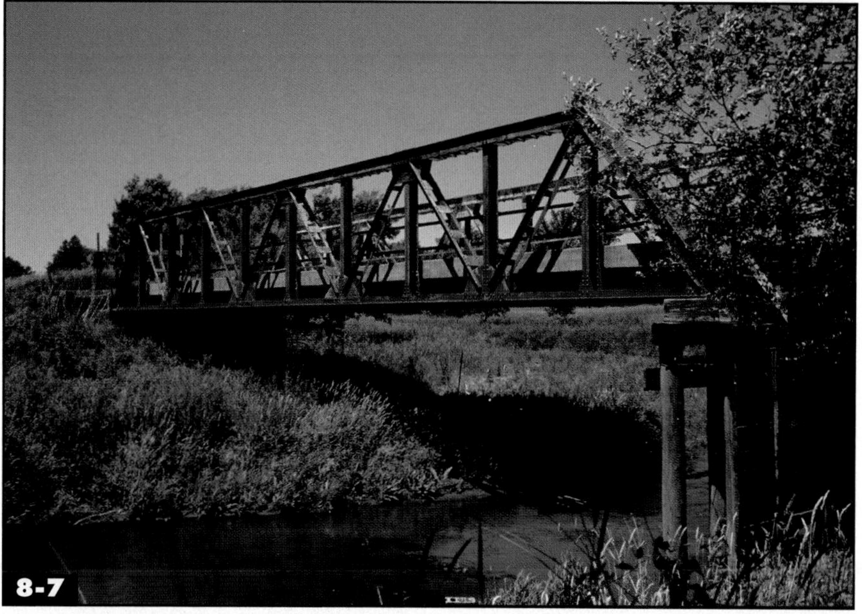

Pony, or half-through, trusses were also popular choices for highway bridges, **8-7**. Several designs were used, with curved-chord Pratt, **8-8**, and Warren structures most common. Many of these are still in service across the country.

As railroad loads increased in the late 1800s and early 1900s, railroads took many of their early truss bridges—iron bridges in particular—out of service. These bridges were still structurally sound but had simply become too light for railroad service. Instead of being scrapped, many found new uses as highway bridges, **8-9** (page 68).

A characteristic of most early highway truss bridges is that they are narrow, especially by today's standards. Many truss bridges built into the 1910s were single-lane bridges, having been built

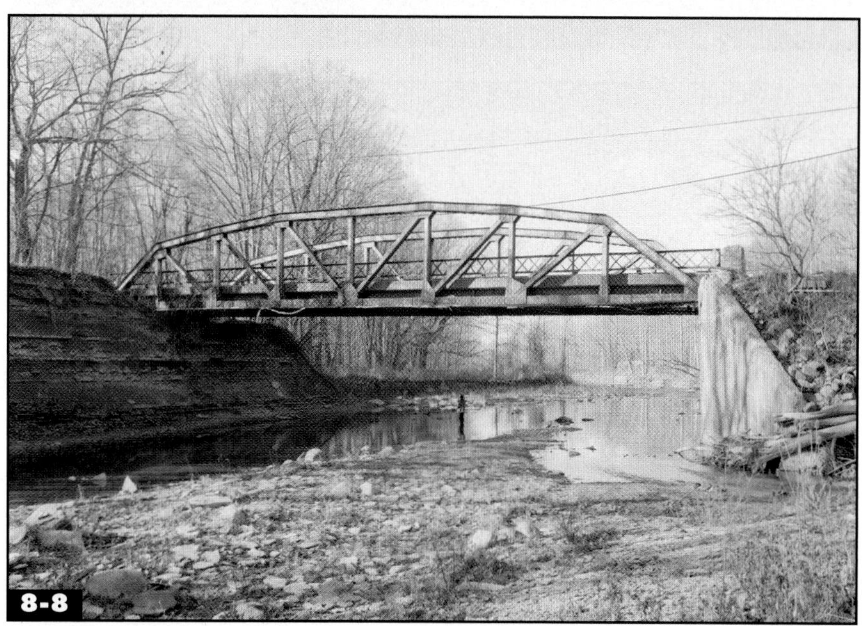

Curved-chord Pony highway bridges, such as this Pratt design, are common. *Historic American Engineering Record; Jet Lowe*

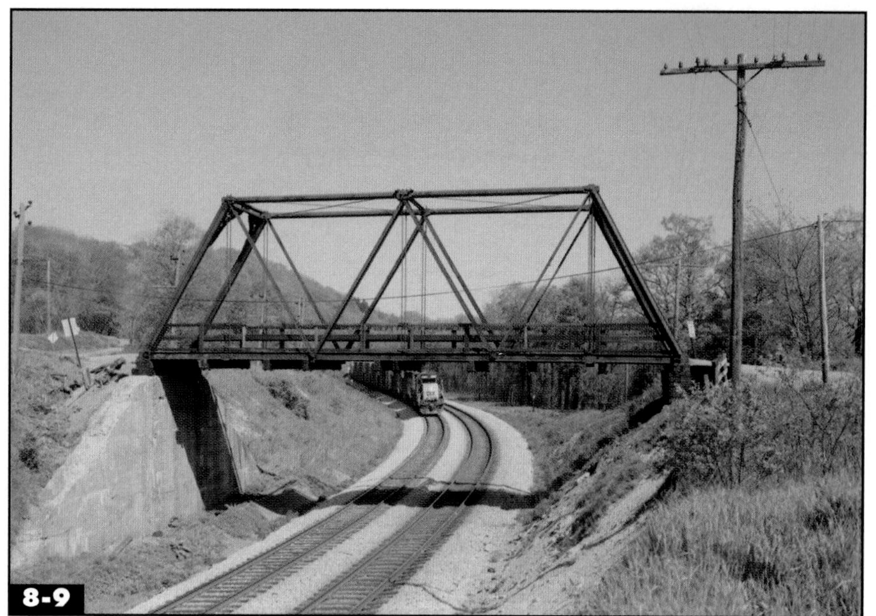

◄ An 81′ iron Warren truss, this former railroad bridge was built in 1871 and converted into a road bridge in 1910. *Historic American Engineering Record; Jet Lowe*

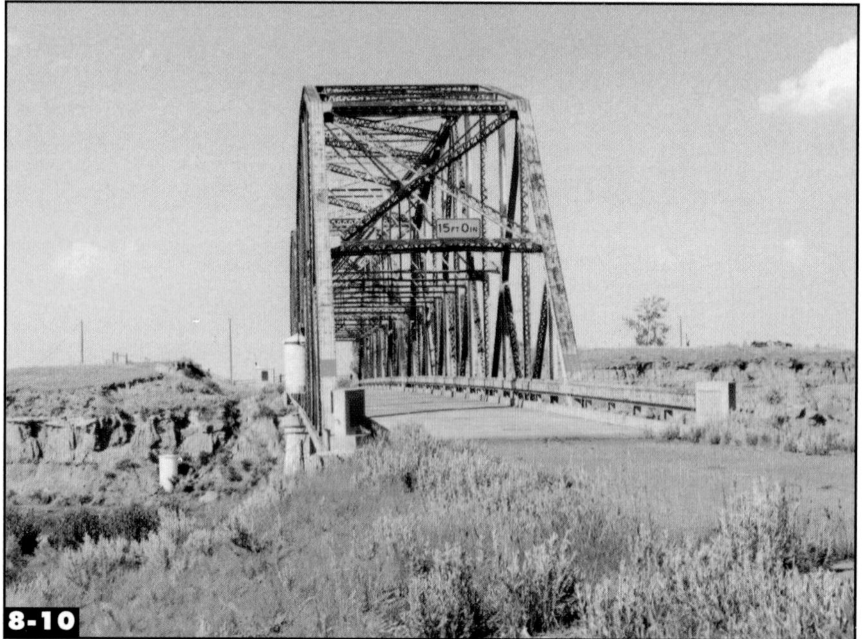

Below left: This Pennsylvania-truss bridge is long, but it certainly isn't wide. It's typical of two-lane truss bridges built in the 1920s and 1930s. *Jeff Wilson*

when horse-drawn wagons outnumbered automobiles, speeds were slow, and traffic volume was low. Although some of these survive in service today, as photo **8-6** (page 67) shows, their numbers are dwindling. Single-lane bridges often have wood decks, although some have metal grating.

Later truss bridges built on major highways from the 1920s through the 1940s typically have two lanes, but they are still usually narrow, with no room for pedestrians and certainly no emergency lanes, **8-10**. Decks are steel grating, asphalt, or concrete.

Stone masonry bridges were sometimes used for highways from the late 1800s into the early 1900s. As with other early bridge types, these can still be found, but almost exclusively on secondary routes nowadays.

Concrete became the material of choice for highway bridges in the 1920s and 1930s, **8-11**. These bridges were fairly simple in design, with concrete abutments and piers, steel or concrete beams spanning the piers, concrete decks, and concrete side railings.

These components followed many different designs. Piers were round or square posts made of steel or concrete, with a large concrete cap on top. The railings were distinctive details on many of these bridges (early examples in particular) and may be a combination of concrete posts with wrought-iron rails, **8-12**, or ornate concrete designs, as in photo **8-11**.

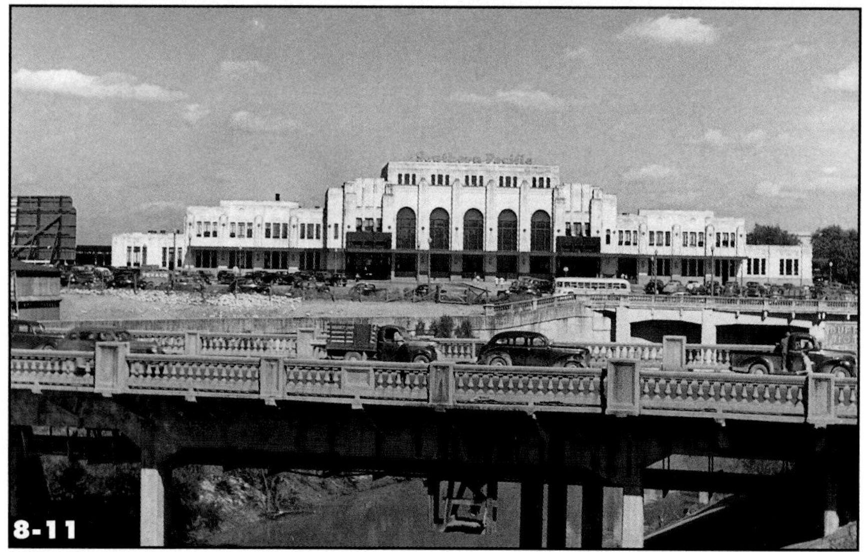

Early concrete highway bridges often had distinctive ornamental concrete guardrails. *LeRoy Wilkie*

▶ Wrought-iron railings and fancy streetlights were often found on early concrete bridges. *Jeff Wilson*

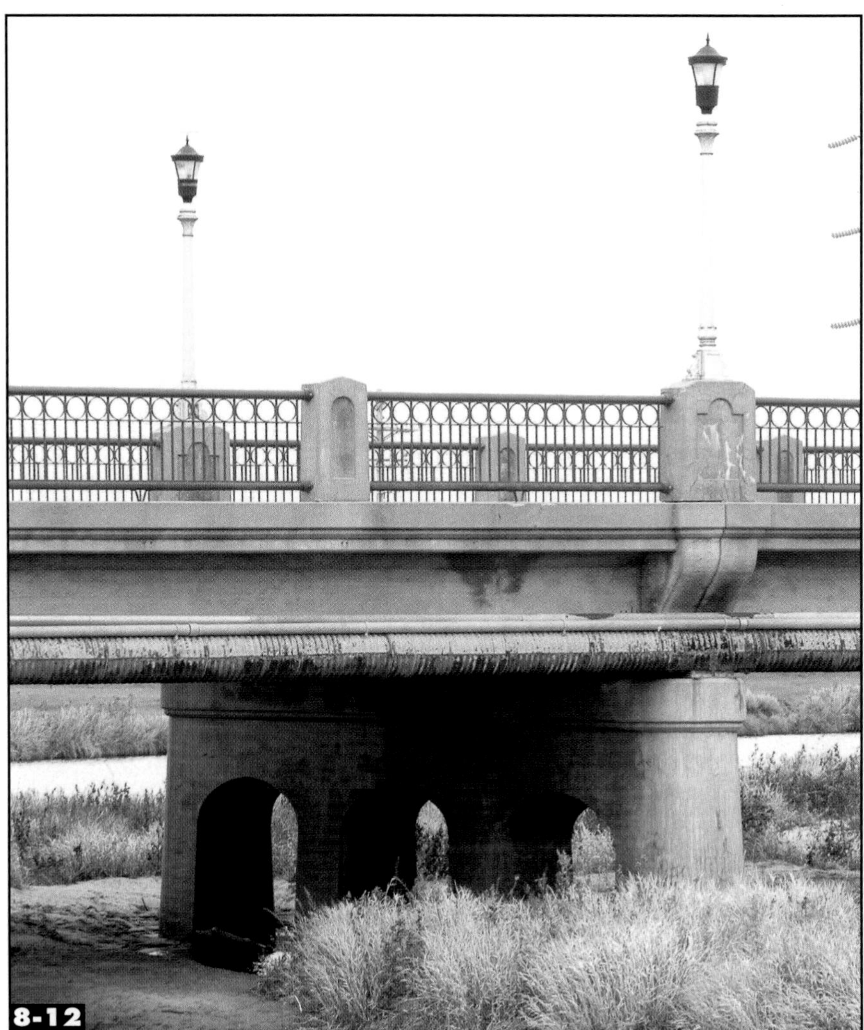

Early concrete bridges don't have to be large to be distinctive. One of my favorites is the bridge in photo **8-1** (page 65), built by the town of Tama, Iowa, for the then-new Lincoln Highway.

Concrete and steel continue to be the materials of choice for modern highway bridges, **8-13**. Current designs tend to be more utilitarian than on early bridges. Guardrails are often constructed of plain concrete, and the bridge decks are wider, usually with sidewalks on one or both sides.

Modeling

Several nice models are available for highway bridges in N and HO scales (see the list of available kits starting on page 86).

Rix offers an injection-molded styrene kit in HO scale for a wood highway overpass. You can also use stripwood to scratchbuild a wood highway bridge in much the same way as wood railroad trestles, described in Chapter 3.

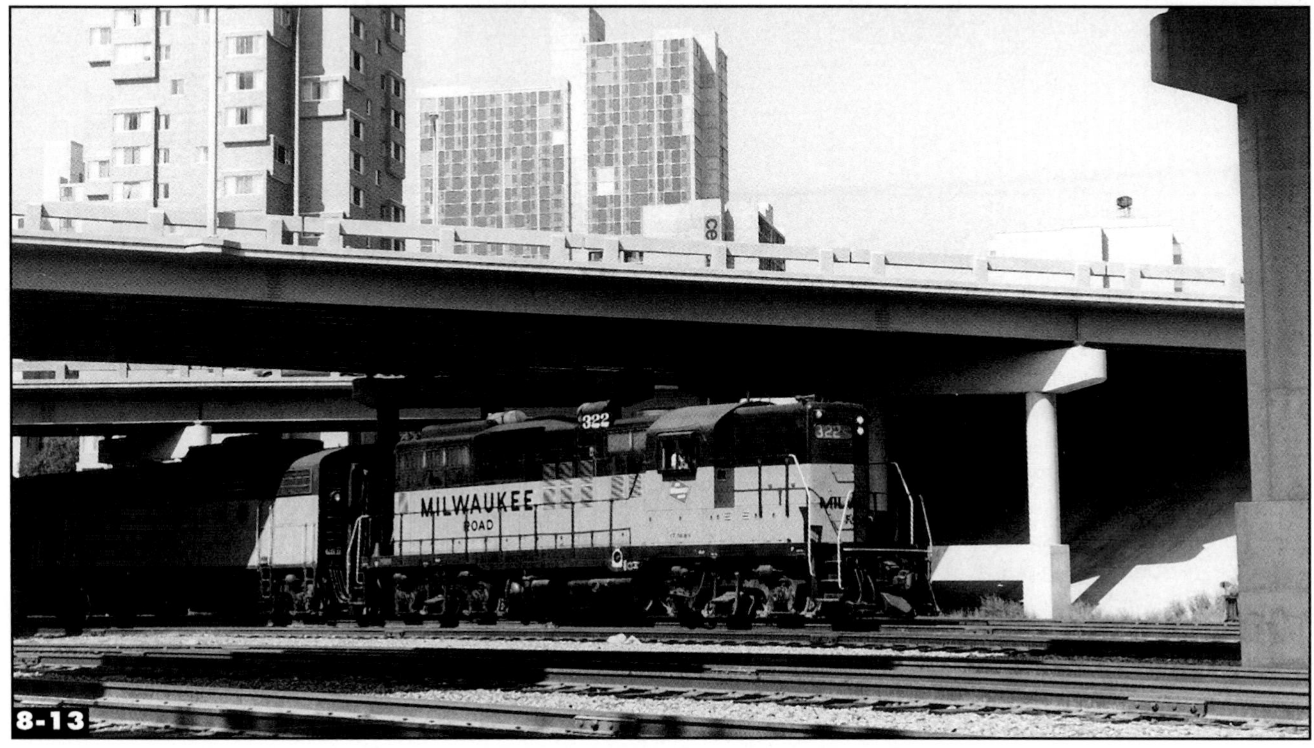

Many modern bridges use steel beams with concrete decks and railings and concrete piers of various designs. *Stan Mailer*

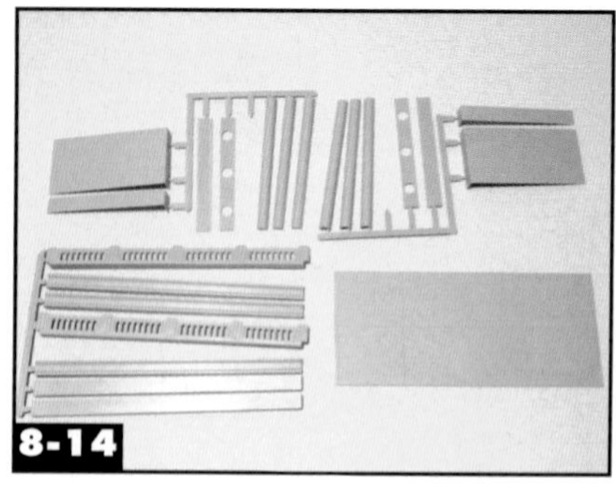

▲ Rix offers a line of easy-to-assemble injection-molded bridge kits in HO (shown) and N scales. Rix also offers a wood overpass kit, listed in the appendix at the end of this book. *Jeff Wilson*

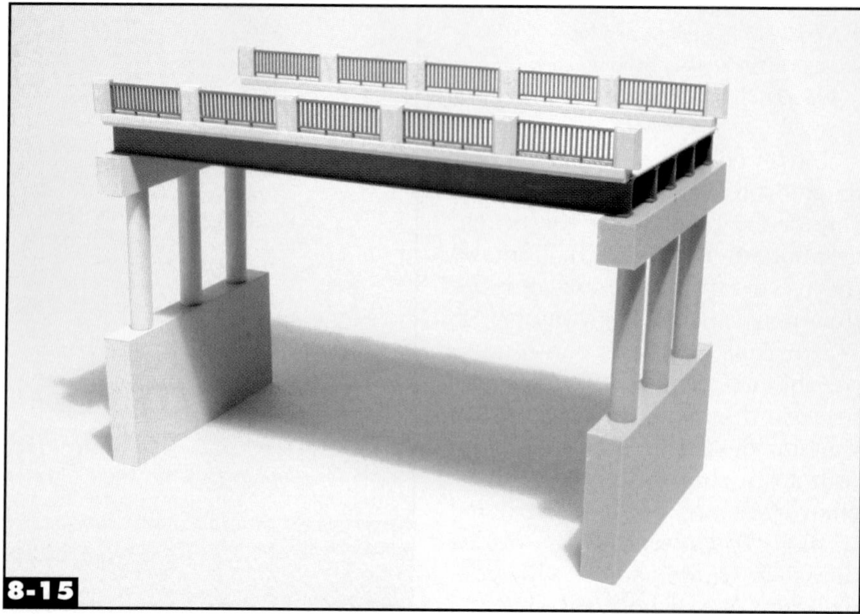

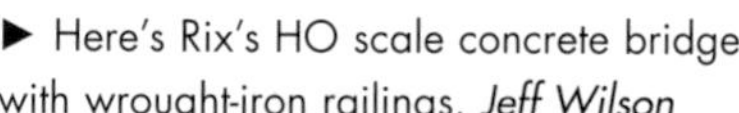

► Here's Rix's HO scale concrete bridge with wrought-iron railings. *Jeff Wilson*

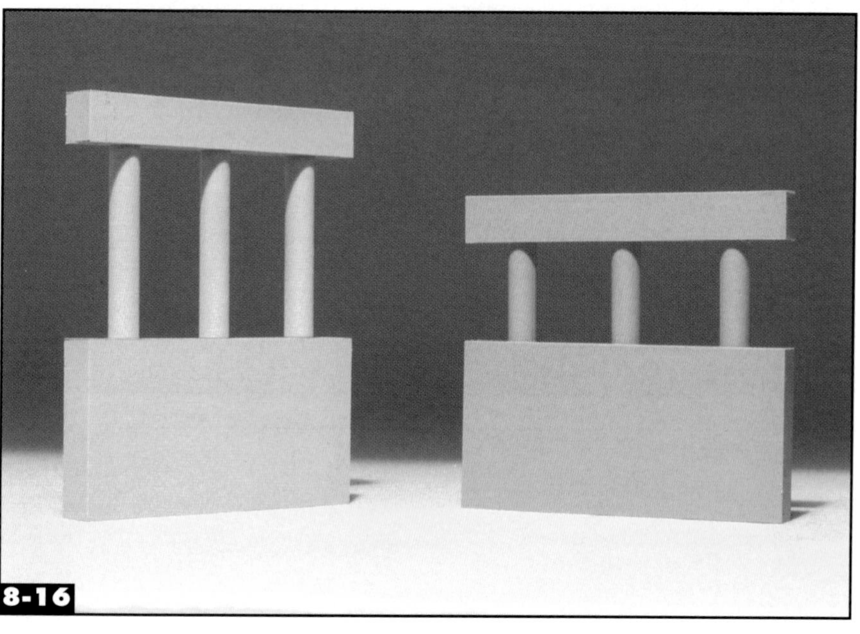

◄ The configuration of the Rix pier is easily altered by changing the length of the vertical posts. *Jeff Wilson*

▼ Omitting the base gives the pier a different look. The outboard posts can be angled outward as shown. *Jeff Wilson*

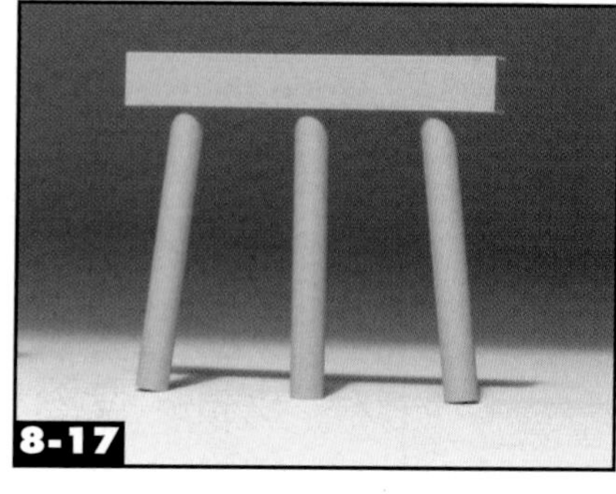

Rix also has a line of injection-molded styrene models of steel and concrete bridges available in N and HO scales, **8-14**. These easy-to-assemble kits also make great raw materials for kitbashing. All follow the same basic pattern, with a 50′ bridge deck, concrete-post piers, either steel I-beam or concrete girders, and railings in concrete/wrought iron, ornamental (old style) concrete, or modern concrete versions.

Photo **8-15** shows a finished HO scale Rix concrete and steel bridge. Like all of Rix's bridge kits, this one is modular in design, making it easy to join two or more to form a longer bridge. I like to look at these bridges as raw materials; it's easy to alter or kitbash the various components to make a unique-looking bridge that fits the specific needs of your layout.

All of the Rix kits come with a basic pier structure, **8-16**. It includes a plastic base, three posts, and a concrete cap. The simplest way of altering the bridge is to shorten the posts, as the photo shows, by simply cutting them.

Another option is to use the cap and posts but not the base piece, **8-17**. The posts can remain straight, or the outer ones can be angled. You can also model heavier bridges by using four or five support posts instead of three.

In order for these road bridges to look realistic, you'll need to follow proper engineering principles when installing them. Much like railroad bridges, the joints between beams always occur directly over a pier.

As is the case with railroad bridges, skewed highway bridges are common. On a multi-span bridge, the beams should be placed with the piers parallel to each other, **8-18**. Resist the temptation to set the piers at various angles for convenience; doing so will result in a very unrealistic appearance.

► Keep beam joints directly above piers as shown, and keep all piers at the same angle to the deck. *Jeff Wilson*

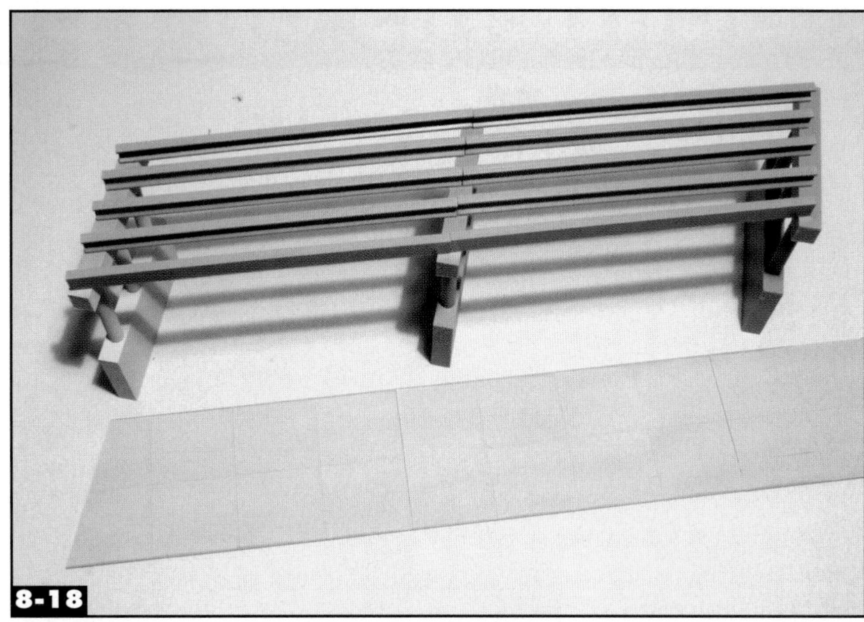
8-18

Painting these bridges correctly will also go a long way toward enhancing the realism of your layout. Follow the process described in Chapter 2 for painting concrete colors.

You can also scratchbuild concrete highway bridges using the techniques described in Chapter 6 for concrete railroad bridges. Bob Smaus used layers of sheet styrene over a plywood base to re-create a concrete-arch highway bridge, **8-19**. The finished bridge is a real attention-getter, **8-20**.

With a bit of care, highway bridges will help establish the time and location of a layout and will give the scene realism-enhancing detail.

► Bob Smaus built this highway bridge to help hide an opening through a backdrop. The bridge has thin plywood sides with styrene layered on top. *Bob Smaus*

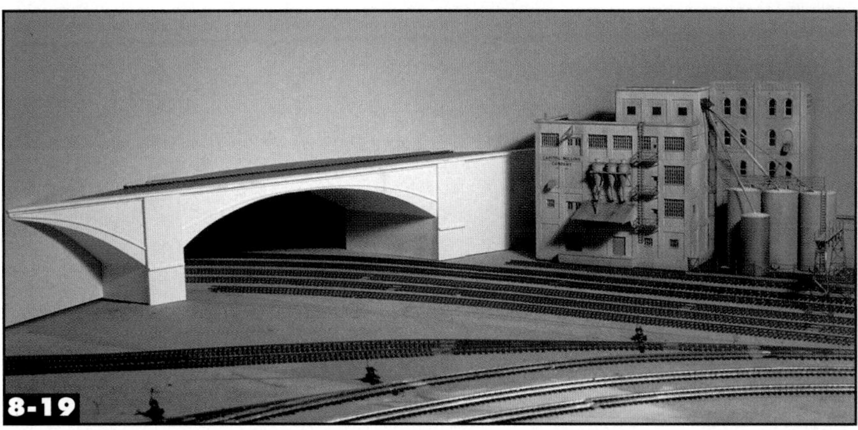
8-19

▼ Bob's finished bridge is attractive and disguises the opening well. *Bob Smaus*

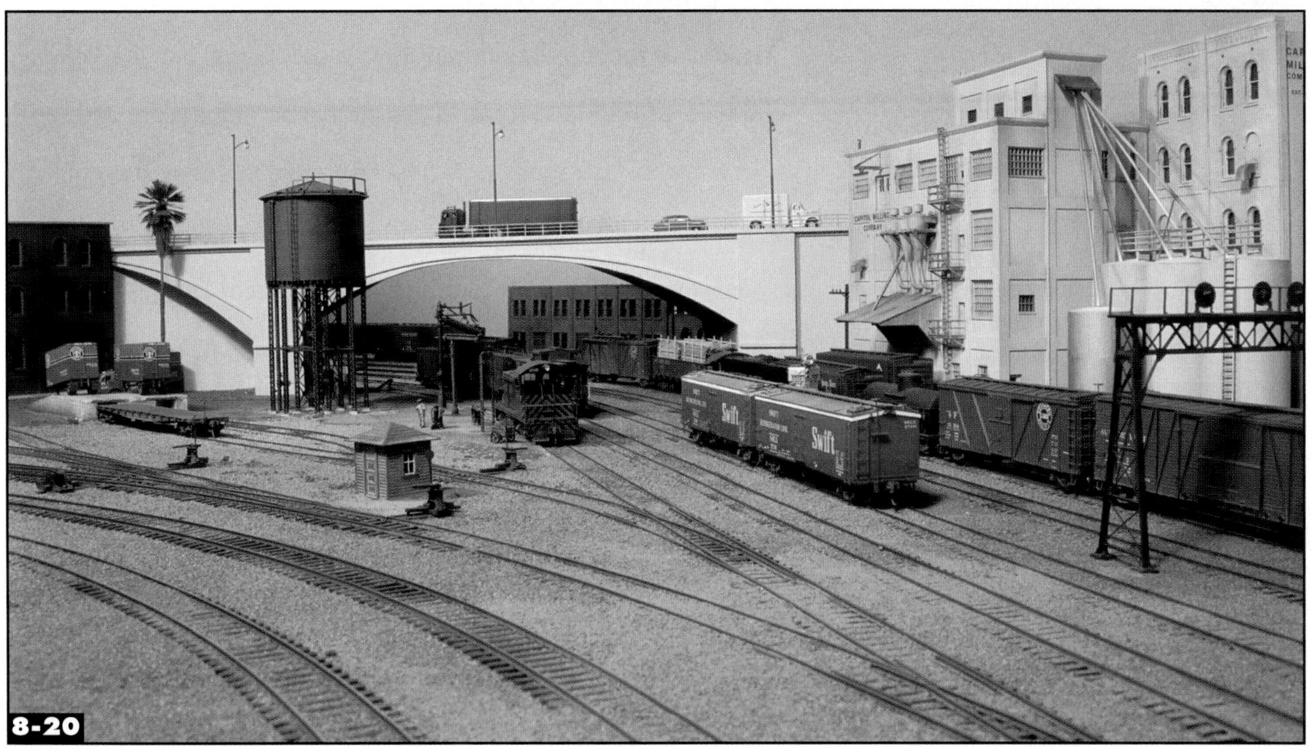

8-20

Abutments and piers

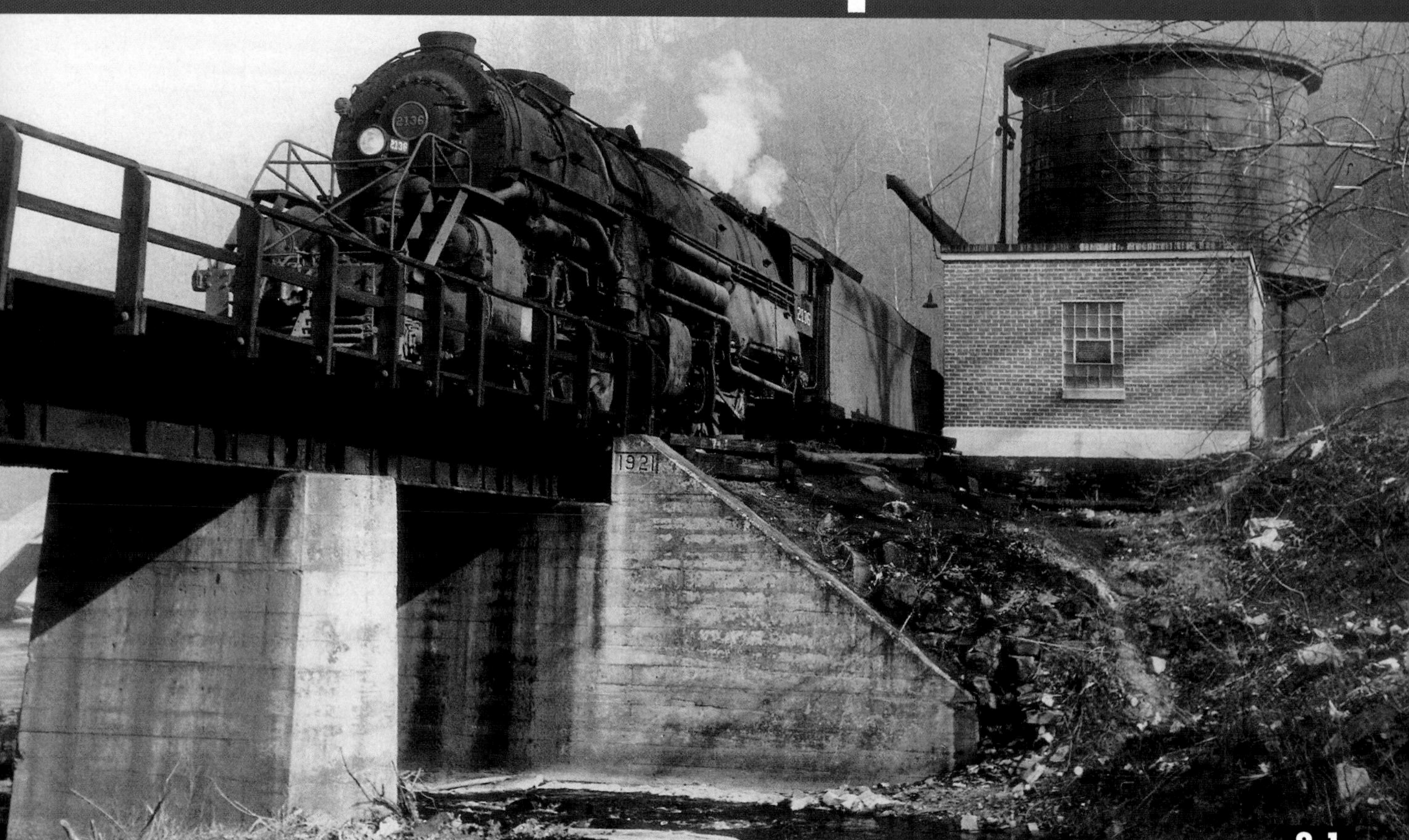

9-1

NINE

Abutments and piers provide crucial support for the main structure of a bridge. The pier shown here has a pointed end (a "cutwater") on the upstream side. The abutment has tapered wing walls. You can see the horizontal marks from the boards used as forms when this concrete pier and abutment were poured. *Bruce R. Meyer*

Oft-neglected areas of bridge modeling are the foundations that support the bridges themselves. In real life, the stability of the entire bridge structure is dependent upon the piers and abutments, so railroads go to a lot of trouble to ensure these structures provide solid footing.

Making sure the piers and abutments are realistic will make your model bridges look better and fit naturally into your layout. Piers and abutments come in a wide variety of styles, some quite ornate. Modeling these items adds supporting detail to a scene and helps capture the look of a specific prototype.

Prototype abutments

Abutments and piers together comprise the bridge substructure; the bridge itself is the superstructure. The substructure's purpose is to transmit the load and forces of the bridge superstructure to the ground.

Abutments are the supporting walls used at the end of a bridge span (or series of spans). Their purpose is twofold: to support and anchor one end of the bridge, and to hold back the adjoining ground. Modern abutments are generally poured concrete, but over the years stone, timber, and steel have also been used. All of these materials can be found on bridges still in service today.

The most common type of abutment is the breast wall with wing walls, **9-1**. The main facing wall is called the breast wall; it supports the end of the bridge. The flat horizontal surface atop the breast wall on which the

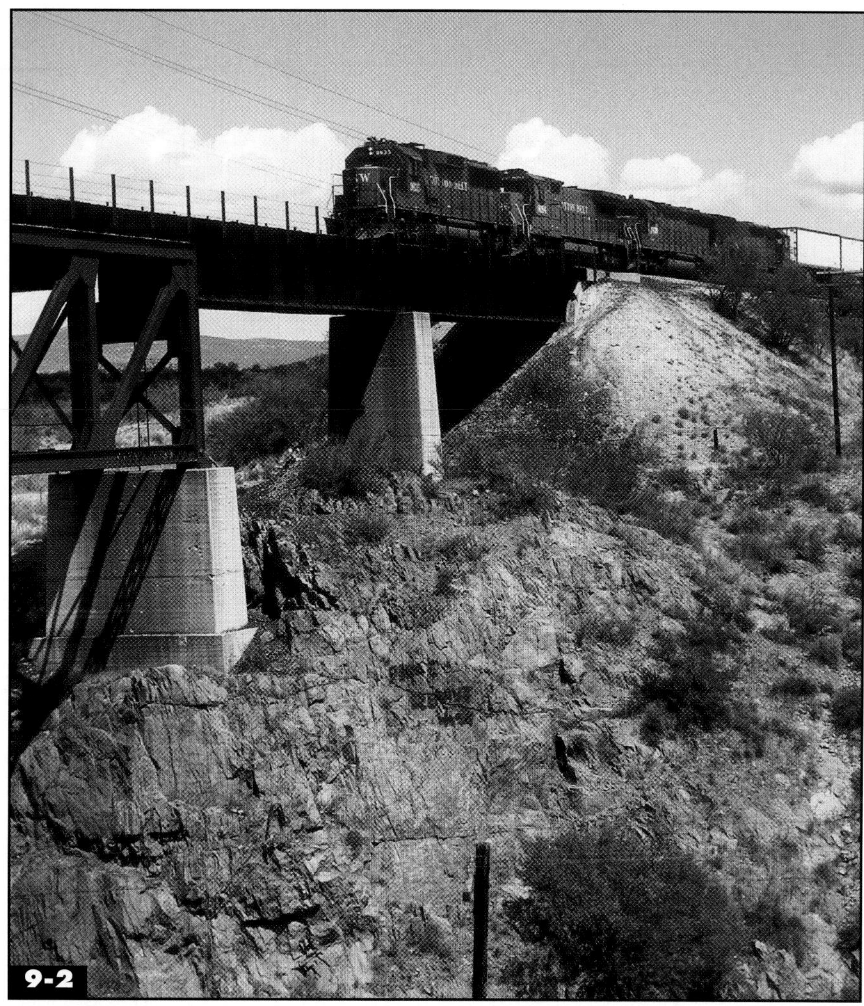

▲ A U-shaped abutment is sometimes used in locations where the surrounding ground slopes away gradually from the abutment. *Jeff Wilson*

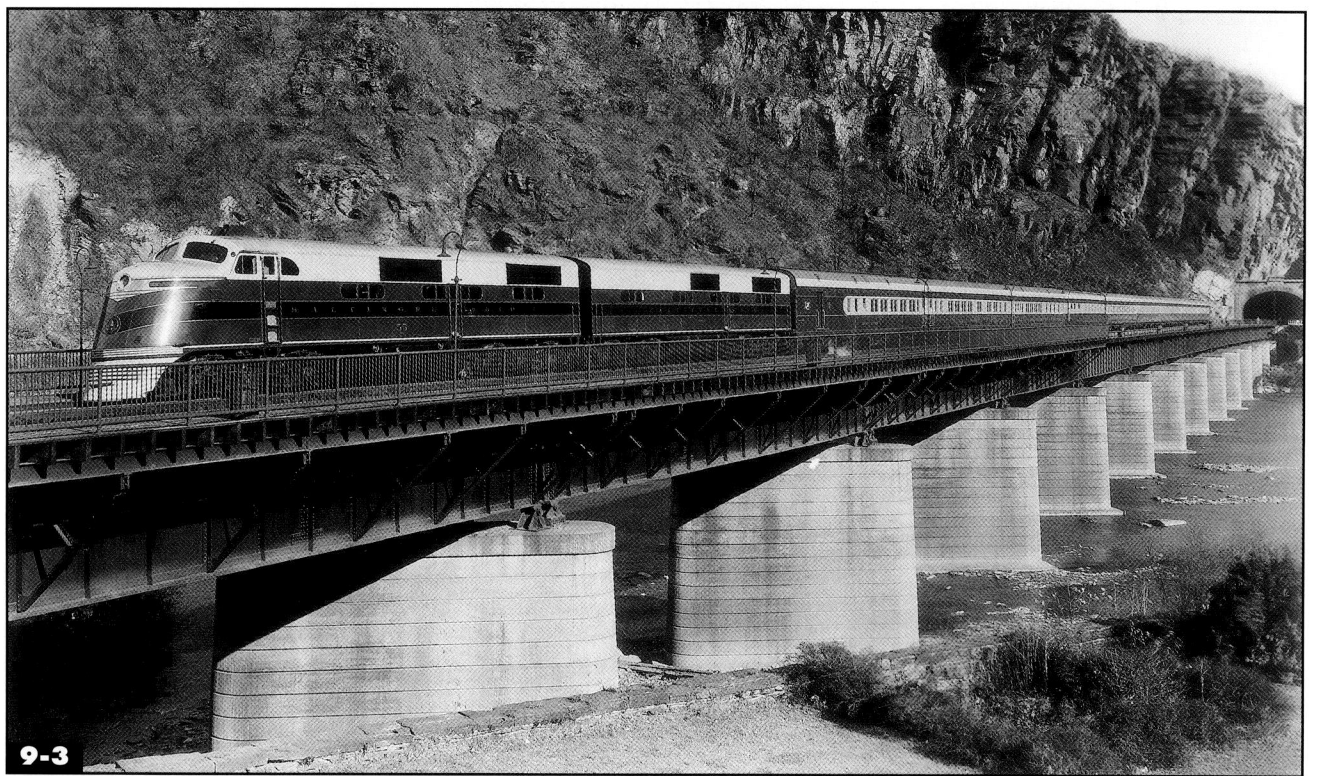

▼ The concrete piers on this Baltimore & Ohio skewed multi-span plate girder bridge over the Potomac at Harper's Ferry, West Virginia, are angled to be parallel with the current flow in the river. *Baltimore & Ohio*

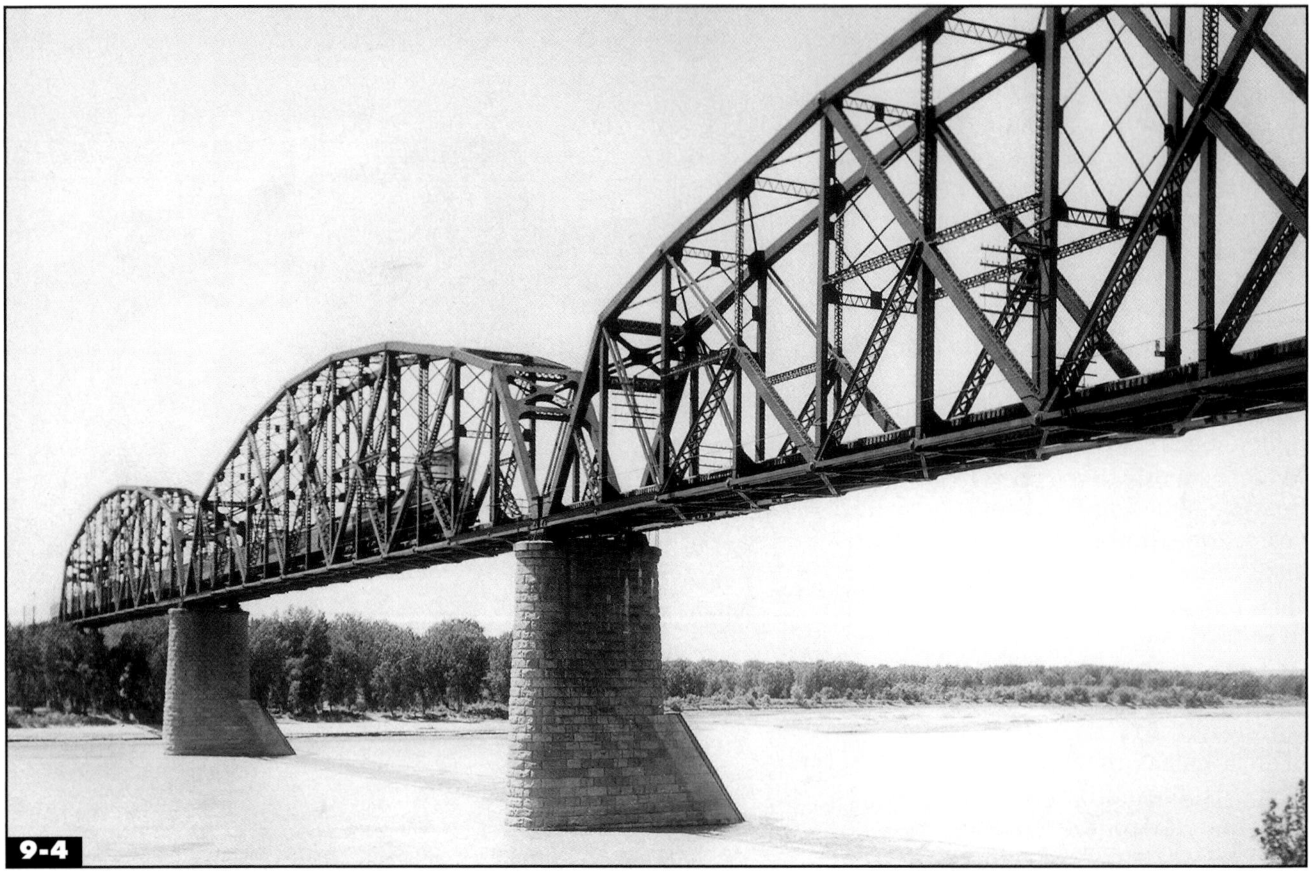

9-4

▲ Stone piers can also have rounded ends. The cutwaters on these piers extend only partway up the pier. These Pennsylvania truss spans are on the Northern Pacific's crossing of the Missouri River at Bismarck, North Dakota. *Northern Pacific*

▼ The stone piers supporting these Warren deck trusses are rectangular. Note the heavier footing and the taper on all corners. *Historic American Engineering Record; Wm. E. Barrett*

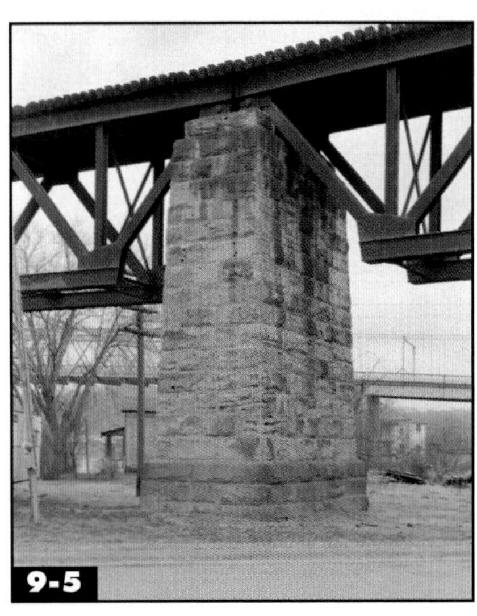
9-5

bridge shoes rest is the bridge seat. The back wall is the vertical wall at the rear of the bridge seat, and its job is to hold the earth in place behind the abutment.

The wings are the extended walls outside the breast wall. These may taper back at an angle to hold back the surrounding earth, and they also taper downward to follow the shape of the surrounding ground.

A variation of this style of abutment is the plain breast abutment, which omits the wing walls. It is often used where fill covers all but the top few feet of the abutment.

Abutments in U or box shapes are also common, with wings projecting backward at right angles from the face, **9-2** (page 73). Abutments are like icebergs—there's more to them below the ground than is visible above ground. Study the photos in this book, and you'll see many abutments with shapes determined by the bridge type and the surrounding ground and features.

The bridge seat must be wide enough to support the bridge. It should be at least the width of the bridge shoe plates plus 4′ (allowing at least 2′ on each side).

Piers

Piers are stand-alone structures that provide intermediate support at the joints of multiple spans, **9-3** (page 73). As with abutments, the top surface—the bridge seat—must be the proper size. The width of the seat should be 3′ greater than the span of the bridge feet or bearing plates (18″ on each side). The long dimension of the seat should be at least 4′ longer than the span of the bridge shoes (2′ on either side). The seat is usually made of concrete, even on stone piers.

Piers are generally wider at the base than at the top, with a slope or "batter" of about ½″ per 12″. A heavy footing, or caisson, is sometimes visible but may be hidden below water level. Piers can be rounded at the ends, like the concrete piers in **9-3** or the stone piers in **9-4**, or they can be rectangular as in **9-5**.

The 275′-tall concrete piers on the Southern Pacific's continuous-truss bridge over the Pecos River near Langtry, Texas, were made by slip-casting. A segment of the pier is cast, then the form is "slipped" up to cast the next higher section of the pier. *Historic American Engineering Record; E. B. Elliott*

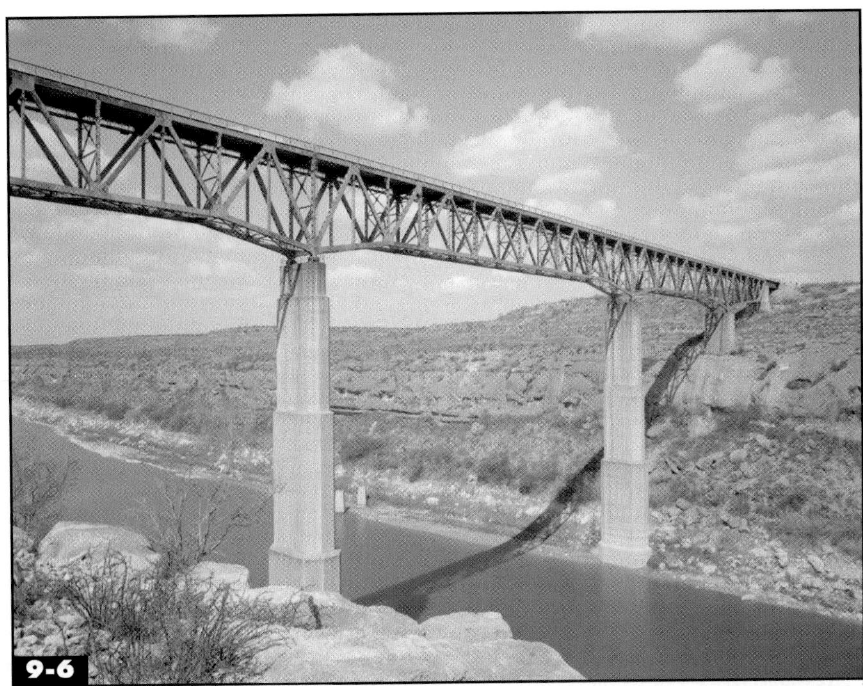

Piers in waterways are usually oriented to be parallel with the flow of water to lessen the effect of the water's force on the bridge structure (see **9-3**). For this reason, skewed spans are often used when multiple spans cross waterways at other than right angles.

A characteristic of many in-water (or near-water) piers is a pointed end on the upstream side (see **9-1**, page 72, and **9-4**). Called a "cutwater," the end deflects ice and other debris in the water, lessening the risk of damage to the pier. The cutwater sometimes runs the entire height of the pier (as in **9-1**) or sometimes only on the lower part of the pier up to the high-water mark, as **9-4** shows.

Concrete piers are cast in place. Depending on the forms used, the piers may have a smooth surface or the distinctive look of the forming planks (see **9-1**).

Piers can be quite tall, **9-6**, and are now usually made from concrete. Wood or steel piers are also common, **9-7**. Wood piers resemble trestle bents but have more posts. They are often doubled up and connected by cross bracing. Steel-frame piers are also found in many locations, especially under plate-girder bridges, **9-8** (page 76).

Where piers are located at the junction of two bridges of different types or sizes, the seat must often have two levels to accommodate both bridges, **9-9** (page 76). This can be done when the pier is built, or it may be done later if the bridges are replaced, as on the

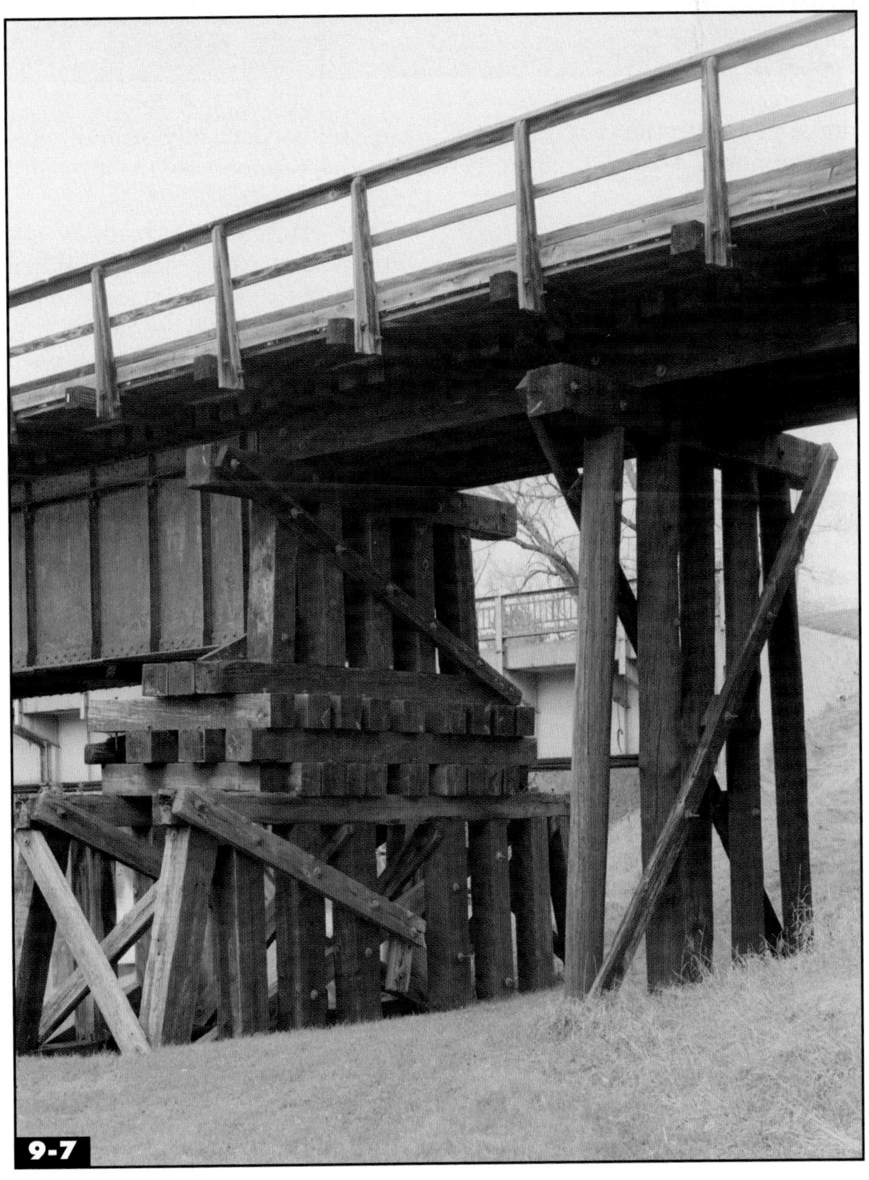

Wood piles are sometimes used to support steel bridges, especially if the bridge has a wood trestle approach. This bridge spans the Eagle River on the Chicago & North Western in Eagle River, Wisconsin. *Historic American Engineering Record; John N. Vogel*

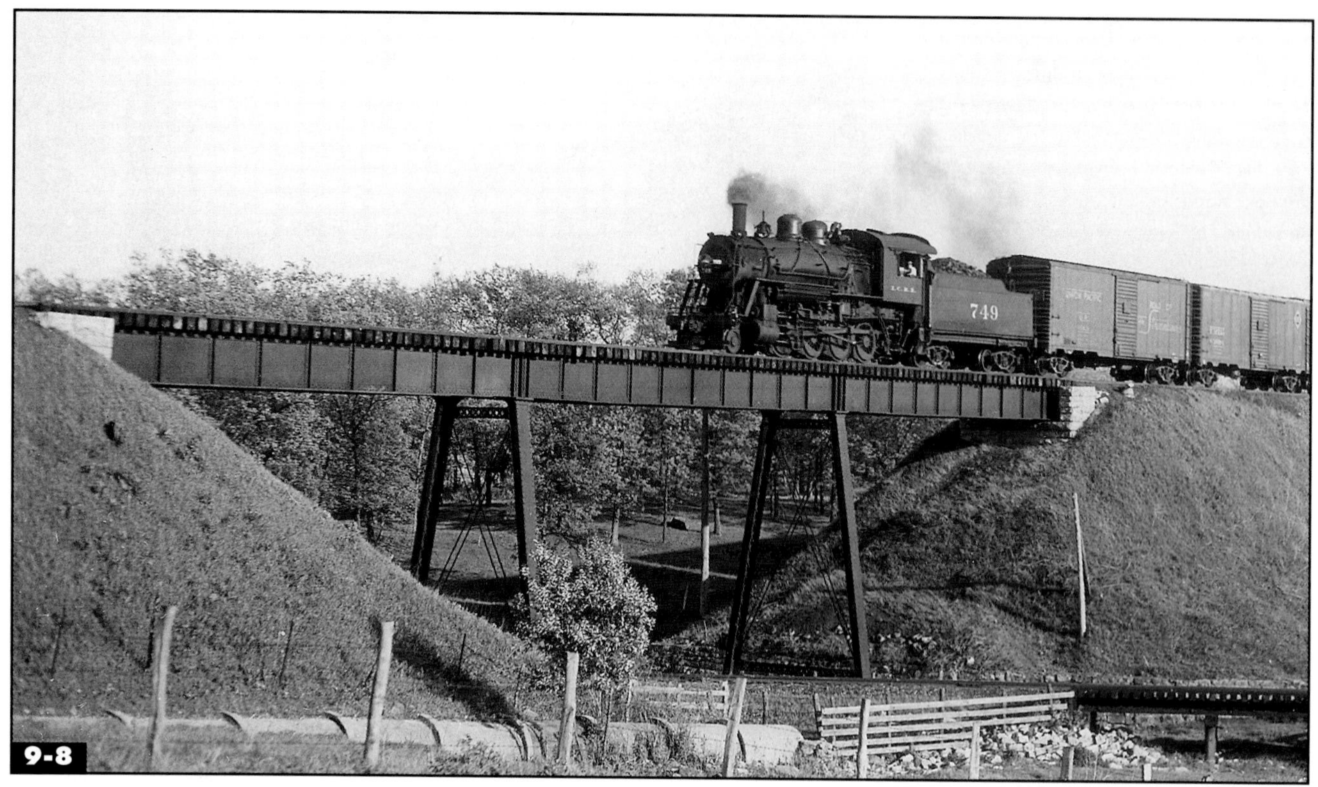

Steel-frame piers are sometimes used to support plate-girder bridges, as on the Illinois Central near Summit, Wisconsin. *Stan Mailer*

stone pier with the concrete addition in photo **4-23** in Chapter 4.

Modified piers

Bridges are frequently replaced or modified to improve the strength of a span. Sometimes the bridge level is raised; other times, spans are lengthened or more spans are added. Where the existing piers are still structurally sound, they may be retained as the base for the new spans.

Sometimes new bridges are built next to existing spans. When the new bridge is in place, the old bridge is usually removed for scrap, but the piers are left in place—as long as they don't interfere with waterway traffic, **9-10**.

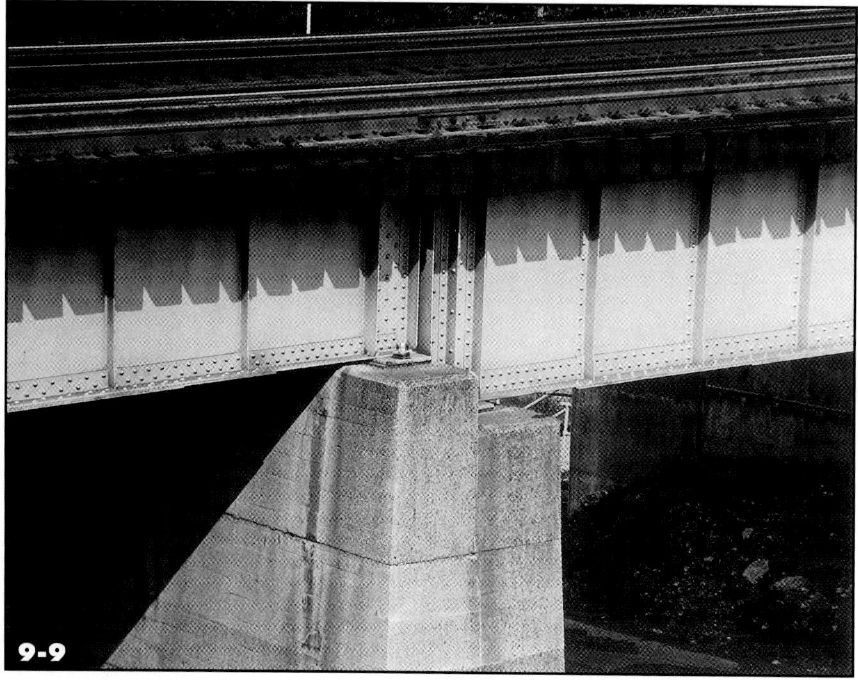

Steps are built into piers where bridges of differing sizes meet. *Harold Russell*

Modeling a set of abandoned piers may add the extra bit of verisimilitude your layout needs.

A similar, realism-enhancing detail worth modeling is a spot where a timber pile trestle has been replaced by a bridge. The old trestle is removed by cutting off the pilings, and these are sometimes visible above the water line as shown in photo **1-1** in Chapter 1.

Modeling

Modeling piers and abutments is easy, thanks to the wide variety of ready-made products available in N and HO scales. Many sizes and styles are offered, including simulated concrete, stone, and timber abutments from companies such as AIM Products and Chooch, **9-11**. Models of cut-stone piers with plain and cutwater ends can also be found, **9-12**. (See the list of available kits starting on page 86.)

You might want to make your own abutments and piers, either to match a specific prototype or to

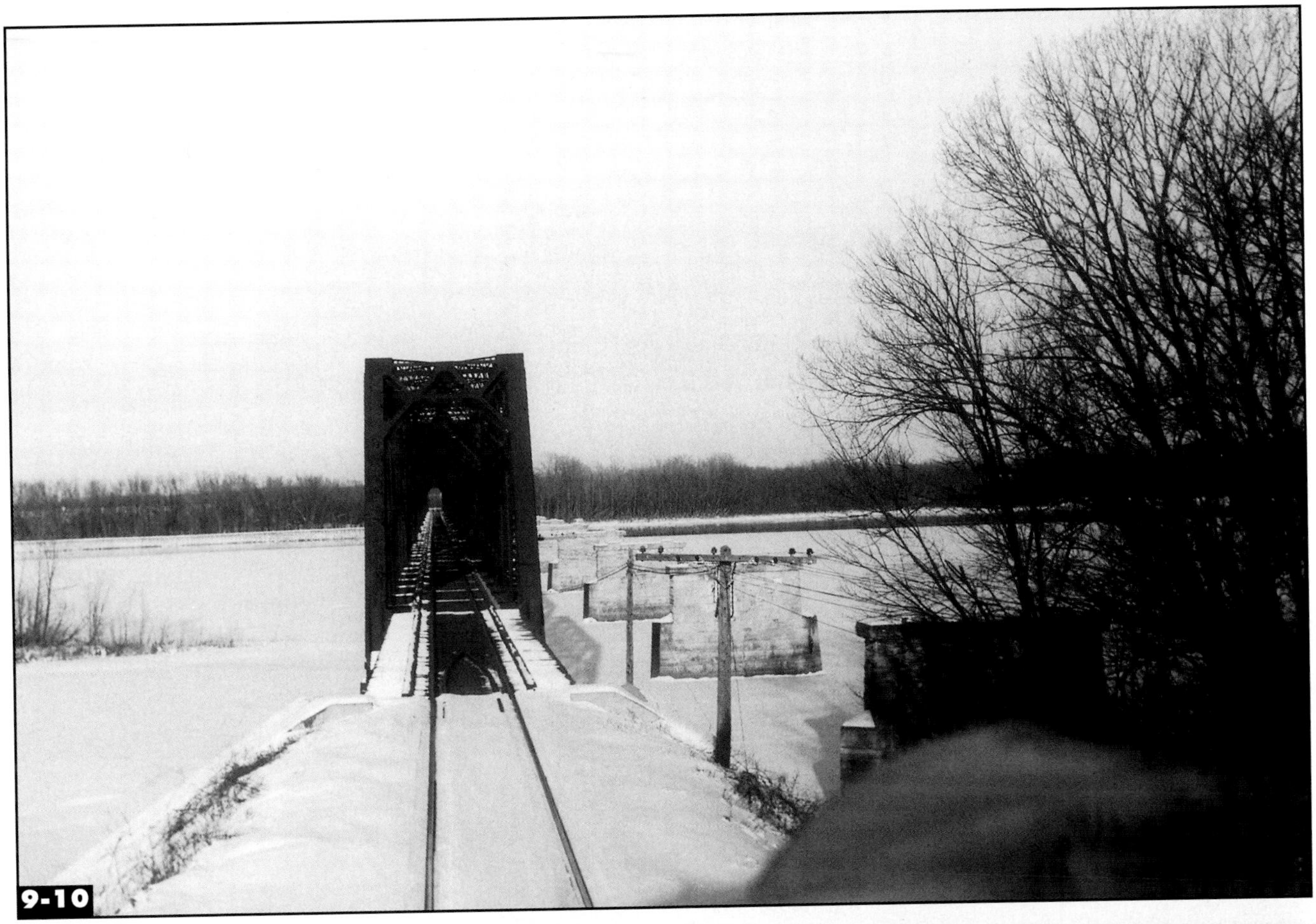

▲ When an old bridge is replaced by a neighboring span, the original bridge's piers are often left in place. This is on the Minneapolis & St. Louis at Keithsburg, Illinois. *Robert H. Milner*

fit the unique needs of your layout.

Sheet styrene is a great material for modeling poured concrete abutments and piers. I followed the techniques shown in Chapter 6 to build a pair of HO scale models based on the prototype piers in **9-13** (page 78). These are simple structures, but a recessed archway design gives them a unique look.

Start by making a scale drawing of the pier, using the dimensions of

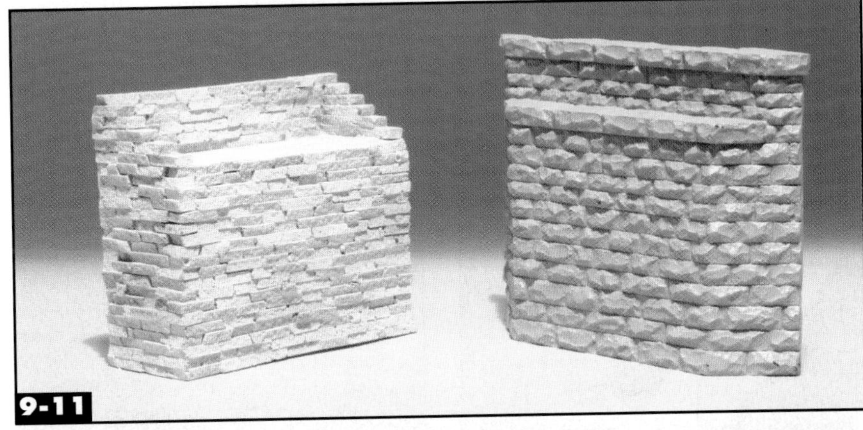

Above right: Available HO abutments include a shelf-type stone model from AIM (no. 718) and a tapered stone model from Chooch (no. 8460).

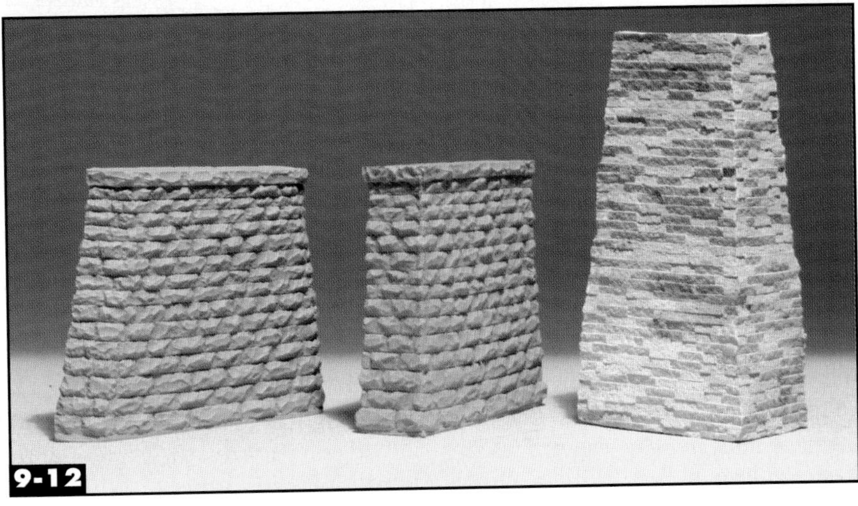

▶ Commercial HO pier models include (left to right) these stone cutwater (no. 8430) and rectangular (no. 8431) piers from Chooch and a tall cut stone pier (no. 735) from AIM Products.

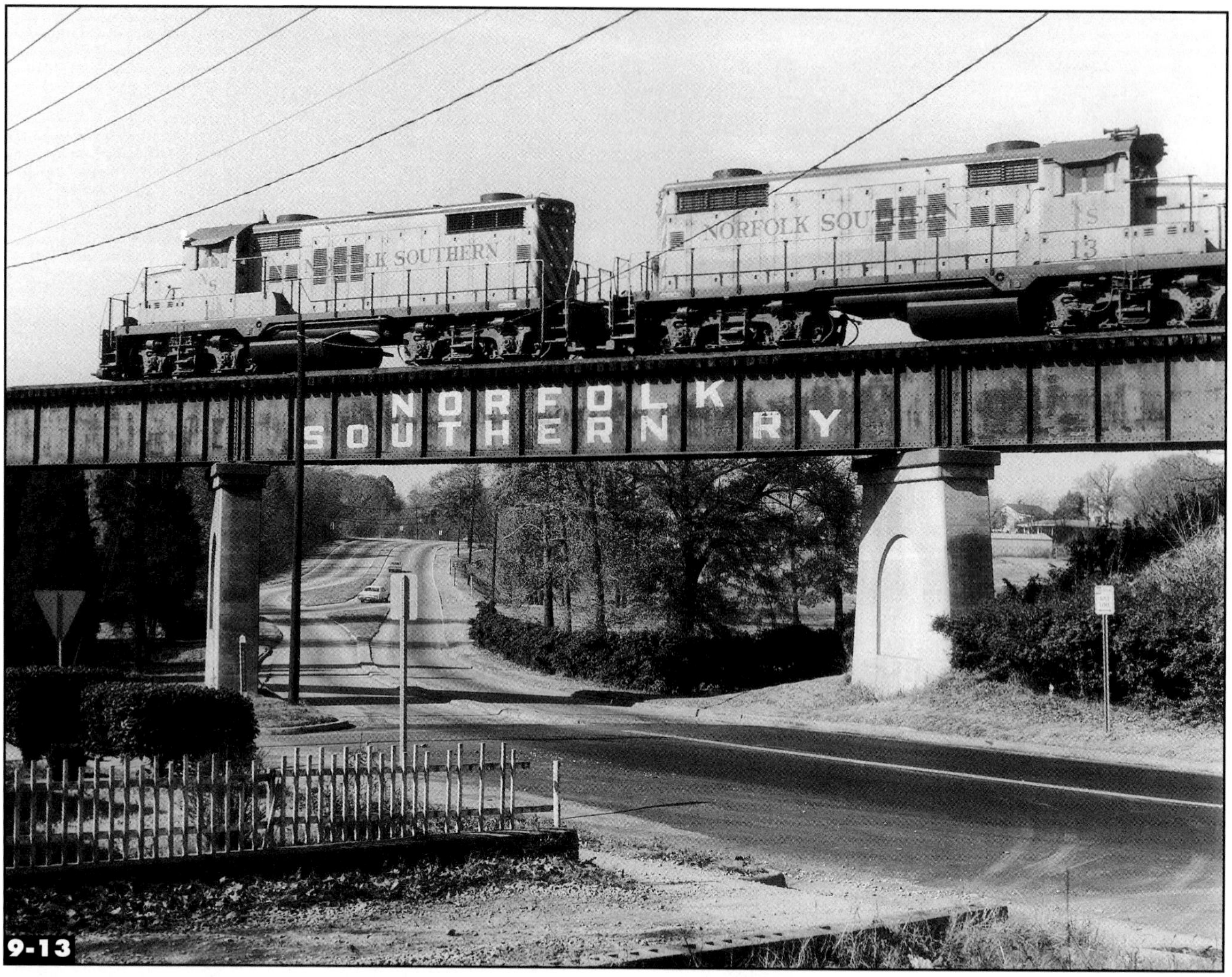

9-13

The eye-catching arch-pattern concrete piers under this skewed Norfolk Southern plate girder bridge would make distinctive scratchbuilt models. *Curt Tillotson, Jr.*

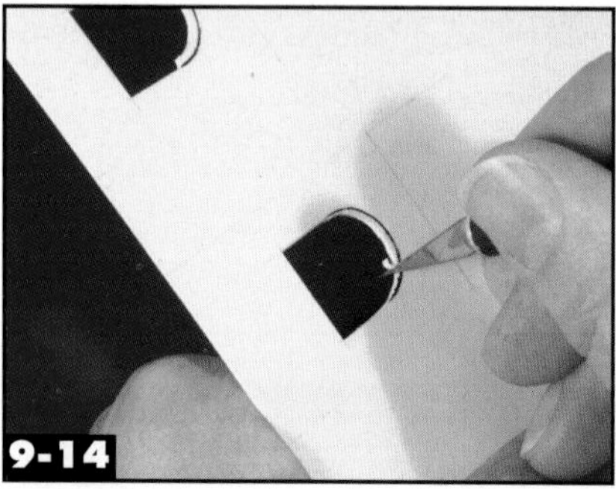

9-14 Draw the arch pattern on the styrene, then use a drill bit to start the curve. Carve out the rest of the curve with a sharp hobby knife. *Jeff Wilson*

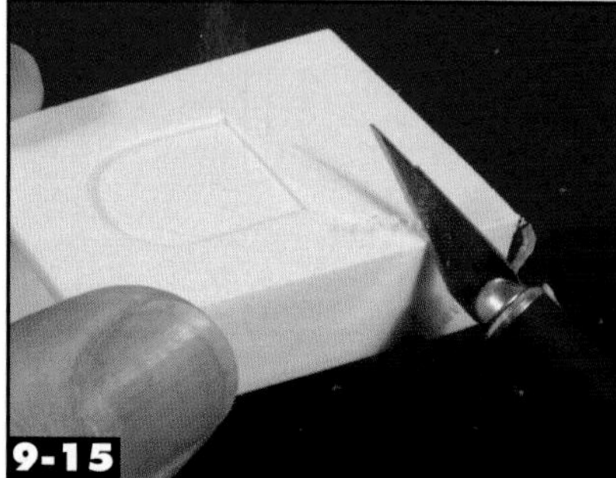

9-15 Corners must be glued tight, with no gaps. After the glue has dried, bevel the edges slightly with a hobby knife. *Jeff Wilson*

your model bridges and the needed height as starting points. The assembly process is essentially making a styrene box. The faces with the arches are cut from sheet styrene then glued to a backing layer of styrene. Cut the arches by first drilling a hole with a curve close to the required curve contour of the arch with a spade bit at low speed. Trim the remaining material from the arch with a knife, **9-14**.

The corners of the box must be glued tightly, with no gaps. Sand all edges square, then glue with liquid plastic cement. When the glue dries, scrape the joints smooth with a hobby knife, **9-15**. Corners on real concrete are slightly beveled; do this with the hobby knife as well. The stepped bridge seats on my models are simply pieces of .10″ styrene cut to fit and glued in place.

The finished piers are shown in **9-16**. You can use this technique to make almost any type of concrete pier or abutment.

Piers using stone sheets

Cut-stone piers can be modeled with the same technique, but by using embossed sheets instead of plain styrene. Embossed brick sheets are available from Plastruct and other companies.

Cut the sides and ends as described above for plain styrene piers. Stone sheets can't be simply butted together like plain styrene. You have to make sure the stone

▶ If the joints were glued tightly, painting will hide any seam marks at the corners of the piers. *Jeff Wilson*

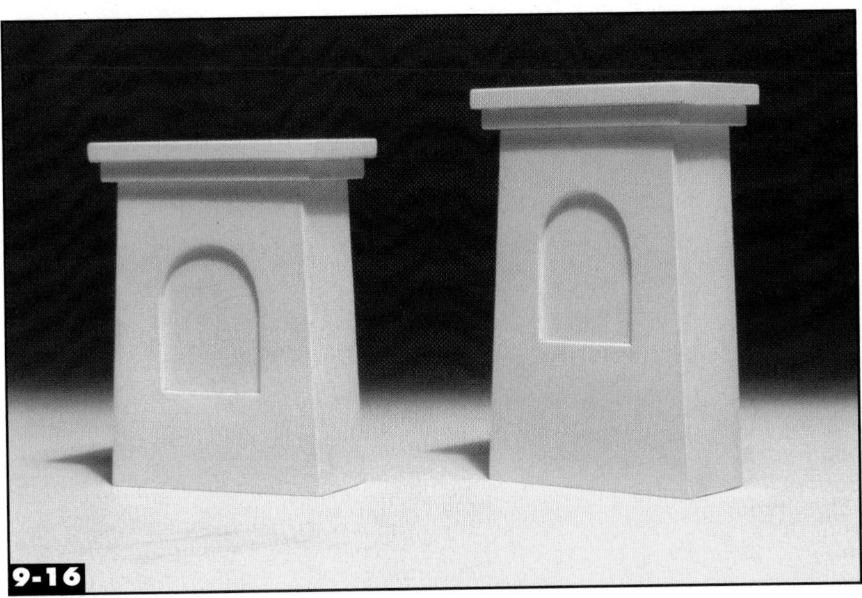

courses match on all four sides, then bevel the mating edge of each side, **9-17**. The photos show Plastruct N scale stone used to model a pair of N scale piers. Positioning the piece at the edge of a block of wood makes it easier to scrape the bevel evenly. Scrape (don't try to cut) the edge with a hobby knife blade until the entire edge is beveled. The angle doesn't have to be exact.

Glue the walls together. A piece of square styrene in the corner will help stabilize the joint. Photo **9-18** shows a pair of completed piers, one with a cutwater. A piece of plain styrene across the top serves as a concrete cap.

They might not draw as much attention as bridges, but piers and abutments are important details, worthy of some time and effort to model them accurately.

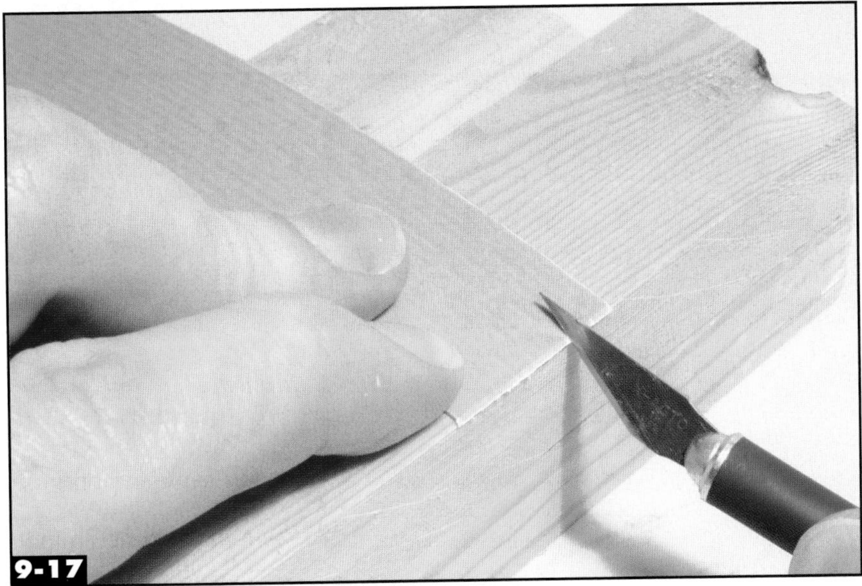

▶ Bevel the mating edges of the stone sheets by scraping with a hobby knife. Use a piece of scrap lumber to support the sheet. *Jeff Wilson*

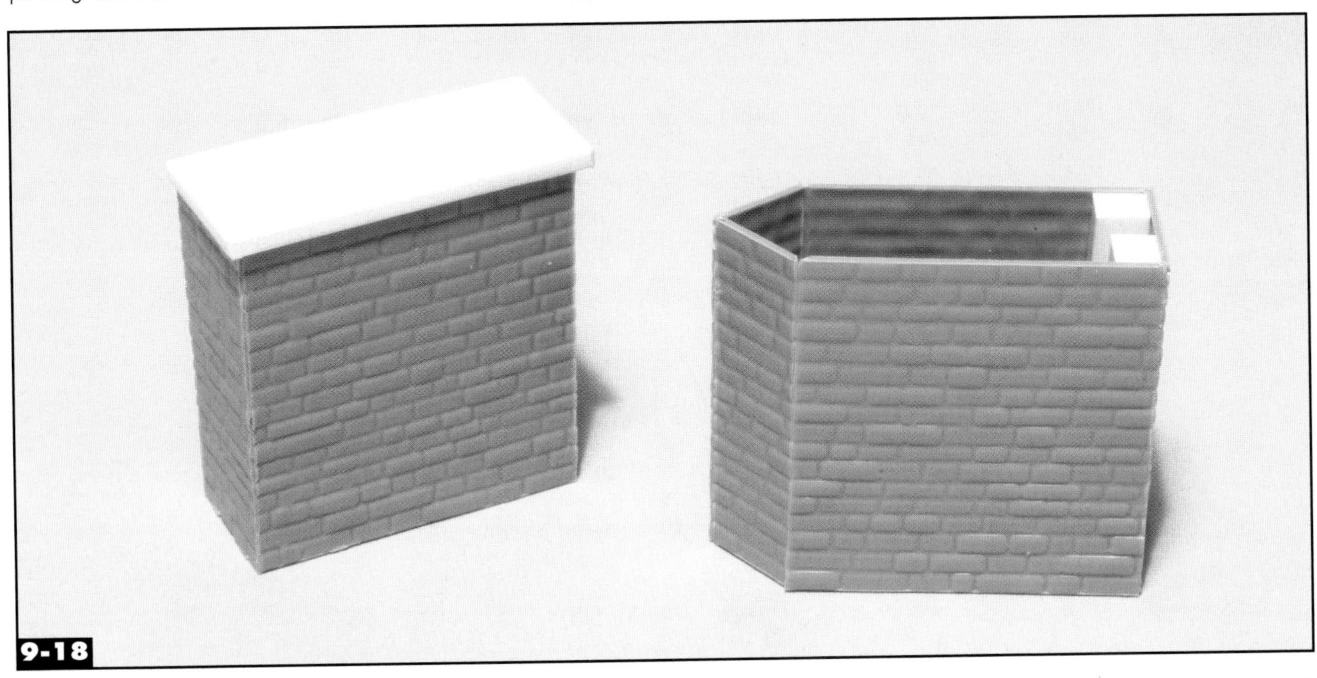

▼ Glue the pieces together and add a bridge seat; the piers are now ready for painting. *Jeff Wilson*

Tunnel portals

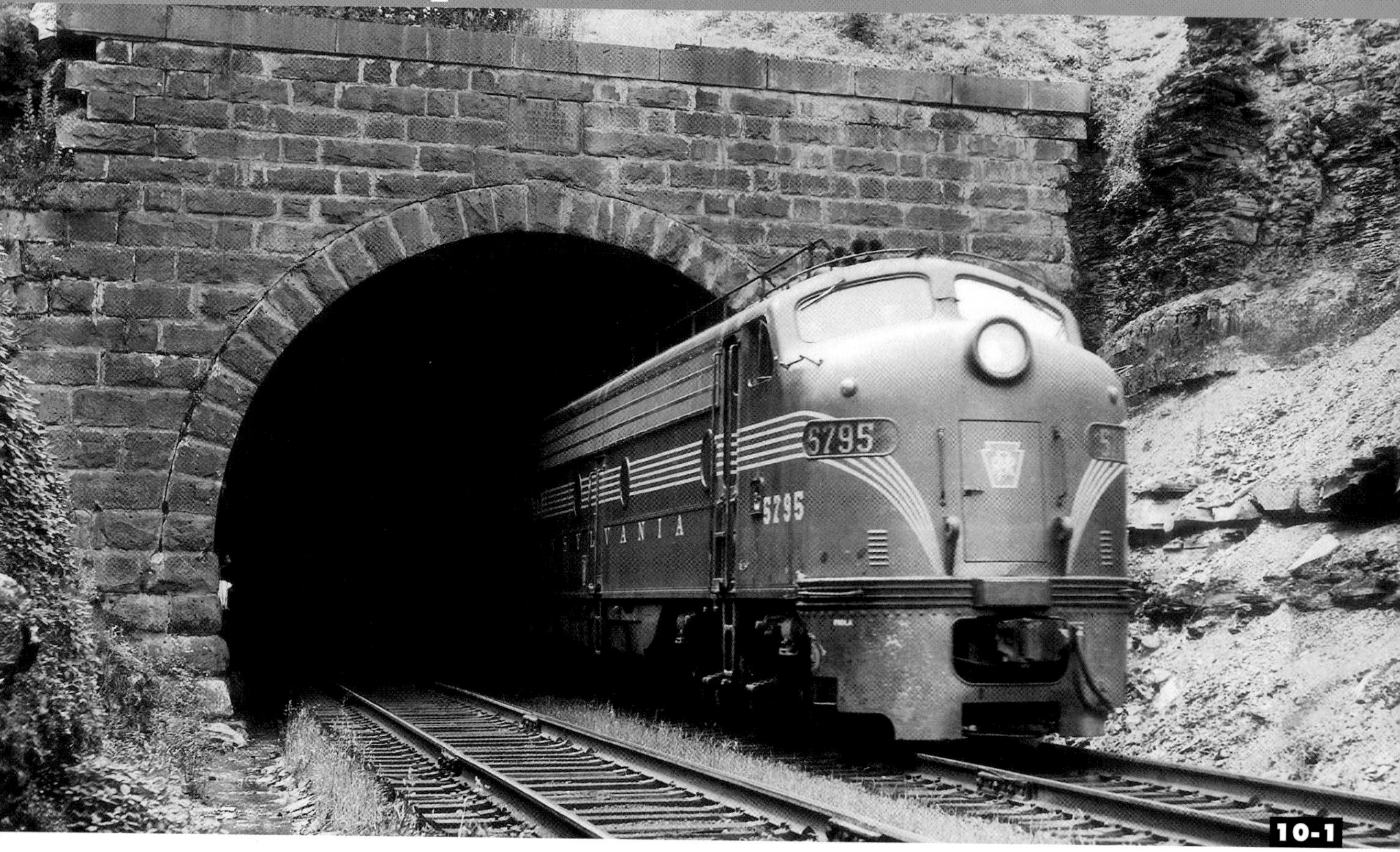

TEN

Tunnels allow railroads to go through mountains rather than over or around them, saving many miles of track. Stone portals, like this one on the Pennsylvania Railroad, are built in much the same fashion as stone bridges, with a row of tapered stones called "voussairs" around the arched opening. *Don Wood*

Tunnels serve important purposes on real railroads, allowing them to go beneath mountains, hills, and cities, shortening routes and avoiding steep grades, as well as dangerous, delay-causing weather conditions, **10-1**. Tunnels are frequently found in scenic locations, which means one is often the focal point of one of the more dramatic areas of a layout's landscape.

Tunnels play an important role on model railroads. Along with being visually appealing scenic elements, they offer modelers a method of hiding track, providing a way for a main line to get to under-table staging areas. Tunnels also can be used to cover openings through walls, or to allow tracks to pass unseen from one area of a layout to another.

► Timber portals, common on tunnels through the late 1800s, were prone to deterioration. *Dick Houghton*

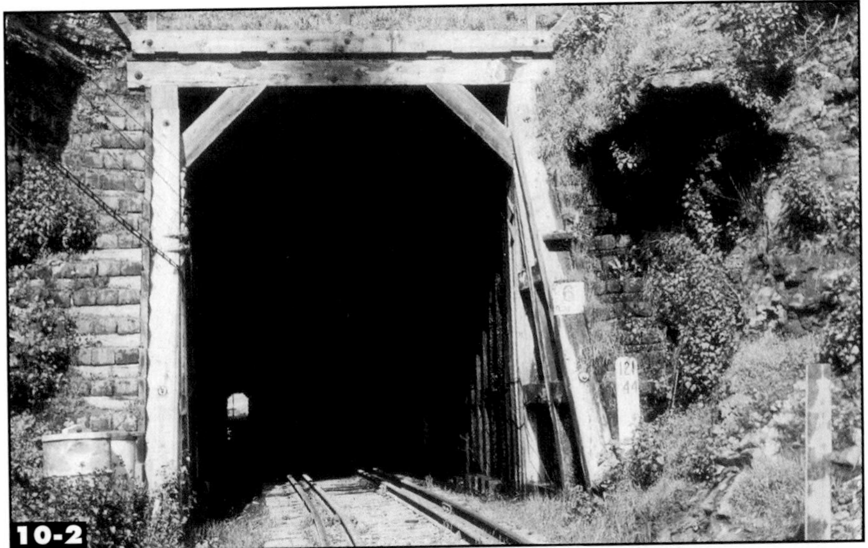

Prototype tunnels

Boring a tunnel through a mountain (or under a city) is an expensive proposition. Railroads do it only when routing track around or over the obstruction would be more expensive or operationally impractical. Because of the expense involved, most tunnels are single-tracked. Only main lines carrying the heaviest traffic can justify the expense of a two-track tunnel.

Tunnels have been a prominent part of the railroad scene almost from the beginning. By the mid-1940s, there were more than 1,500 in the United States. Railroads try to keep tunnel length as short as possible; about two-thirds are 1,000′ or less.

Since they are the only exposed part, portals are the most visible element of a tunnel. Portals have been built from wood, stone, and concrete. Wood portals were common in the early days of railroading through the late 1800s, **10-2**. Most were replaced by the early to mid-1900s.

Stone portals became predominant in the late 1800s (see photo **10-1**), and many stone portals built into the early 1900s are still being used. They follow the same basic design principles as stone arch bridges, with a row of stones (voussairs) forming an arch around the opening. They can be found with many styles and sizes of wing walls and adjoining retaining walls.

Concrete became the portal material of choice around the turn of the 20th century, **10-3**. Some concrete portals are quite plain; others are ornamented with faux stone cuts or emblazoned with their construction dates, names, or the name of the railroad operating the tunnel.

Some tunnels are cut into a face of hard rock; these don't require portals, **10-4**.

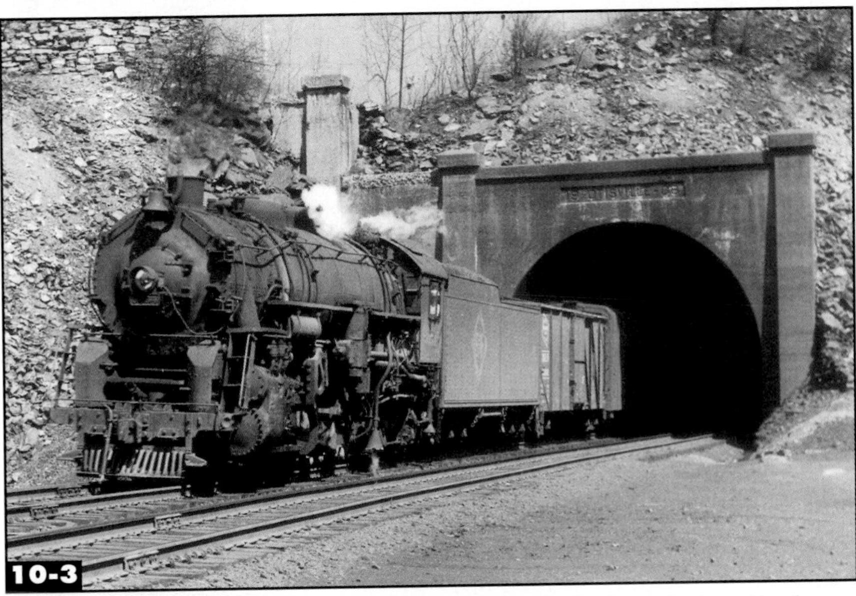

The concrete west portal of Erie's Otisville (New York) tunnel is fairly simple, but with pilasters and the inscription "19–OTISVILLE–08" in embossed lettering overhead. *Wayne Brumbaugh*

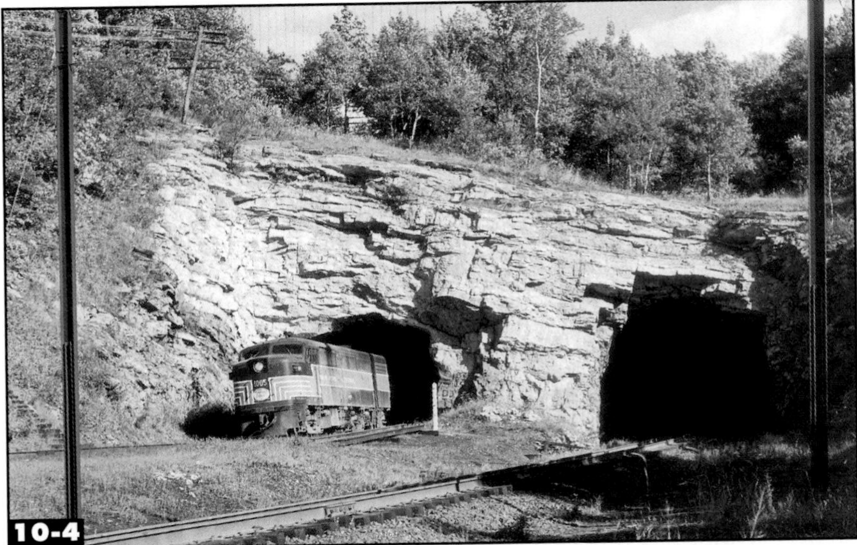

Tunnels bored into solid rock don't require portals. These are on the New York Central's Boston & Albany line near Canaan, New York. *Jim Shaughnessy*

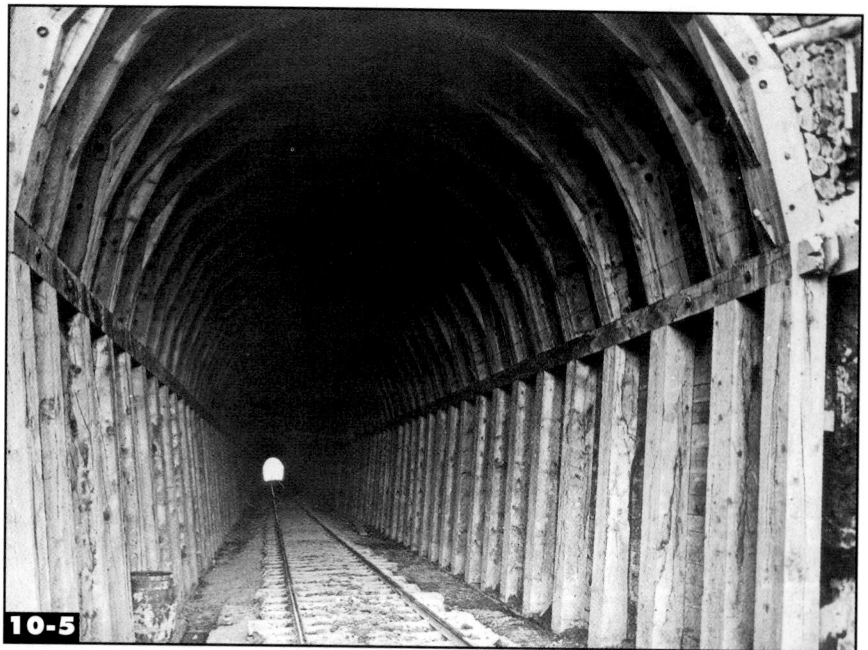

◀ Timber lining was common in the early days of tunnel construction, but risk of fire and other factors brought about a switch to stone. *David P. Morgan Library collection*

Lining

In any tunnel, the stability of the tunnel roof and walls is of prime importance. Obviously, the tunnel must be free from falling rocks and debris to be safe. This is accomplished by lining the tunnel walls and roof.

Some tunnels bored through solid rock require no lining, but these are not common—about 8 percent of all tunnels in service. By the late steam era, about 40 percent of tunnels were lined with concrete (as with portals, the material of choice from the early 1900s on), 12 percent with timber, 20 percent with stone or brick, and about 18 percent with a combination of materials.

Timber lining was common in the 19th century, **10-5**, but the risk of fire—especially with steam locomotives—and the deterioration of material caused wood to fall from popularity.

Stone and brick became popular, as they are durable and fireproof. However, installation was labor-intensive and expensive, especially for long tunnels.

Concrete became an economical choice around 1900, and by the 1940s, it was used almost exclusively for lining new tunnels. Concrete was also used to re-line many existing stone, brick, and timber tunnels, **10-6**.

Remember that tunnels aren't located exclusively in the mountains. They are sometimes used to cut under cities as well, **10-7**.

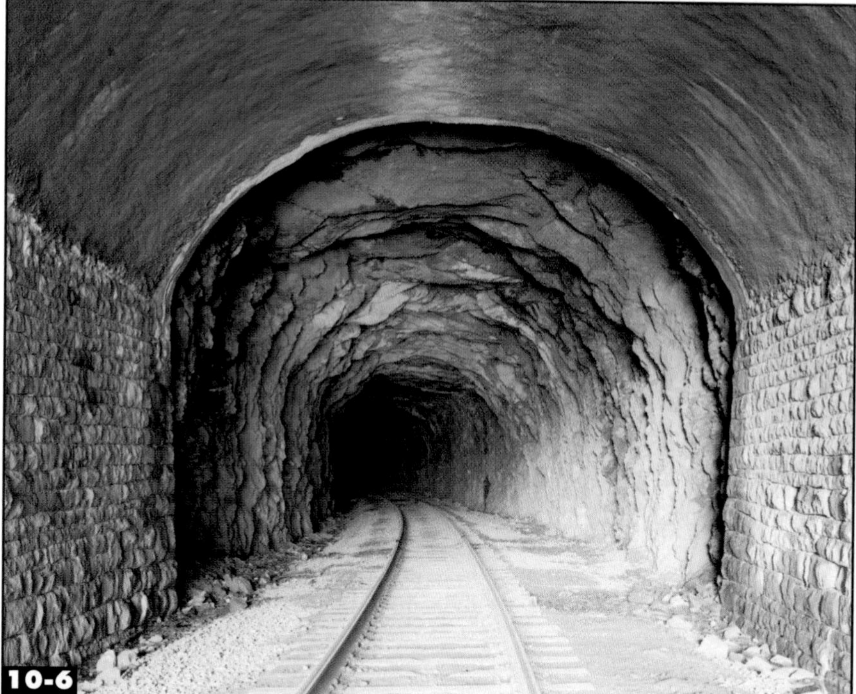

▲ The lining of this tunnel is stone (lower walls) and concrete (upper walls, ceiling) near the entrance, then changes to natural rock farther inside. *Historic American Engineering Record*

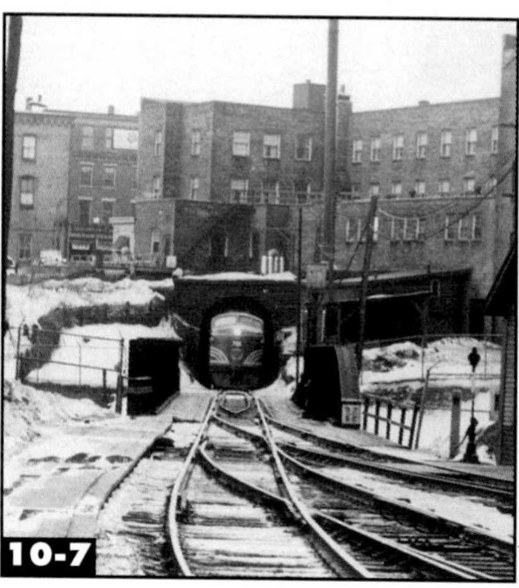

◀ Tunnels pass under cities as well as mountains. This one is on the Boston & Maine at Bellows Falls, Vermont. *David K. Johnson*

Ventilation

Ventilation is a prime concern in tunnel construction. Some type of artificial ventilation is usually used on tunnels longer than 2,500′. In the steam era, locomotives produced a lot of smoke and gases, especially when working hard. These gases collected at the top of the tunnel and could be strong enough to asphyxiate train crews and passengers. They can be a problem even with modern diesel locomotives.

Tunnel ventilation is usually accomplished by large fans placed at one end of the bore. They either blow against the train direction, carrying the gases out behind the locomotive, or with the direction of the train, pushing gases out ahead of the locomotive.

These can be spotted by the presence of a fan house, a building housing the fans and controls. Through the early 1900s these fans were usually controlled by operators on site; later systems worked automatically, using track circuits much like signaling systems.

Modeling

Fortunately, modelers don't have the same concerns as real railroads. The only details that modelers really need to worry about are the tunnel portals themselves, along with a few scale feet of tunnel lining inside the opening.

A wide variety of portals is available from companies such as AIM Products, Chooch, CM Shops, Model Railstuff, Pre-Size Model Specialties, and Woodland Scenics (see the list of available kits starting on page 86).

Several European companies, including Faller and Noch, also offer portals. Be aware, however, that these portals follow European styling—namely tapering the sides of the portals outward from the base—not commonly used in North America.

Available models include all styles of prototype portals, including timber, **10-8**, random and cut stone portals, **10-9**, and concrete portals, **10-10**. Many of these are available with dates embossed in the portals—a common detail on prototype portals.

Some companies offer models based on specific well-known prototype tunnel portals, including Model Railstuff's east and west Moffat Tunnel portals, and AIM's

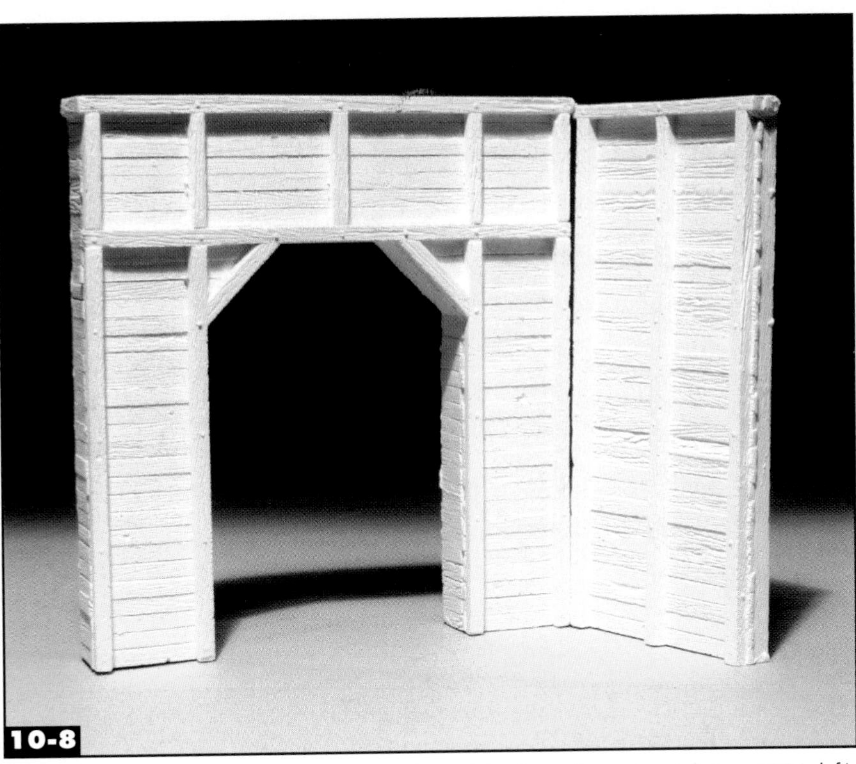

10-8

Woodland Scenics offers cast-plaster HO scale models of wood tunnel portals (no. 1254, left) and retaining walls (no. 1260). N scale versions are available as well. *Jeff Wilson*

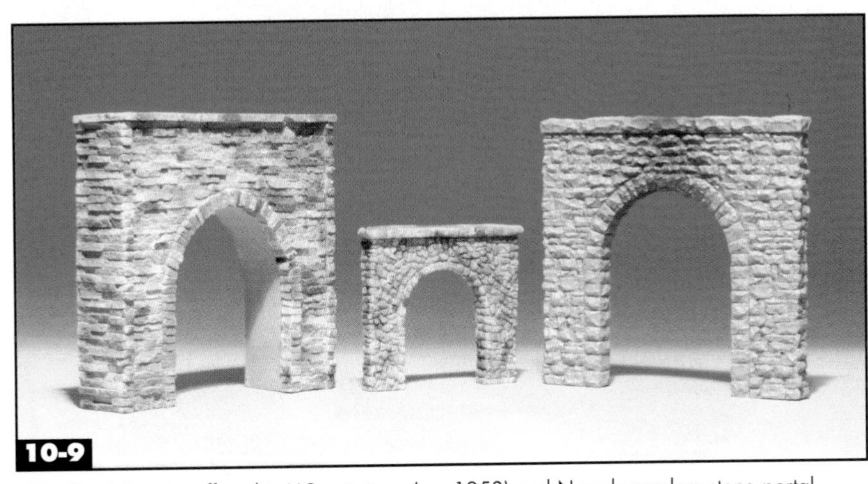

10-9

Woodland Scenics offers this HO cut stone (no. 1253) and N scale random stone portal (no. 1155), and Chooch has this random stone model (no. 8360). *Jeff Wilson*

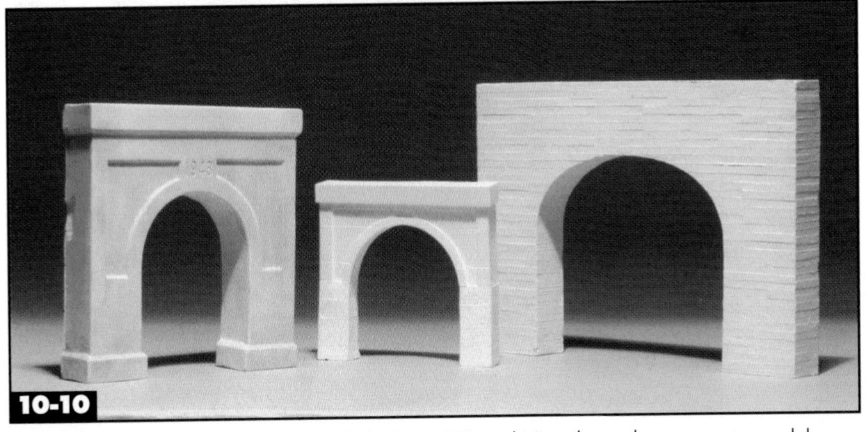

10-10

Concrete portal models from AIM include these HO and N scale modern concrete models (nos. 133 and 218) and a board-formed double-track portal (no. 129). *Jeff Wilson*

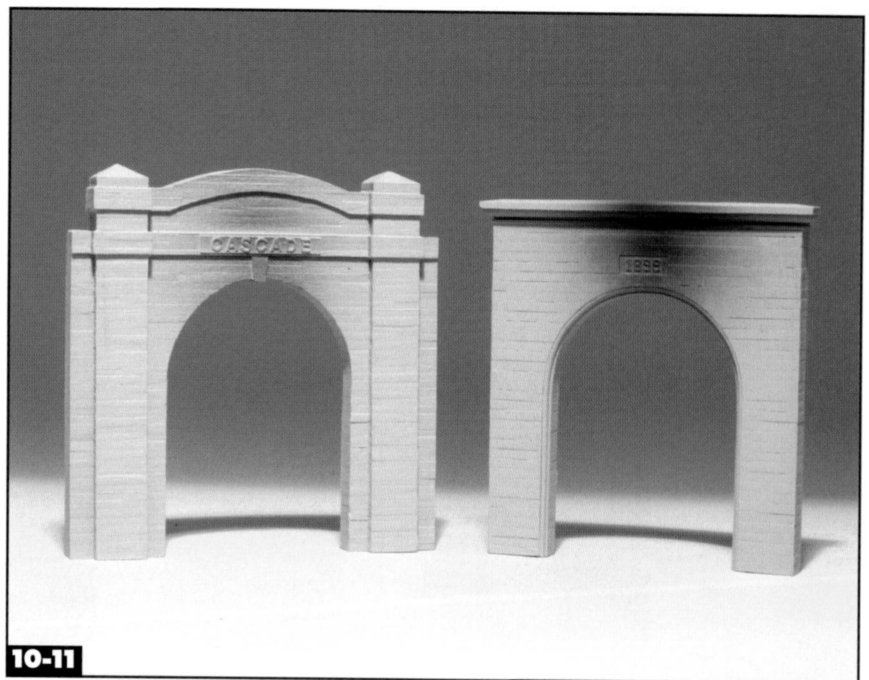

Chooch offers this HO model of a Cascade Tunnel portal (no. 8321) as well as a dated concrete portal (no. 8320). *Jeff Wilson*

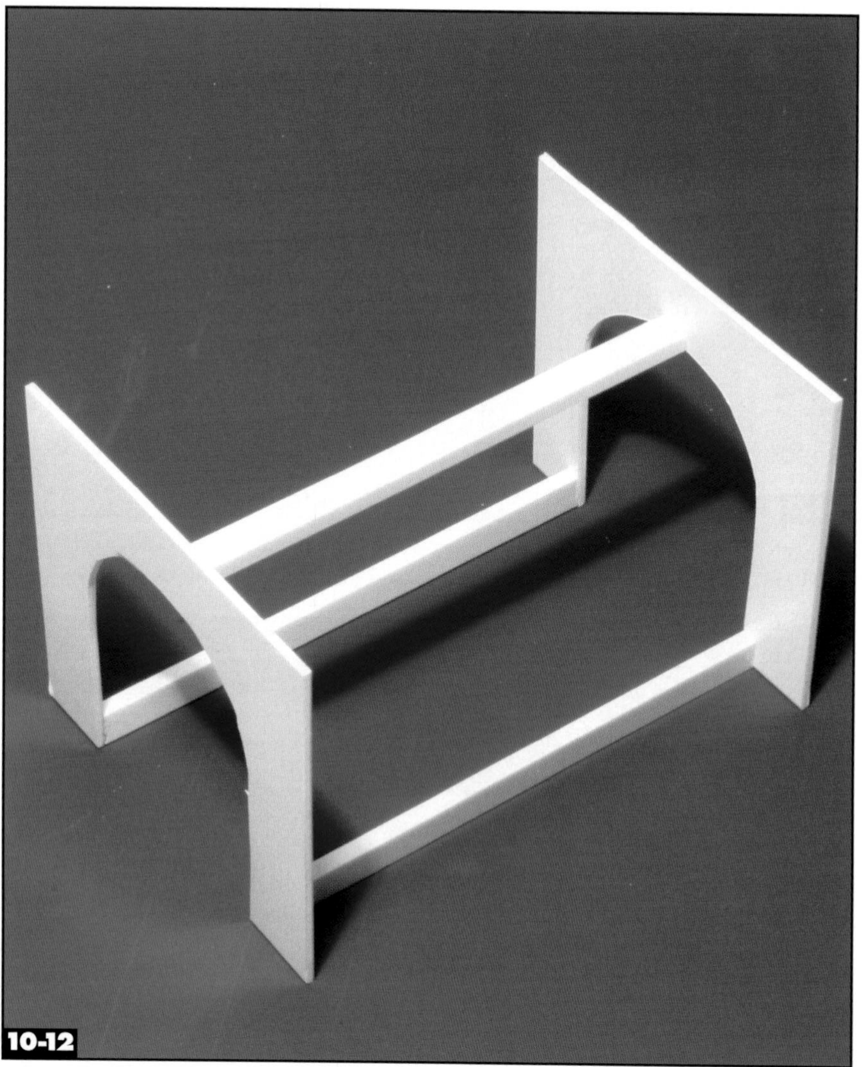

Make a frame from sheet and strip styrene to hold a plastic tunnel liner in place. *Jeff Wilson*

model of one of the Cascade Tunnel's portals, **10-11**.

If you're trying to model a specific prototype portal, you can either modify a commercial model, or you can try building it from scratch. Concrete portals are relatively easy to build from plastic, and can be built following the styrene construction guidelines in Chapters 6 and 9.

Tunnel linings

Model railroad tunnels aren't actually bored through rock, but it's important to disguise their openings. Viewers should not be able see plaster cloth, plywood, or an open area inside.

One solution is to build a partial tunnel lining, as I did for an N scale AIM portal. To build one, start by tracing the outline of the tunnel portal onto a piece of .060" sheet styrene. Use a hobby knife to cut the opening slightly outside the outline. You'll need two or three of these depending upon the length of your tunnel lining.

Connect these pieces with strips of thick styrene, **10-12**. The exact dimension of this bracing isn't critical, but it must be heavy enough to hold the liner material in position. Glue the strips in place with styrene cement, making sure the bottom strips are lined up flush with the bottom of the arched openings. Add more strips for more additional strength and stability if necessary. Let these dry thoroughly before proceeding.

Make the frame long enough to block the normal view looking into the tunnel. I suggest a minimum of 3" to 4", and a maximum of 8" or 9"—anything longer and accessing derailed equipment becomes a problem. The one shown in **10-12** is about 6" long.

Next, make a tunnel liner to match the portal. For the frame shown here, I used Plastruct stone-textured sheet styrene. Cut the material slightly longer than the frame, test-fit it, and trim it as needed. Begin gluing it in place at one corner of the front of the

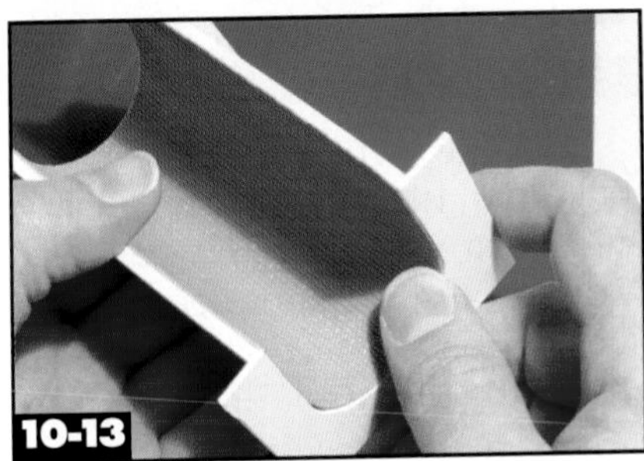

10-13

Glue one side of the liner and clamp it, then wait for it to dry before clamping and gluing the other side. *Jeff Wilson*

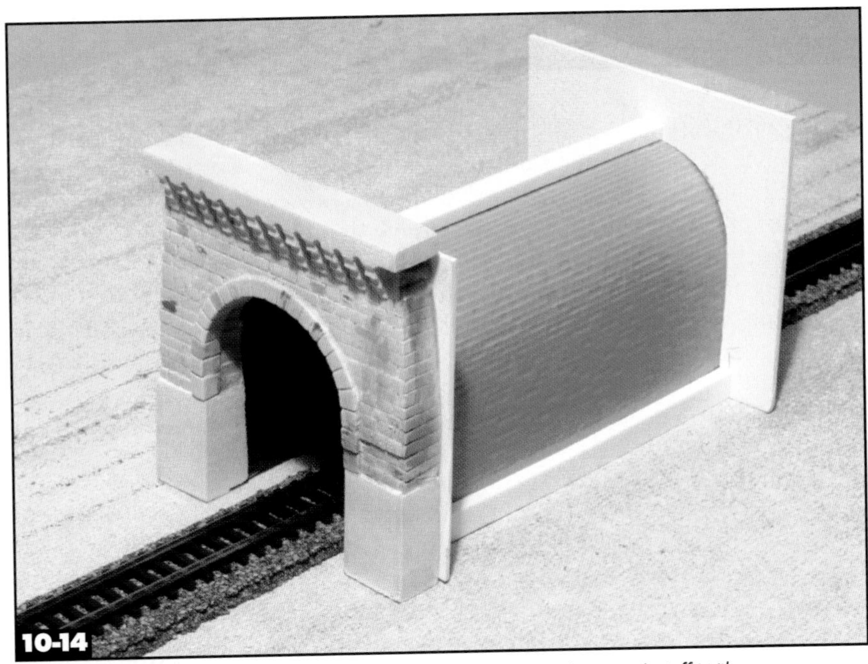

10-14

The finished liner will give people a more realistic view into the tunnel. *Jeff Wilson*

frame, **10-13**. Clamp it in place until the glue sets. Clamp the other side in place, add glue, and set it aside again until the glue dries.

Paint the interior a dark, flat color—grimy black or dark gray are almost always good choices for stone, rock, and brick, **10-14**.

To simulate a concrete-lined tunnel, use plain styrene painted a dark concrete color. For natural rock texture, use aluminum foil. Crumple the foil, flatten it out, and glue it to the styrene sheet lining. After it's painted, it will look just like rock.

Once the portal and liner are done, finish the area with standard scenery methods. Ballast the track as far into the tunnel as will be visible when the tunnel is installed on the layout. Ballasting before adding the liner frame and scenery is usually easier.

Painting plaster

Many simulated stone portals, piers, abutments, and retaining walls are cast in plaster. Plaster is porous, so it takes paints and stains well. Mix your own colors using model or artist's acrylic paints, as described in Chapter 3, use ready-to-apply colors like the Woodland Scenics color kit, which includes various rock and earth colors.

Start by painting some individual stones with various colors, then follow this with a wash of a darker rock.

To make a wash, thin a color with water, then test it on the rear of the casting to make sure the wash is strong enough to give the effect you're looking for. Apply the wash liberally over the surface with a wide brush, working it into all the cracks and crevices. You can come back later to highlight individual stones or to apply another wash (either darker or a different color).

Photos **10-9** (page 83) and **10-14** show a few samples painted with this technique. It's easy to vary the color and intensity of a wash to match specific prototype examples.

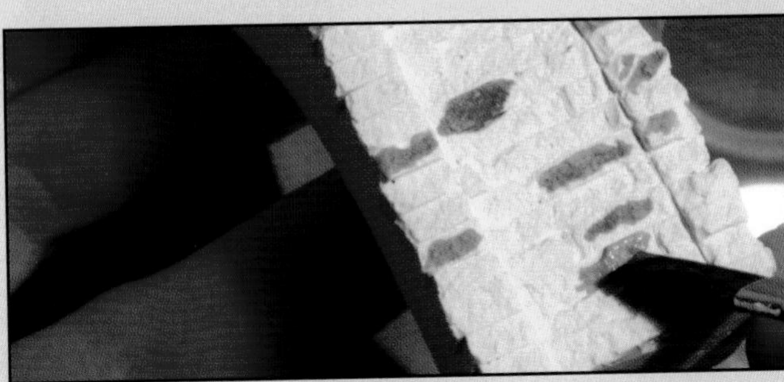

Start painting a plaster tunnel portal by painting a few random stones with various earth tones. *Jeff Wilson*

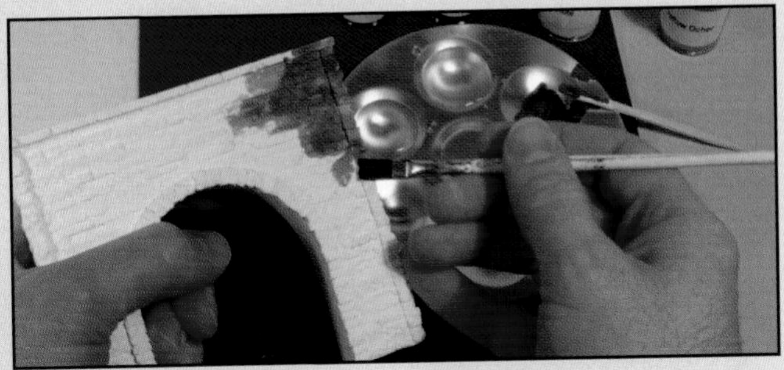

Finish the portal with a medium to dark-gray wash. *Jeff Wilson*

List of available models

Space prohibits listing all models and all variations that have been produced. Space also precludes a detailed assessment of each model: Some are very close to specific prototypes, others have details that are not accurate. Some of the models listed may have gone out of production recently but are still included as a reference. Many hobby shops and dealers still have models in stock that haven't been produced recently, and Internet sites such as eBay are also good places to track down out-of-production models.

Note: Dimensions in this list given in inches are the actual size of the model; dimensions given in feet represent scale feet.

HO scale

Bridges

Prototype/description	Mfr./ Item Number
Wood truss, Howe, $14\frac{1}{2}$"	Campbell 305
Wood truss, Howe, $11\frac{7}{8}$"	Midwest 3054
Wood deck truss, 50'	Campbell 761
Wood deck truss, $9\frac{7}{16}$"	Midwest 3052
Wood pony truss, 70'	Campbell 762
Wood pony truss, $11\frac{7}{8}$"	Midwest 3053
Wood, covered, $14\frac{5}{8}$"	Campbell 306
Deck truss, Warren, 9"	Atlas 591
Pony truss, Warren, 9"	Atlas 590
Through truss, Warren, 20"	Walthers 933-3185
Through truss, Warren, 125'	Campbell 763
Through truss, Warren	Plastruct 1002
Through truss, Pratt, 150'	Central Valley 1902
Through truss, double-track Warren, 20"	Walthers 933-3012
Through truss, double-track Warren, 125'	Campbell 764
Truss bridge kit, multiple options	Three Brothers 1161
Swing bridge, truss, 27"	Walthers 933-3070
Bascule bridge, truss, 34" ($21\frac{1}{2}$" span)	Walthers 933-3070
Rolling bascule bridge, girder, 18"	Faller 120490
Plate girder, through, 9"	Atlas 592
Plate girder, through, 50'	Micro-Engineering 75520
Plate girder, through, double-track, 50'	Micro-Engineering 75521
Plate girder, through, 70'	Campbell 766
Plate girder, through, 72'	Central Valley 1903
Plate girder, double-track, 72'	Central Valley 1904
Plate girder, deck, 30'	Micro-Engineering 75502
Plate girder, deck, 50'	Micro-Engineering 75501
Plate girder, deck, 70'	Campbell 765
Plate girder, ballasted deck, 30'	Micro-Engineering 75508
Plate girder, ballasted deck, 50'	Micro-Engineering 75507
Steel viaduct, 150'	Micro-Engineering 75513
Steel viaduct, 210'	Micro-Engineering 75515
Steel viaduct, city-style, 90'	Micro-Engineering 75509

Prototype/description	Mfr./ Item Number
Steel viaduct, city-style, two-track, 90'	Micro-Engineering 75510
Steel viaduct, city-style, 150'	Micro-Engineering 75511
Steel viaduct, city-style, two-track, 150'	Micro-Engineering 75512
Stone viaduct, two-arch, 7"	Faller 120545
Stone arch, single, $11\frac{1}{2}$"	Monroe Models 2001
Stone arch, tall viaduct	Peco 121135
Culvert, timber	Woodland Scenics 1265
Culvert, brick	Model Railstuff 430
Culvert, masonry arch	Woodland Scenics 1263
Culvert, stone	Model Railstuff 431
Culvert, stone	Mountains in Minutes 204
Culvert, small stones	Rix 651
Culvert, large stones	Rix 652
Culvert, stone with pipe	Pre-Size 122
Culvert, random stone	Woodland Scenics 1264
Culvert, cut stone arch	Pre-Size 123
Culvert, concrete	Pre-Size 124
Culvert, concrete	Woodland Scenics 1262
Culvert, concrete twin	Pre-Size 126
Culvert, concrete with pipe	Pikestuff 2
Concrete, three-pier, $9\frac{1}{4}$"	Monroe Models 2002
Concrete Art Deco, two-track, 14"	Monroe Models 2003
Beam bridge, 4"	AM Models 301
Trestle, 4"	AM Models 302
Trestle, 6"	AM Models 303
Trestle, ballasted deck	BTS 27103
Trestle	Brawa 504
Trestle	Bar Mills 404
Trestle, pile	Blair Line 167
Trestle, frame	Blair Line 171
Trestle, ballasted deck pile	Campbell 301
Trestle, pile	Campbell 302
Trestle, curved	Campbell 303
Trestle, curved, tall	Campbell 304
Trestle, tall	Campbell 751
Trestle, tall	JV Models 2014
Trestle, tall curved	JV Models 2016
Trestle, tall	Midwest 3051

Prototype/description	Mfr./ Item Number

HO scale (cont'd)

Bridges (cont'd)

Prototype/description	Mfr./ Item Number
Highway, wrought iron, 50′	Rix 121
Highway, concrete, old style	Rix 101
Highway, concrete, modern	Rix 112
Highway, concrete arch	Walthers 933-3196
Highway, wood	Rix 200
Highway, wood covered	Walthers 933-3602

Abutments

Prototype/description	Mfr./ Item Number
Timber	Pre-Size 141
Field stone	AIM Products 101
Random stone	AIM Products104
Cut stone	AIM Products 102
Cut stone	Chooch 8440
Cut stone, tapered	Chooch 8460
Cut stone, double-track	Chooch 8450
Cut stone stepped walls	Chooch 8400
Cut stone	Pre-Size 143
Concrete, wide	Walthers 933-3185
Concrete wing walls	Walthers 933-1042
Concrete	AIM Products 118
Concrete stepped walls	Chooch 8420
Poured concrete	AIM Products 124
Old concrete	Pre-Size 144
Concrete, smooth	Pre-Size 145

Piers

Prototype/description	Mfr./ Item Number
Split stone	AIM Products 735
Split stone with cutwater	AIM Products 836
Cut stone with cutwater	Chooch 8430
Cut stone	Chooch 8431
Cut stone	Pre-Size 131
Stone viaduct footings	Model Railstuff 1400
Random stone	Pre-Size 130
Granite block, oval	Pre-Size 135
Granite block, rectangular	Pre-Size 136
Concrete	AIM Products 135
Concrete, wide	Walthers 933-1041
Concrete with cutwater	AIM Products 125
Concrete, old	Pre-Size 132
Concrete, smooth	Pre-Size 133
Concrete viaduct footings	Model Railstuff 1410

Components

Prototype/description	Mfr./ Item Number
Box girder sections	Central Valley 19025
Plate girder sections	Central Valley 19031
Bridge tie sections	Central Valley 19032
Viaduct tower, 10″	Micro-Engineering 75169
Bridge shoes	Three Brothers 4400
Rivet sheet	Three Brothers 4000
Bridge track	Walthers 948-886, -899
Bridge flextrack	Micro Engineering 11101

Tunnel portals

Prototype/description	Mfr./ Item Number
Timber	AIM Products 121
Timber	Campbell 351
Timber	Pre-Size 101
Timber	Woodland Scenics 1254
Timber, double-track	Pre-Size 102
Brick	Mountains in Minutes 101
Cut stone	AIM Products 110
Cut stone	Chooch 8340
Cut stone	Pre-Size 105
Cut stone, double-track	Pre-Size 106
Cut stone	Woodland Scenics 1253
Cut stone, double-track	Woodland Scenics 1257
Cut stone	Mountains in Minutes 102
Random stone	AIM Products 112
Random stone	Chooch 8360
Random stone, double-track	Chooch 8370
Random stone	Woodland Scenics 1255
Eroded limestone	AIM Products 130
Hoosac Tunnel west portal	Mountains in Minutes 104
Blasted rock	Pre-Size 117, 118
Blasted rock, double-track	Pre-Size 119, 120
Natural rock	AIM Products 109
Concrete, grooved face	AIM Products 116
Concrete	AIM Products 128, 134
Concrete, modern	AIM Products 133
Concrete	Chooch 8320
Concrete, Cascade Tunnel	Chooch 8321
Concrete, tall	Chooch 8322
Concrete, double-track	Chooch 8330
Concrete arch	CM Shops 2001
Concrete arch, double-track	CM Shops 2002
Concrete, square opening	CM Shops 2011
Concrete, square opening, double-track	CM Shops 2012
Concrete	Model Railstuff 690
Concrete, Moffat Tunnel west portal	Model Railstuff 1271
Concrete, Moffat Tunnel east portal	Model Railstuff 1270
Concrete	Pre-Size 113
Concrete, double-track	Pre-Size 114
Concrete	Woodland Scenics 1252
Concrete, double-track	Woodland Scenics 1256

N scale

Bridges

Prototype/description	Mfr./ Item Number
Truss, through Warren double-track	Walthers 933-3242
Truss, through 120′	Plastruct 2002
Truss, through Warren, $9^3/_4$″	Kato 20434
Truss, through Warren double-track, $9^3/_4$″	Kato 20438
Truss, deck Warren, 5″	Atlas 2547
Truss, pony Warren, 5″	Atlas 2546
Truss, timber pony, $5^1/_4$″	Campbell 760

N scale (cont'd)

Bridges (cont'd)

Prototype/description	Mfr./ Item Number
Plate girder, through, 5″	Atlas 2548
Plate girder, through, 5″	Heljan 662
Plate girder, through, $7\frac{5}{16}$″	Kato 20454
Plate girder, deck, $4\frac{7}{8}$″	Kato 20464
Plate girder, deck, 40′	Micro Engineering 75151
Plate girder, deck, 80′	Micro Engineering 75150
Plate girder, 40′ ballasted deck	Micro Engineering 75153
Plate girder, 80′ ballasted deck	Micro Engineering 75152
Rolling lift, plate girder	Faller 272-222584
Steel viaduct, five-span	Micro Engineering 75518
Stone arch	Faller 222588
Stone arch	Monroe Models 9001
Stone viaduct	Faller 222585
Stone viaduct, curved	Faller 222586
Concrete, art deco double-track	Monroe Models 9003
Concrete beam	Monroe Models 9002
Concrete arch	N Scale Architect 10200
Timber trestle, 4″	Bar Mills 304
Timber trestle, $5\frac{5}{8}$″ pile and frame	Blair Line 71
Timber trestle, $5\frac{5}{8}$″ pile	Blair Line 67
Timber trestle, 11″	Campbell 752
Timber trestle, 12″	JV Models 1014
Timber trestle, 13″	Walthers 933-3217
Timber trestle, curved, $5\frac{1}{2}$″	Campbell 753
Timber trestle, tall curved	Campbell 754
Culvert, brick	Model Railstuff 1330
Culvert, stone	Model Railstuff 1331
Culvert, concrete	Model Railstuff 1340
Culvert, masonry arch	Woodland Scenics 1163
Culvert, concrete	Woodland Scenics 1162
Culvert, random stone	Woodland Scenics 1164
Culvert, timber	Woodland Scenics 1165
Highway, concrete, modern, 50′	Rix 161
Highway, concrete 1930s, 50′	Rix 151

Abutments

Prototype/description	Mfr./ Item Number
Cut stone	AIM Products 200
Cut stone wings	AIM Products 202
Cut stone	Chooch 9840
Cut stone, tapered	Chooch 9860
Cut stone, double track	Chooch 9850
Cut stone, stepped	Chooch 9820
Random stone	AIM Products 204
Concrete wings	AIM Products 216

Piers

Prototype/description	Mfr./ Item Number
Cut stone, cutwater	Chooch 9830
Cut stone, rectangular	Chooch 9831

Components

Prototype/description	Mfr./ Item Number
Concrete footings	Model Railstuff 2150
Plate girders, 80′	Micro Engineering 80170
Plate girders, 40′	Micro Engineering 80171
Bridge flextrack	Micro Engineering 11110

Portals

Prototype/description	Mfr./ Item Number
Cut stone	AIM Products 210
Cut stone double-track	AIM Products 213
Random stone	AIM Products 212
Random stone double-track	AIM Products 211
Concrete	AIM Products 214
Concrete	Chooch 9720
Concrete, double-track	Chooch 9730
Cut stone	Chooch 9740
Cut stone, double-track	Chooch 9750
Random stone	Chooch 9760
Random stone, double-track	Chooch 9770
Concrete double-track	AIM Products 215
Concrete, modern	AIM Products 218
Clarksburg double-track	AIM Products 619
Timber	Pre-Size 201
Timber, double-track	Pre-Size 202
Random stone	Pre-Size 203
Random stone, double-track	Pre-Size 204
Cut stone	Pre-Size 205
Cut stone, double-track	Pre-Size 206
Concrete	Pre-Size 213
Concrete, double-track	Pre-Size 214
Concrete	Model Railstuff 2110
Concrete	Woodland Scenics 1152
Concrete, double-track	Woodland Scenics 1156
Cut stone	Woodland Scenics 1153
Cut stone, double-track	Woodland Scenics 1157
Timber	Woodland Scenics 1154
Random stone	Woodland Scenics 1155
Concrete	Woodland Scenics 1158

O scale

Bridges

Prototype/description	Mfr./ Item Number
Truss, through Pratt	Atlas O 7920
Truss, through	Plastruct 3002
Truss, through Pratt double-track	Atlas O 7921
Truss, Howe wood pony	Midwest 3060
Plate girder, through	Atlas O 7923
Plate girder, through	K-Line 41814
Timber trestle	JV Models 4014
Timber trestle, curved	JV Models 4016